About the author

Patrick **Holford** BSc, DipION, FBANT, NTCRP is a leading spokesman on nutrition in the media, and is author of over 30 books, translated into over 20 languages and selling over a million copies worldwide, including *The Optimum Nutrition Bible, The Low-GL Diet Bible* and *Optimum Nutrition for the Mind*.

Patrick Holford started his academic career in the field of psychology. In 1984 he founded the Institute for Optimum Nutrition (ION), an independent educational charity, with his mentor, twice Nobel Prize winner Dr Linus Pauling, as patron. ION has been researching and helping to define what it means to be optimally nourished for the past 25 years and is one of the most respected educational establishments for training nutritional therapists. At ION Patrick was involved in groundbreaking research showing that multivitamins can increase children's IQ scores – the subject of a *Horizon* documentary in the 1980s. He was one of the first promoters of the importance of zinc, antioxidants, essential fats, low-GL diets and homocysteine-lowering B vitamins.

Patrick's revolutionary low-GL diet has been successfully followed by thousands of people with diabetes since it was first published in 2004. People who have used it have been able to greatly reduce or completely stop medication for diabetes, cholesterol and blood pressure. Since then, Patrick has further refined the perfect diet for stabilising blood sugar, backed up with supplements and lifestyle changes to reverse type-2 diabetes as quickly as possible.

Patrick is director of the Food for the Brain Foundation, an educational charity, and director of the Brain Bio Centre, the Foundation's treatment centre. He is an honorary fellow of the British Association of Nutritional Therapy, as well as a member of the Nutrition Therapy Council.

By The Same Author

100% Health
500 Top Health and Nutrition Questions Answered
Balance Your Hormones
Beat Stress and Fatigue
Boost Your Immune System (with Jennifer Meek)
Food GLorious Food (with Fiona McDonald Joyce)
Hidden Food Allergies (with Dr James Braly)
How to Quit Without Feeling S**t (with David Miller and Dr James Braly)
Improve Your Digestion
Natural Highs (with Dr Hyla Cass)
Optimum Nutrition Before, During and After Pregnancy (with Susannah Lawson)
Optimum Nutrition for the Mind
Optimum Nutrition for Your Child (with Deborah Colson)
Optimum Nutrition Made Easy
Say No to Arthritis
Say No to Cancer
Say No to Heart Disease
Six Weeks to Superhealth
Smart Food for Smart Kids (with Fiona McDonald Joyce)
Solve Your Skin Problems (with Natalie Savona)
The 10 Secrets of 100% Healthy People
The Alzheimer's Prevention Plan (with Shane Heaton and Deborah Colson)
The Feel Good Factor
The H Factor (with Dr James Braly)
The 9-day Liver Detox (with Fiona McDonald Joyce)
The Little Book of Optimum Nutrition
The Low-GL Diet Bible
The Low-GL Diet Counter
The Low-GL Diet Cookbook (with Fiona McDonald Joyce)
The Optimum Nutrition Bible
The Optimum Nutrition Cookbook (with Judy Ridgway)
The Perfect Pregnancy Cookbook (with Fiona McDonald Joyce)

patrick
HOLFORD

Say No to Diabetes

piatkus

PIATKUS

First published in Great Britain in 2011 by Piatkus
Copyright © Patrick Holford 2011
Reprinted 2011

ℚ is the registered trademark of Holford & Associates Ltd

A CIP catalogue record for this book
is available from the British Library.

ISBN 978-0-7499-5589-2

Typeset in Plantin Light by Phoenix Photosetting, Chatham, Kent
Printed and bound in Great Britain by CPI Group (UK), Croydon, CR0 4YY

Papers used by Piatkus are from well-managed forests
and other responsible sources.

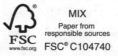

MIX
Paper from
responsible sources
FSC
www.fsc.org   FSC® C104740

Piatkus
An imprint of
Little, Brown Book Group
100 Victoria Embankment
London EC4Y 0DY

An Hachette UK Company
www.hachette.co.uk

www.piatkus.co.uk

Acknowledgements

I am especially indebted to Dr Fedon Lindberg, who wrote the foreword, checked the manuscript and taught me so much about diabetes from his experience of running clinics in Norway. Dr Lindberg and Professor Charles Clarke, here in the UK, are my two favourite diabetes specialists flying the low-GL flag. Sincere thanks to medical journalist Jerome Burne, who assisted me in researching some of the cutting-edge topics and helped write the chapter on reprogramming your genes. I am indebted to nutritional therapist Nina Omotoso, my research assistant, to Fiona McDonald Joyce for her delicious recipes, to Jo, my wonderful executive assistant, and Gaby, my wife, for their support and creating the space for me to focus on this book. As ever, I am deeply grateful to the team at Piatkus, especially Jillian Stewart and Jan Cutler, for their painstaking attention to detail in the editing process. Most of all I am indebted to my clients with diabetes who have proven the principles in this book and remained free from diabetes ever since.

Contents

Guide to Abbreviations and Measures

Conversions

European and American laboratories use different measures to record test results. The measurements in this book are in mmol/l and pmol/l (the European measures). If necessary, your results can be easily converted to those used in the book by using the following:

To convert **blood glucose** readings: multiply the mg/dl (US) by 0.0555 to get mmol/l (UK).

To convert **glycosylated haemoglobin (glycated haemoglobin A1, A1C, HbAIC)** readings: multiply 'proportion of total haemoglobin' by 100 to get 'per cent of total haemoglobin'.

To convert **insulin** readings: multiply the μIU/mL (US) by 0.6945 to get mmol/l (UK).

To convert **total cholesterol**, **HDL** and **LDL** readings: multiply the mg/dl (US) by 0.0259 to get mmol/l (UK).

To convert **triglyceride** readings: multiply the mg/dl (US) by 0.0113 to get mmol/l (UK).

Abbreviations and measures

Vitamins

1 gram (g) = 1,000 milligrams (mg) = 1,000,000 micrograms (mcg, also written as μg)

Most vitamins are measured in milligrams or micrograms. Vitamins A, D and E used to be measured in International Units (iu), a measurement designed to standardise the various forms of these vitamins, which have different potencies.

6mcg of beta-carotene, the vegetable precursor of vitamin A is, on average, converted into 1mcg of retinol, the animal form of vitamin A. So, 6mcg of betacarotene is called 1mcgRE (RE stands for retinol equivalent). Throughout this book beta-carotene is referred to in mcgRE.

1mcg of retinol (1mcgRE) = 3.3iu of vitamin A
1mcgRE of beta-carotene = 6mcg of beta-carotene
100iu of vitamin D = 2.5mcg
100iu of vitamin E = 67mg
1 pound (lb) = 16 ounces (oz)
2.4lb = 1 kilogram (kg)
1 pint = 600 millilitres (ml)
1¾ pints = 1 litre
In this book 'calories' means kilocalories (kcals)
Some food measurements are given as cups: 1 cup = 250ml (9fl oz)

References and Further Sources of Information

In each part of the book, you'll find numbered references. These refer to research papers listed in the References section on page 306, and are there for readers who want to study this subject in depth. More details on most of these studies can be found on the Internet, at PubMed, a service of the US National Library of Medicine, which includes over 18 million citations dating back to 1948. This is where you can access most of the studies mentioned (see http://www.ncbi.nlm.nih.gov/pubmed/).

On page 324 you will find a list of the best books to read to enable you to dig deeper into the topics covered. You will also find many of the topics touched on in this book covered in detail in feature articles available at www.patrickholford.com. If you want to stay up to date with all that is new and exciting in this field, we recommend you subscribe to Patrick Holford's 100% Health newsletter, details of which are on the website.

Foreword

The diabetes epidemic is upon us. More than 230 million people world-wide have diabetes and, according to the World Health Organization, that number will increase to 333 million by 2025. The numbers for the UK alone are no less frightening, with approximately 3 million people diagnosed with the disease. In Norway, where I practise, there are around 200,000 people with diabetes, in a country with a population of 4.5 million. Of the 200,000, only about 30,000 have type-1 diabetes, while the rest have type-2 diabetes.

Type-1 diabetes (formerly called 'insulin dependent') occurs mainly in children and adolescents and is characterised by the body's inability to produce enough insulin (insulin deficiency). With type-2 diabetes (formerly called 'non-insulin dependent') the body's insulin no longer functions normally and too much is produced. Type-2 diabetes used to affect mostly people aged over 60 but, increasingly, younger individuals are affected and the disease is becoming more common in children. It is mainly the rise in cases of type-2 diabetes that is fuelling the worldwide diabetes epidemic.

So what causes type-2 diabetes? Genetic predisposition, poor diet, physical inactivity, not enough sleep, chronic stress and obesity are the main contributors. However, obesity appears to be one of the main drivers of the rise in the level of type-2 diabetes. Eighty per cent of sufferers are or have been overweight. In fact, it wouldn't be overstating the role of obesity if we were to call it a 'diabesity' epidemic.

One of the most alarming features of the rising tide of diabetes is the fact that 50 per cent of all those who have the disease do not know that they have it. This is a potential time bomb and makes it doubly important that people become aware of the risk factors and how to prevent the disease. This book will help you do that.

Diabetes is a serious – and costly – disease

Many people mistakenly believe diabetes is a 'bit player' when compared to the big killer diseases such as heart disease and cancer, yet it is intimately connected with these diseases and implicated in a wide range of others. Cardiovascular disease is the most common complication for people with diabetes and also the leading cause of death in industrialised countries. Approximately 50 to 80 per cent of deaths in people with diabetes are due to cardiovascular disease. Behind every four premature deaths in developing countries you will find diabetes. The disease is also the leading cause of blindness and vision loss, disease-related amputations and chronic renal failure. Sadly, it does not stop there. Diabetes and obesity are associated with a greater risk for several cancers (including breast and colon cancer), osteoarthritis, migraines, psoriasis, asthma and other inflammatory diseases. In addition, far more people with diabetes develop depression and Alzheimer's disease.

And, of course, let's not forget the cost. Worldwide, diabetes care costs between £100 and 180 billion annually – and that doesn't include indirect costs due to disability and other such consequences. The price tag is paid by us all. Seventy per cent of drug costs are paid by the public – that's you and me. Medications and insulin are big business – insulin is among the 20 bestselling drugs – so there is little incentive for the pharmaceutical industry to find a less costly solution. Thankfully, that solution already exists – and it doesn't involve a new drug.

Food and exercise are better than insulin

A Norwegian study, conducted by Aker University Hospital and published in 2005, concluded that lifestyle change is better than insulin therapy for type-2 diabetics. Several international studies have come to the same conclusion. In the Norwegian study, one group with type-2 diabetes was treated with insulin injections, while another group was treated with dietary advice and exercise. The aim was to achieve weight loss and better insulin sensitivity and blood sugar control. The latter group lost 3kg of weight in 12 months and saw an improvement in blood sugar, blood pressure and triglyceride levels. (The weight loss might not sound particularly impressive but the diet used was the more traditional low-fat and high-carbohydrate diet – but low in sugar and high in fibre – and not a low-glycemic/low-carbohydrate diet, which can achieve much more impressive results.) In contrast, the insulin group increased their weight by 4.9kg and had worsened metabolic parameters such as triglyceride levels.

Given that heart disease is the biggest cause of death in type-2 diabetics, and increased triglycerides increases the risk of heart disease, insulin treatment is obviously not the best choice! Nevertheless, the number of people with type-2 diabetes receiving insulin therapy has skyrocketed over the last two to three decades. The reason for this lies with the health-care system, which is simply not designed to help people improve their lifestyle and take care of their own health. It is a 'sick-care' system, not a health-care system. I believe most doctors and other health professionals would welcome the opportunity to raise awareness, convey knowledge and motivate diabetes patients to change their lifestyle habits, but they simply don't have the time required to do this successfully.

Could incorrect advice be making things worse?

According to food and health authorities and the diabetes charities, diabetics should eat plenty of starch and cut down on fat – essentially the same guidelines as the general public. The assumption seems to be that diabetes patients should not feel different and that they should be able to continue to eat like everyone else. Yet the fact that starch increases blood sugar is undeniable. People who get type-2 diabetes, not the insulin-dependent type, are by definition what we call glucose intolerant, not fat intolerant. For years, they have failed to tolerate the modern carbohydrate-rich diet and, as a result, eventually developed diabetes. Instead of recommending that they reduce what has caused the problem, our authorities recommend eating more of the same or that they cut down even further on their fat intake. Incredible! Instead of all diabetics eating 'healthily', they just eat as badly as everyone else, hence the number of people with non-insulin dependent diabetes who must resort to insulin.

Health professionals and authorities can help to reverse the trend, but they must be open to new ideas and brave enough to change the advice they give, when it proves to be wrong. They must dare to admit that some official dietary advice may have contributed to more health problems. There is new knowledge that must be taken into consideration. The results of large studies from the US and Finland do not tally with the general healthy eating advice given to diabetics to eat plenty of starch. These new studies show that eating more fish, vegetables, berries, nuts and pulses; less sugar, starches (bread, potatoes, rice, pasta) and red meat; and choosing healthy fats can dramatically reduce the risk of diabetes.

The nutrition debate has been lively in recent years and has increased awareness of the importance of a healthy diet in preventing and treating disease and improving well-being. At the same time, many people are understandably confused by the substantial differences in what various experts advocate as being healthy. For the time being we will have to live with this confusion and evaluate the different arguments with an open mind.

For some readers, this book may seem eye-opening, and to others shocking, because it may turn upside down their perception of what is healthy and unhealthy in relation to an appropriate diabetes diet. Patrick Holford has been an important and courageous voice in the UK and internationally, and has dared to challenge the establishment. However, it is important to understand that the challenge is a credible one because the thrust of this book ties in with what the latest research is beginning to show.

So, what should you make of all the conflicting advice and what can you do to help yourself? I hope my experience will inspire you.

The key is mastering change

At my clinic I have treated thousands of patients with obesity and type-2 diabetes since 1999, focusing on lifestyle change. The results are astounding. Most people manage to quit insulin completely or reduce their dose sharply, while they lose weight and achieve normal blood sugar, blood pressure, cholesterol and triglyceride levels. This means that they reduce their need for medication and dramatically improve their quality of life. What does this require? Essentially the answer is change: re-organising meals to follow a low-GL diet, taking more exercise, sleeping better and reducing stress. That sounds simple enough but changing habits is not always easy. In my practice, I have learned that people have very different coping skills. For some, it is easier to take extra medication or insulin, than to change dietary and lifestyle habits – but the latter means a healthier and longer life. The choice to me seems obvious.

If you suffer from diabetes, or have a relative with diabetes, this book will give you the knowledge to make the appropriate changes to diet and lifestyle. I would also like to think that it will be read by people who wish to reduce their risk – after all, prevention is vital if we are to halt this epidemic. There are many paths to reach the goal of better health and blood sugar control. I believe that eating a diet that is more in line with what our ancestors ate in the Stone Age is wise, because our genes are the same now as then. Of course we do not live in the Stone Age and that means that most need to figure out their own way of eating and living that is more in line with their genetic make-up, while taking into account the realities of the 21st century. There is no one path that is optimal for all – some people with diabetes can tolerate more carbohydrate than others, but the low-fat, carbohydrate-rich diet recommended by the authorities is, in my opinion, misguided. The approach of this book is much more in line with what studies are now telling us is the best approach and I have no doubt it will help you to achieve better blood sugar control, reduce your risk of disease and live a long and healthy life!

Fedon Lindberg, Physician, Specialist in Internal Medicine

Introduction – Freedom from Diabetes

Whether you have diabetes, or you know someone who has, or if you want to do whatever is possible to avoid developing it in the future, this book is essential reading. The good news is that type-2 diabetes (which accounts for 90 per cent of all diabetes cases) is not only completely preventable but is also reversible. The vast majority of people with diabetes can achieve perfectly stable blood sugar balance, even without the need for medication, by following the advice in this book.

You may have been told that this isn't possible and that you'll need medication for the rest of your life. Don't believe it. There is a way out. Over the last 30 years I have worked with thousands of people who are suffering from ill health as a direct result of blood sugar imbalances, which if untreated will lead to diabetes and all the problems connected to this serious illness. I have introduced them to the benefits of a different lifestyle and diet that, far from being a daunting prospect where they feel that they have to give up everything they like, opens the door to good health, a lighter spirit (as well as a trimmer waistline) and, mostly importantly, freedom from the grip of diabetes.

For every three people who have been diagnosed with diabetes there's another person who has it but doesn't know,[1] and ten people who have pre-diabetes – increasing insulin resistance and metabolic syndrome (which I'll be explaining all about later). If you are over 40, you have a one-in-three chance of developing diabetes type-2 – often described as 'age-onset diabetes'. If you are significantly overweight, your odds are more like one in two. If you already have diabetes type-2, you can reverse it. If you haven't, but you are concerned for your health, now is the time for you to act to avoid suffering with this condition, because ignorance is not bliss. The very same advice that I would give to someone who has diabetes is the advice that will stop you getting it, and is what I follow every day to stay healthy, slim and full of energy. By the way, in case you have the rarer type-1 'insulin-dependent' diabetes, my advice is just the same and by following it you will at least halve your requirement for insulin.

Understanding diabetes, in a nutshell

Diabetes is the end result of eating a diet and living a lifestyle that repeatedly keeps your blood sugar at too high a level. As a consequence, the body produces a hormone, called insulin, which floods into the bloodstream to take the glucose out of the blood and into the liver and muscles. The glucose is first converted to glycogen, but when our glycogen stores are full it turns it into fat and stores it. High insulin increases fat storage both from dietary carbohydrate and fat. If your blood glucose levels keep going too high, over time, and if you are genetically susceptible, you become insensitive to insulin and develop what's called insulin resistance. When that happens, you have even more blood sugar highs, and you produce even more insulin to cope. Too much glucose, and too much insulin, damage all kinds of tissues – arteries, eyes, kidneys and brain to name a few. Your whole system tips into a state of inflammation, which means that you start experiencing more pain and more health problems – from heart disease to painful joints. Up goes LDL ('bad') cholesterol, triglycerides and blood pressure; down goes your energy, HDL ('good') cholesterol and your mood – and your memory suffers too.

This pattern of problems is called metabolic syndrome. I call this change in your body's biology 'internal global warming' and I'm going to show you how to cool down, not only for diabetes reversal but also to prevent a whole host of other common 21st-century diseases, from high blood pressure to low mood.

My proven way forward

I started working with people with diabetes in the 1980s. In 1984 I founded the Institute for Optimum Nutrition, a training college for nutritional therapists to learn how to treat the many common Western diseases, not with drugs but with diet and nutrition. There are now thousands of trained nutritional therapists all over the world helping thousands of people with diabetes become free from the disease. The chances are there is one near you.

The real breakthrough came in 2000 when we started experimenting with what's called a low-glycemic load (GL) diet. This is the most precise way to eat for blood sugar control, and not only did our results with people who had diabetes take a quantum leap but so did our weight-loss results. This culminated in a book, *The Holford Low-GL Diet*, now called *The Low-GL Diet Bible*, which thousands of people have successfully used, often achieving weight loss of 6.4kg (14lb/1st) a month, as well as perfect blood sugar control in *weeks*.

A different way forward

My low-GL diet is not a low-fat or a low-calorie diet and, as such, was originally viewed as heresy. After all, haven't we all been told that the only way to lose weight while improving our health is to eat fewer calories and to exercise more? Since fat has more calories, we were told to eat less fat, but from the 1980s as people started eating less fat they began to eat more carbohydrates – after all, you have to eat something! In my opinion, this fat phobia has been a fatal mistake and one of the main reasons why diabetes has hit epidemic proportions. This is because people have increased their intake of carbohydrates (which, as I will explain, affect the blood sugar levels in the body) in the place of fatty foods, and their weight and blood sugar levels have suffered as a result. Over the last 25 years in the US, for example, fat intake has gone down, carbohydrate intake has gone up and the number of obese people has more than doubled. A consequence of this is the rise of a host of other serious illnesses, including heart disease and cancer.

The great diabetes disaster

In most developed and developing countries, roughly one in six people over 40 already has diabetes.[2] But this is only the tip of the iceberg. Worldwide, we've gone from 30 million people with diabetes 25 years ago to 300 million right now, and a conservative projection of something close to half a billion people (that's a lot more than the population of America) with diabetes by 2030, according to the International Diabetes Federation.[3] We can see how conservative that figure might be by looking at some parts of the world that have rapidly shot into the high-sugar fast lane of Western foods; in the United Arab Emirates, for example, many schools are reporting that 15 per cent of their teenagers already have diabetes.

In the UK there are currently about 3 million people diagnosed with diabetes,[4] costing the National Health Service £1 million an hour.[5] This figure could easily double in the next 30 years. That's the equivalent of a new diagnosis every three minutes in the UK!

Maybe that's what a 'developing' country means – developing diabetes, and the host of other completely preventable and reversible man-made modern disease disasters, from breast and prostate cancer to heart disease and Alzheimer's. These are the diseases that ruin and shorten your life unnecessarily. They are the diseases that simply didn't exist in pre-industrial man. So much for progress!

Exploding the myths

As I sit here writing this book I am drowning in evidence, very good evidence, that shows two things: (1) much of what you are told about treating diabetes is wrong, and (2) there really is a way to reverse diabetes and return to good health. Here are a few examples:

- Being obese causes diabetes. WRONG

- You should be eating a low-fat, low-calorie diet. WRONG

- People with type-2 diabetes should be taking insulin or insulin-promoting drugs. WRONG

- Supplements are a waste of time. WRONG

- You have to be on medication to control your blood sugar levels. WRONG

I've also interviewed a range of doctors and diabetes experts. Some say 'you can't reverse diabetes and must be on drugs for life'. Others say 'diabetes type-2 is completely reversible, without the need for medication'. Which ones would you rather listen to? I've spent time with the ones that get the best results and learned their secrets. Here are what some of the specialists say:

Professor Charles Clarke, Fellow of the Royal College of Surgeons of Edinburgh says, 'There is a simple cure for the obesity and diabetes epidemic, but everyone is looking in the wrong place.' Norway's leading diabetic expert, Dr Fedon Lindberg, says, 'With the right advice and lifestyle changes type-2 diabetes is reversible, even if you are currently injecting insulin.' In America, Dr Mark Hyman says, 'Diabetes and pre-diabetes *are* reversible. New science shows that it's possible, through an aggressive approach of lifestyle, nutritional support, and occasionally medications.' Another successful American doctor, Julian Whitaker, says 'ninety per cent of all cases of diabetes can be treated and reversed naturally'.

These guys get good results. The proof is out there if you look for it; for example, reporting in *The New England Journal of Medicine*,[6] Dr Walter Willett and his team from the Harvard School of Public Health demonstrated that 91 per cent of all type-2 diabetes cases could be prevented through the kind of improvements in lifestyle and diet that I'm going to tell you about.

It's not only about freedom from diabetes

The great news is that it really isn't difficult to prevent and reverse diabetes, and the strategy that achieves it, which boils down to a delicious and practical diet, daily supplements and an active lifestyle, is exactly the same recipe for increasing your energy, mood and memory and massively cutting your risk of cancer, heart disease and Alzheimer's. In a nutshell, this means you have everything to gain, and nothing to lose except, in most cases, all that unwanted fat, especially around your middle. If you follow the regime in this book, you can, and you will, get your life back, cheating the system that made you ill in the first place and sending back those drugs you don't like taking. And you will reclaim a life that's worth living.

The six-week diabetes reversal challenge

To make a point, I challenged ITV's *This Morning* programme to give me a person with type-2 diabetes and allow me six weeks to completely reverse their condition. I should point out again that it is type-2 diabetes that is the most common. (Type-1 diabetes is an autoimmune disease which responds to exactly the same strategy but is not completely reversible.)

Kyra was ITV's volunteer. She had been diagnosed with type-2 diabetes a year before I met her. Her blood sugar was much too high (11mmol/l – it should be below 6) and so too was her glycosylated haemoglobin at 7.8 per cent. Put simply, when your blood sugar goes too high your red blood cells get sugar-coated, or 'glycosylated'. Glycoslyated haemoglobin (also called HbA1c) is the best single indicator of a risk of diabetes, reflecting how many blood sugar peaks you have had over the past couple of months. You want to get your level below 6 for that as well. I'll be explaining about important tests such as these in Part 1, Chapter 1.

When Kyra was diagnosed, her doctor had put her on a double dose of the drug metformin and told her she'd be on drugs for life (but this is wrong), referring her to the specialist diabetes unit. En route, she saw a dietician who told her to stop eating pumpkin seeds because they are high in fat (wrong again), to stop drinking cola and switch to diet cola and not to have more than five pieces of fruit a day (although this is good advice, there's a world of difference between certain fruits – berries and a banana, for example – as I'll be explaining). The diabetes specialist said that she could reverse diabetes and come off medication, if she did all the right things. The trouble is that no one told her what those things were, so she continued to have high blood sugar levels, hovering between 7 and 8, even with the drugs – although she had managed to lose a stone in weight by exercising every day and eating what she thought was a well-balanced diet.

That's when we met. I put her on my very precise low-GL diet, explained in this book, and four daily supplements, taken twice a day. She continued her exercise.

Six weeks later was the 'reveal', live on TV. Since Kyra's blood sugar had completely stabilised within three weeks she was now medication-free. Her blood sugar level was 5.5, which is close to perfect. Her glycosylated haemoglobin was 6.2 per cent and she was feeling fantastic. 'My energy is much better. My skin is clearer, my mood more stable and I've lost 12lbs [5.4kg] in a month. I feel in control of food instead of it being in control of me.' She said, 'I am really thrilled to have been able to come off medication and still have a stable blood sugar.'

One year on her blood sugar averages 5 and her glycosylated haemoglobin is 5.2, which is perfect, and she's lost another 12.7kg (2 stone/28lb). Point proven.

The GL revolution

GL stands for glycemic load and is a precise measure of what a food or a meal will do to your blood sugar level. It's a critical cornerstone for preventing and reversing diabetes and other common diseases. I will explain exactly how to eat in this way and why it is totally sustainable and completely delicious. I will also introduce you to the top eight anti-diabetes food groups, the super-fibres that you can add to any meal to help keep your blood sugar level as flat as a pancake, and the vitamins, minerals and the spices that cut your need for insulin, because the key to diabetes prevention and reversal is producing *less, not more*, insulin, and making sure the insulin you are producing works really efficiently. If you have type-1 diabetes, and are dependent on insulin injections, your need for insulin will considerably reduce.

Put this lot together and you have something more powerful than any combination of drugs, and the beauty is that it doesn't only reverse diabetes: it improves your mood, protects your heart, and stops sugar cravings and constant hunger. Here are just a few of the many people who have benefitted and made themselves diabetes-proof:

'I lost 7 stone [44.5kg/100lb] in seven months. My blood pressure is normal and I am off all medications,' said Eamon from Dublin, Ireland.

'I lost 5 stone [31.7kg/70lb] in five months. The weight literally fell off me, I have lots of energy, I'm not depressed and life has become very, very good,' said Fiona from Glasgow, Scotland, who quit all medications.

'I started the Low-GL diet last year, only 12 months ago, and I've lost 5 stone [31.7kg/70lb]. This is the first time in my life that I've had so much energy to play with. My blood sugar level has levelled right out. I don't crave sweet things anymore. It's changed my life. The recipes are amazing and I will never go back to eating any other way,' said Jennifer from Cardiff in Wales.

'My doctor advised the Holford Low-GL diet. I am a totally changed person. I feel incredible. I no longer get any gout at all. I've lost 84lbs [38kg/6 stone] in six months and ten inches [25cm] off my belly. After a month on the diet my blood sugar was stable – never above 6. Generally, it ranges from a normal 4.2–5.5. It's amazing. It's totally changed my life,' said Adrian from South Africa who had previously been significantly overweight at 145kg (22 stone 11lb/319½lb).

Adrian had followed every diet that's ever come out, year after year, but he still gained weight. A medical check-up identified that he had diabetes with a whoppingly high blood glucose level of 19.8. 'Before, I didn't have a cut-off switch. I could just eat and eat and would still be hungry throughout the day. After two months on your diet I now feel full and can leave food on the plate because I'm full,' he says.

The wrong approach

You might be surprised to learn that it isn't high blood sugar that does all the damage in diabetes. It's also insulin, the hormone that lowers high blood sugar levels. You might therefore think that if you had *more* insulin you'd have *lower* blood sugar levels, and less risk of disease. Well, that's actually wrong, because insulin itself, in high amounts, raises the risk of many of the diseases and complications we associate with diabetes – from heart disease to cancer. Insulin is as bad for you as sugar! That's why drugs that are designed to raise your insulin levels as the means to lower your blood sugar are missing the point, and I'll be discussing this in detail in the following chapters.

How to use this book

If you are driving along in your car and a red light starts flashing on the dashboard, what do you do? Do you stop, get out some black tape and put it over the light? No. You get out the manual and work out what your car needs.

Instead of taking anti-inflammatory painkillers, anti-cholesterol and anti-diabetes drugs you need to find out what's going on under your bonnet, and that's what I'm going to explain in **Part 1** of this book: what diabetes is, how you get it, how you know if you're at risk, how to reverse insulin resistance and metabolic syndrome, which are the precursors for type-2 diabetes, and the truth about the drugs you might be offered. I'll also explain how you develop type-1, the rare kind of diabetes, and what to do about that too.

In **Part 2** you'll discover the ten ways to prevent and reverse diabetes. Exactly what you need to eat, which supplements to take depending on your current condition (the worse you are the more you will need, and the healthier you become the less you'll need), and which lifestyle changes really make a worthwhile difference.

Part 3 is your Action Plan for saying no to diabetes, and **Part 4** gives you enough recipes to get started on the road to a better life – free from the need for drugs or with a greatly reduced need, free from disease, and with a lot less weight (if you need to lose it) and a lot more energy.

My dietary advice is good for anyone, because it is a healthy diet that will give your body what it needs to keep well. If you have diabetes, it is life-saving. If you have pre-diabetes (and I'll show you how to find out), it'll make you diabetes-proof. You really *can* say NO to diabetes.

Wishing you the best of health,
Patrick Holford

ONE WORD OF CAUTION If you are on diabetes medication, your need is likely to become less as your blood sugar level stabilises once you start following the recommendations in this book. If you start having too low blood sugar, go to your doctor who will, or should, recommend you lower or stop your medication. Please don't change your medication dose without consulting your doctor.

PART ONE

The Causes of Diabetes and its Treatments

No treatment of diabetes is ultimately going to be effective if it doesn't directly address the cause – and the cause is obviously not a deficiency of drugs. By truly understanding how diabetes develops, the secret to its undoing is revealed.

1

What is Diabetes?

Put simply, a person with diabetes has an excess of glucose and a deficiency of functioning insulin. Since insulin is the hormone that takes excess glucose out of the bloodstream, the net result of this imbalance is a high blood glucose level.

The two types of diabetes

There are two kinds of diabetes. Type-1 diabetes – the rarer kind – is primarily caused by the destruction of cells in the pancreas that make the hormone insulin. It is called an autoimmune disease because the body mistakenly makes antibodies that attack the cells in the pancreas. Once the majority of these cells are destroyed, a person cannot function without insulin. It used to be called 'insulin-dependent diabetes'. This usually develops in childhood and hence was also called 'child-onset diabetes'. I'll talk more about what causes this rarer kind of diabetes and what you can do about it, if that's what you've got, in Chapter 4 of this part.

Type-2 diabetes accounts for over 90 per cent of all diabetes. Unlike people with type-1 diabetes, who have low levels of insulin, type-2 diabetics almost always have very high levels of insulin. The trouble is that the insulin isn't doing its job of lowering blood glucose levels. This is because the underlying cause of type-2 diabetes is that insulin receptors in cells in the artery walls and in other cells in muscles and the liver shut down so that you become insulin insensitive or insulin resistant. The net result is a lack of functioning insulin, so the body tends to make more and more, but it doesn't work, so blood glucose levels continue to stay too high.

Normally, your blood sugar level should stay pretty even. It goes up a little when you eat carbohydrates, which are broken down into glucose in the gut then absorbed into the blood. But insulin is then released, bringing it back down again.

Your blood sugar balance should look like a gently rolling landscape (see the illustration below). Once it looks like hills or mountains, with higher peaks and deeper troughs, this shows you are losing blood sugar control – called dysglycemia – and that you are becoming increasingly insulin resistant. This can get worse and worse over years, and even decades, before you develop diabetes. I'll explain how this happens, how you can know how far you are along the track, and how to put yourself into reverse gear later in this part in Chapter 3.

> **NOTE** From this point on, unless I specify that I am talking about type-1 diabetes, when I refer to diabetes I am talking about type-2 diabetes, because this is by far the most common kind.

Blood sugar balance: normal, dysglycemia, diabetes

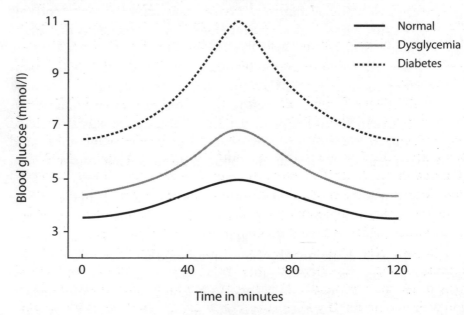

The symptoms of diabetes

Although there are tests to diagnose diabetes, there are also symptoms that some people suffer with. These include:

- Excessive thirst

- Excessive hunger and carbohydrate or sugar cravings

- Frequent urination

- Unusual changes in weight (either way)

- Increased tiredness

- Blurred vision

- Itchy skin or cuts and sores that take a long time to heal

But you can have none of these and still be diabetic.

Diagnosing diabetes

There are two ways to diagnose diabetes. The first is by testing your blood glucose level. If it is often above 7mmol/l before you've eaten, that's too high and you have diabetes. Ideally, it should be around 5. Your blood glucose level, however, does depend on what and when you've eaten.

You can take a fasting blood glucose test, taken with a simple pinprick of blood which is put onto a stick then inserted into a device. You can also have a urine test for glucose levels, because if glucose is not being filtered out of the blood by your kidneys you've got a problem. (One of the hallmarks of more advanced diabetes is kidney damage. Poor kidney function, coupled with too much glucose to filter, overloads the ability of the kidneys to filter out glucose. The urine actually tastes sweet, which is how it was diagnosed in the old days.)

You can also have a 'challenge' test. This involves ingesting an amount of sugar equivalent to what you'd get in a can of a sweetened fizzy drink such as a cola. That's about ten teaspoons of sugar. Then you wait two hours. If your insulin is working properly your blood glucose level shouldn't go above 7. If it isn't, you get a blood sugar spike: your levels rise significantly.

Diabetes is really hyper-glyc-aemia – high sugar in the blood.

What should your blood glucose level be?

	Healthy	Not great	Mild hyperglycemia	Diabetes
Fasting				
UK (mmol/l)	less than 5	5–5.4	5.5–6.4	6.5+
US (mg/dl)	<90	90–99	100–119	120+
2 hours after eating (postprandial)				
UK	less than 6.6	6.7–7.9	8–10.9	11+
US	90	125	145	200+

Now, the problem with all of these tests is that they only tell you what's happening the very second you test the blood. They don't really tell you if you are generally in the hills (dysglycemia) or the mountains (diabetes).

Remember Kyra, who took part in the six-week reverse-diabetes challenge? Her fasting glucose was 11, which dropped to around 7 with medication, then dropped to 5.5 six weeks after starting her nutrition regime, then to 5 after a year, which is in the healthy range.

A second way to test for diabetes is through a more long-term test that's becoming increasingly popular; it measures glycosylated haemoglobin. Technically, this is also called HbA1c, so that's what you might see on your blood test results. You may remember that this is when your blood sugar goes too high so your red blood cells get sugar coated, or 'glycosylated'. Sometimes this is called glycated haemoglobin – it's the same thing. Now, red blood cells (called haemoglobin or Hb) live for about three months, and once they are glycosylated they stay that way. So, the greater the percentage of red blood cells that are glycosylated, the more sugar spikes you must have had over the past three months. If I could only run one test, this is the one I'd go for. You can also do it yourself on a home test kit called the GLCheck (see Resources) and I'll be explaining how to do the test in Chapter 2.

What should your glycosylated haemoglobin level be?

	Healthy	Not great	Dysglycemia	Diabetes
(per cent)	5.5 or less	5.6–6.5	6.5+	7+

If you have a glycosylated haemoglobin score above 7 per cent, the chances are you have diabetes or will soon develop it. Kyra's glycosylated haemoglobin started at 7.8 per cent, then dropped to 6.2 per cent after six weeks. It was 5.2 per cent after a year, which is in the healthy range. Six weeks is too short a time to 'normalise' glycosylated haemoglobin completely, because red blood cells live for 12 weeks. In other words, half her red blood cells would have been 'old' red blood cells when she scored 7.8 per cent, and half would have been 'new' red blood cells, benefiting from her low-GL diet. So it's best to retest your glycosylated haemoglobin three months after starting the Anti-diabetes Action Plan that I'll be explaining in this book.

Kyra's blood glucose and glycosylated haemoglobin

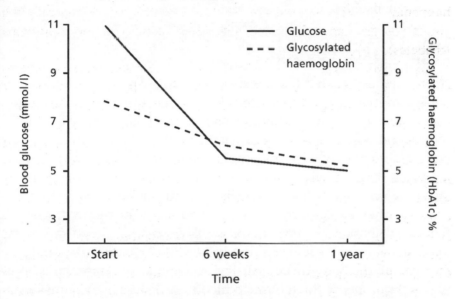

The consequences of diabetes are:

- Heart disease, including high blood pressure and high cholesterol, and an increased risk of thrombosis or stroke
- Kidney disease
- Nerve disease, called neuropathy, leading to loss of feeling and coldness in the extremities, sometimes so severe that limb amputations are necessary

continued

- Eye disease, called retinopathy, and other problems, from glaucoma to macular degeneration and blindness
- Obesity
- Periodontal disease (gum and teeth degeneration)
- Memory loss and Alzheimer's disease
- Depression
- Fatty liver disease
- Joint stiffness

In Part 3, I'll explain how to undo the damage caused by diabetes, once you've stopped the problem getting worse by stabilising your blood sugar and insulin levels.

Sugar makes you AGE

As we saw earlier, red blood cells get damaged by sugar by becoming sugar-coated, or glycosylated. Sometimes this is also called glycation. But it isn't just red blood cells that get damaged, it's all cells, including those in the arteries, the kidneys, the eyes, the joints and the brain. This is because too much glucose in the blood turns into what are called advanced glycation end-products, or AGEs for short. These attach to proteins, such as haemoglobin, and stop them working properly. So, when AGEs form in the eye your eyesight worsens, when in the skin your skin becomes more wrinkly, or when they form in the joints they become stiffer. AGEs are almost like handcuffs, gradually gripping all the body tissue, causing ageing and stiffening until nothing works properly. So, too much blood sugar does literally make you age.

Glucose effectively handcuffs together collagen and other molecules in the blood-vessel wall, making the arterial wall stiffer and less elastic. This means that more pressure is required to get the blood around the body, creating high blood pressure, which creates stress in the arteries. The result is more damage and inflammation (an essential process in the body that stimulates repair but which will, if unchecked, itself start causing damage). Inflammation eventually leads to narrowed arteries in which a blood clot could get stuck. This causes thrombosis, or a heart attack or stroke – hence the link between sugar, diabetes and heart attacks.

The beauty of the glycosylated haemoglobin test is that it not only tells you about your blood sugar control but it also reflects the amount of AGEing happening in your body. Now, you might think that you don't want to know, but if you do know, then you can do something about it – anything that brings your glycosylated haemoglobin score closer to 5 per cent.

It's insulin that does the damage

Most people think the problems and complications of diabetes I've listed above are all caused by too much sugar in the blood, but actually it's having high insulin that does a lot of the damage. Insulin itself, in high amounts, raises the risk of many of the diseases and complications we associate with diabetes. If you have metabolic syndrome your insulin levels are already likely to be raised, and many of its symptoms are caused by high sugar levels and the damage created by too much insulin.

- Too much insulin promotes fat storage and stops your body breaking down fat, so you gain more and more weight.

- It increases your cholesterol level and the level of fat, called triglyceride, in your blood and thereby increases your risk of heart disease.

- It causes your kidneys to retain both water and salt, which increases your blood pressure.

- The combination of too much insulin and too much glucose damages your arteries and raises your blood pressure, both of which make thrombosis, heart attacks and strokes more likely. Your kidneys start to fail. Eyesight deteriorates rapidly and the weight keeps piling on.

At this stage you would probably be taking drugs to control your blood sugar, your blood pressure and your kidney function, but the bottom line is that the best way to lower your insulin and your blood sugar is with diet and nutritional supplements, not drugs.

By now you might be thinking, *How on earth did I get into this mess?* I am going to tell you all the factors that contribute towards developing diabetes. But, rest assured that you can also get out of this downward spiral more quickly than you got into it. Obviously, the further down you are the longer it's going to take to get all the way back up to health, but you'll get there.

The problem with drugs and type-2 diabetes

As I explained in the Introduction, drugs that are designed to raise your insulin levels as the means to lower your blood sugar are missing the point. An example is sulfonylurea drugs, given for type-2 diabetes, including Amaryl, Euglucon and Diamicron. These stimulate the beta cells in the pancreas to produce even more insulin. In the short term this does bring blood sugar under control, but in the long term this is really bad news, because it speeds up the progression of the disease.

Another family of anti-diabetes drugs, called glitazones, were touted a few years ago as the next best thing, driving down insulin levels, but now glitazones are being actively discouraged due to their link with increased heart disease risk.[1] One such drug, Avandia, has recently been banned.[2] Drugs are not the answer to producing a healthy balance of glucose and insulin. There is much research to prove this point.

A big trial by the National Heart, Lung, and Blood Institute in the US, involving ten thousand people with diabetes, had to be halted because more people with diabetes on the drug cocktail designed to aggressively lower blood glucose were dying than those in the control group. Some were getting both insulin shots and glitazones.[3]

Another study from Denmark reports that those injecting insulin have a 50 per cent higher risk of cancer.[4] There's growing evidence that quite a few insulin-promoting drugs also increase cancer risk (except metformin, which is probably the best of the drugs).[5] In fact, there is growing evidence that metformin actually reduces cancer risk.[6]

In Part 2, Chapter 2 I'll explain the different drugs on offer, their advantages and disadvantages, the ones that aren't so bad and the ones you really want to avoid – and how to get off them.

Diabetes and high insulin levels go hand in hand. That's because the precursor for developing diabetes is 'insulin resistance'. As I've already explained, the more often your blood sugar level goes high the more insulin you make. The more you make, in time, the more insensitive you become to it. So now you have to make even more. Since insulin's job is to get glucose out of the blood, your blood sugar level goes up higher before the torrents of insulin you produce eventually bring it back down, sometimes too low. So, that's why before you develop diabetes you get blood sugar imbalances (dysglycemia), which make you grumpy, tired and hungry, and crave sweet foods. Eventually you end up with type-2 diabetes.

If you have type-2 diabetes and you've ended up needing insulin, your disease has been mismanaged. You should never have got to this point, but don't worry, you can get off insulin too – it'll just take closer to six months to achieve than six weeks, unless you are willing to follow an even stricter carbohydrate-controlled diet, which should only be undertaken with medical supervision.

Insulin resistance and blood sugar highs and lows are two of the attributes of a condition called metabolic syndrome, as I mentioned earlier. Another one is high cholesterol. One in four people have some degree of insulin resistance or metabolic syndrome, putting them at risk of diabetes.[7]

The road to developing diabetes

Although you'll often read that the most common risk factors for developing type-2 diabetes are being overweight or having a large waist, being aged over 40 (or over 25 for black and South Asian people), and having a close relative with diabetes, there are in fact many causes and contributory factors that lead to diabetes. You may recognise some or even several of them.

Consuming, and craving, sugar and sugary drinks This doesn't just mean sugar. It includes honey, raisins, sweets, pastries, even bananas, dates and grapes, which contain sugars that are released quickly in the blood, hence they're called 'fast-releasing'. Particularly bad are drinks sweetened with glucose or high-fructose corn syrup – that includes most fizzy drinks.

Consuming, and craving, too many refined carbs This includes bread, cereals, pastries, pasta and white rice. Although these are all obviously worse if you choose the white, refined variety, there's an awful lot of processed cereals and bread that are technically 'brown' or claim to contain 'wholegrain' but are actually still high in fast-releasing sugars – I'll be explaining about the slow- and fast-releasing carbohydrates later. Refined carbs are also devoid of the important mineral chromium. Often, people who try to follow a low-fat diet, choosing foods labelled as low fat, unfortunately end up eating more carbohydrates instead.

Inactivity If you neither exercise nor are particularly active at home or at work, this increases your risk of both weight gain and diabetes.

Chronic stress and poor sleep Both of these raise the adrenal hormone cortisol, which makes you more insulin resistant, and it can also contribute to overeating.

Gaining weight, especially around your middle Excess blood sugar is dumped by insulin into the liver, which then converts it into fat, stored most easily around your middle. So, if you are gaining inches around your girth that's a bad sign.

Smoking This is also an independent risk factor for diabetes according to Diabetes UK.

Not eating enough vegetables and fruit High consumers of vegetables and fruit (especially colder-climate fruits like apples, pears and plums, which are naturally lower in fruit sugars), take in a substantial amount of antioxidant vitamins, especially vitamin C, and so cut their risk of diabetes by 62 per cent.

Not eating enough fish As you'll see in Part 2, Chapter 4 a high intake of omega-3 fats, found particularly in oily fish, helps protect you from diabetes.

Not taking supplements As you'll see in Part 2 there are many nutrients, such as vitamin C and the mineral chromium, plus omega-3 fats, that protect you from diabetes.

Taking certain prescription drugs Some drugs increase your risk of diabetes. These include corticosteroid drugs, based on cortisone, which are often given long-term for asthma and also for arthritis, although they are not advised for more than a couple of months. If used for a year or more they certainly mess up hormone balance and cortisol, the adrenal hormone which is intimately linked to blood sugar control. Thiazide diuretics and beta blockers, given for high blood pressure, also increase risk.

Family history and ethnicity If you have a family history of diabetes, your risk is higher but is this due to inherited 'bad' habits or genes, or both? This is really a hard question to answer but there is certainly evidence that certain ethnic groups of African, Hispanic, South Asian and Native American origin have greater risk than, for example, those of Caucasian/European origin. Genetic predisposition appears to be largely to do with genes that control insulin sensitivity. If you have one parent with type-2 diabetes, you have a 40 per cent chance of developing it, and if both parents have it, your risk increases to 80 per cent. But, as you'll see in Part 2, Chapter 10, there's a lot you can do to reverse that inherited risk.

Age It is certainly true that the older you are the greater is your risk of diabetes. But this is true for most disease. Age, as such, is not really a cause of diabetes, it's just an indicator that the above causes have been going on for longer, thus increasing your risk.

Insulin resistance Your greatest risk of all is developing insulin resistance, which can happen many years before diabetes appears. Diabetes is really the end of the road of insulin resistance, which is one of the main attributes of metabolic syndrome – the 'internal global warming' that indicates your body's metabolism has switched into an unsustainable mode of operation.

What is metabolic syndrome?

Metabolic syndrome (previously known as syndrome X) is a cluster of disorders which, when present together, raise your risk of developing type-2 diabetes, as well as coronary heart disease and stroke. Although insulin resistance appears to be the underlying driving mechanism of the syndrome, increased waist circumference, high blood sugar, high blood pressure, high blood fats and low levels of 'good' HDL cholesterol are other identified factors; and having three or more of them will lead to a confirmed diagnosis of metabolic syndrome.

This book provides answers for those with diabetes. People who have many of the causes or contributory factors do have a higher risk, but reading this book will provide you with information to help you identify and reduce those associated risks.

The best way to know if you are at risk of diabetes is to know if you have insulin resistance. This is what the next chapter is all about.

2

Is Your Metabolism Overheating?

Whether you already have diabetes, are concerned about the possibility or are overweight and not feeling great, there's a very good chance that your metabolism is already starting to shift into an unhealthy pattern which, when particularly pronounced, is called 'metabolic syndrome'. This is the precursor for type-2 diabetes. Diabetes is just one of a number of increasingly common health issues of the 21st century that are probably affecting you and members of your family, right now. And to get at the source of the problem it's important to recognise that good health means addressing the other health issues that are connected to it. Have a look at the illustration on the following page – which diseases do you or your close circle of family and friends have? Many of those health issues were extremely rare a hundred years ago, so what has changed to make us more susceptible to them?

Diabetes is part of a wider problem

If you've got quite a few of the health issues listed in the illustration the chances are you have what I call 'internal global warming', because many of the drivers of these problems relate to a shift in your body's biology that is almost inevitable with today's diet and lifestyle. However, I'm going to show you how to buck the trend and undo the damage.

There is a trend in medicine, and in life, to label your biggest problem as some kind of disease, such as diabetes, when in fact what you've got at any moment in time might be a mixture of symptoms – tiredness, weight gain, feeling light-headed if you haven't eaten, low mood and so on. Just being diagnosed as 'diabetic' and treated accordingly doesn't undo all the symptoms you'd rather not have, although some of them do go away.

Of course, you might end up on anti-diabetes drugs, an antidepressant, a cholesterol-lowering pill and something for your high blood pressure. Then you are really in trouble because none of these drugs really address the underlying problem, which is a diet and lifestyle that is completely normal to us but completely alien to the design of the bodies we live in.

Internal global warming

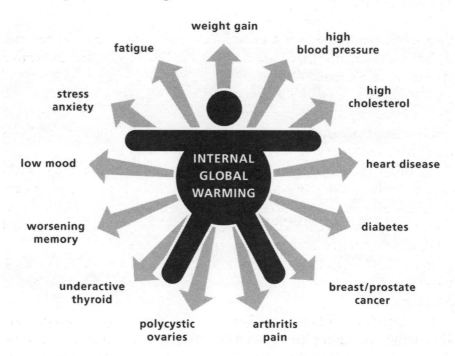

Internal global warming = metabolic syndrome

If you are suffering from internal global warming that means that you have some degree of metabolic syndrome. The cluster of problems illustrated above is being recognised more and more in mainstream medicine as the consequences of metabolic syndrome, originally called 'syndrome X'. Since mainstream medicine prefers objective test results to nebulous 'subjective' symptoms, metabolic syndrome is officially diagnosed when you have three or more of the following:

- High blood sugar or glycosylated haemoglobin

- High blood pressure (above 130/85)

- Increased waist circumference (above 102cm/40in in men or 89cm/35 inches in women)

- High blood fats, called triglycerides (above 3.9)

- Low HDL cholesterol (the 'good' cholesterol – below 1.03 in men and 1.3 in women)

- Insulin resistance

'Metabolic syndrome' is not a disease as such, in the way that diabetes is, but a cluster of symptoms, diseases and test results that indicate a change in one's metabolic processes. If you don't have diabetes but your health is not good you could well have metabolic syndrome, but if you have type-2 diabetes you almost certainly do have metabolic syndrome. (Type-1 diabetes is completely different, however, and you don't have to suffer with metabolic syndrome to have it.)

To discover whether you have most of the above symptoms you will need to make a trip to the doctor for tests. The first two symptoms are relatively easy for you to arrange to have measured yourself, whereas the last three require a blood test. All will be measured in a standard medical screening except, perhaps, insulin resistance.

If you have symptoms such as tiredness, low mood, sugar cravings, thirst and frequent urination, however, these are important for you to take notice of.

Like insulin resistance, or dysglycemia, metabolic syndrome isn't something you either have or haven't got – there are ever-increasing degrees that, if left unchecked, will eventually create the symptoms of diabetes. So, to find out where you are on the scale of metabolic syndrome you need to take into account any tests you have already had as well as your current symptoms. Complete the metabolic syndrome checklist overleaf and add up the two scores. This will give you a useful yardstick to monitor where you are now and your progress as you start to put the strategy I outline in this book into effect.

Questionnaire: Do you have metabolic syndrome?

		Yes	No

Part 1

1 Are you aged 40 or over?

2 Are you or both your parents of African, South Asian, Hispanic or Native American origin?

3 Are you a woman with a waist circumference greater than 89cm (35in)?

4 Are you an Asian man with a waist circumference greater than 94cm (37in)?

5 Are you a white or black man with a waist greater than 102cm (40in)?

(To answer each of the next three questions see Appendix 1 to calculate your BMI):

6 Is your BMI 30 or more?

7 Is your BMI 27 or more?

8 Is your BMI 24 or more?

9 Have your parents or siblings been diagnosed with:

a diabetes?

b heart disease?

c high cholesterol?

d high blood pressure?

10 Are you rarely wide awake within 20 minutes of rising?

11 Do you need tea, coffee, a cigarette or something sweet to get you going in the morning?

12 Do you crave chocolate, sweet foods, bread, cereal or pasta?

13 Do you often have energy slumps during the day or after meals?

14 Is your energy less than it used to be?

		Yes	No
15	Are you gaining weight and finding it hard to lose even though you're not eating more than usual or exercising less?	☐	☐
16	If you exercise for only a short period of time do your muscles feel tired?	☐	☐
17	Are you too tired to exercise?	☐	☐
18	Do you often forget things or have difficulty concentrating?	☐	☐
19	Do you quite often feel down or depressed, sad and defeated?	☐	☐
20	Have you been diagnosed with clinical depression?	☐	☐
21	Do you feel stressed or anxious and tend to overreact to unexpected situations?	☐	☐
22	Do you often feel angry, edgy and irritable?	☐	☐
23	Do you drink alcohol most days?	☐	☐
24	Do you smoke cigarettes every day?	☐	☐
25	Do you smoke at least ten cigarettes each day?	☐	☐
26	Do you eat less than one serving of vegetables each day?	☐	☐
27	Do you eat fewer than five pieces of fresh fruit each week?	☐	☐
28	Do you eat oily fish (salmon, tuna, herring, sardines, mackerel) less than twice a week?	☐	☐
29	Do you eat red meat (lamb, beef), fried foods or crisps?	☐	☐
30	Do you have aching or sore joints or arthritis?	☐	☐
31	Do you suffer from acne, dry flaky skin or eczema?	☐	☐
32	Has your sex drive decreased?	☐	☐
33	Have you been diagnosed with PCOS (women only)?	☐	☐

		Yes	No
34	Do you have difficulty getting or maintaining an erection (men only)?	☐	☐
35	Are you infertile or impotent, or have you been having trouble conceiving?	☐	☐
36	Do you find it hard to fall asleep (generally taking longer than 30 minutes)?	☐	☐
37	Do you wake frequently in the night or very early in the morning and find it hard to get back to sleep?	☐	☐
38	Do you wake up feeling tired and exhausted?	☐	☐
39	Do you feel sleepy during the day or nod off when being driven/in meetings/on the train/in front of the TV?	☐	☐

Score 2 for each 'yes' answer and 0 for each 'no'.

Total score: ☐

Part 2

		Yes	No	Don't know
1	Is your total cholesterol above 6mmol/l?	☐	☐	☐
2	Is your HDL cholesterol below 1.29 (women) or 1.04 (men)?	☐	☐	☐
3	Is your blood pressure greater than 130/85?	☐	☐	☐
4	Is your glycosylated haemoglobin (HbA1c) greater than 5.5% but lower than 7%?	☐	☐	☐
5	Is your glycosylated haemoglobin (HbA1c) greater than 7%?	☐	☐	☐
6	Is your fasting blood sugar level (mmol/l) greater than 5mmol/l (90mg/dl) but lower than 7.0mmol/l (125mg/dl)?	☐	☐	☐
7	Is your fasting blood sugar level (mmol/l) greater than 7.0 mmol/l (90mg/dl)?	☐	☐	☐

Score 2 for each 'yes' answer, 1 for each 'don't know' and 0 for each 'no'.

Total score:

Rating your metabolic-syndrome risk

Less than 20: very low risk
You have a very low metabolic-syndrome risk at present. However, modern living and a hectic lifestyle can easily take their toll on the body. Taking care over your diet, including regular exercise and finding time to relax and recharge your batteries will keep your risk low and help to safeguard your physical and mental health.

21–40: low risk
You have a small metabolic-syndrome risk, so this is the time to make changes to reverse it. Start following a low-GL diet, and make some positive changes to your lifestyle, including regular exercise and finding time to relax and recharge your batteries. Together, these will keep your risk low and help to safeguard your physical and mental health.

41–60: medium risk
This score indicates a medium risk of metabolic syndrome and suggests you have started along the road to poor health. You may have developed a degree of insulin resistance, perhaps experiencing fluctuations in energy and mood on a daily basis. Addressing lifestyle factors, such as eating sugar and the GL level of your diet, as well as high degrees of stress, alcohol and cigarette use, where appropriate, are some of the changes that could have a significant impact on your overall state of well-being.

61 or more: high risk
You have a high risk of metabolic syndrome and may have already been diagnosed with any of the diseases associated with internal global warming, such as diabetes, cardiovascular disease or depression. As you start to make the dietary changes recommended in this book, however, you can greatly reduce your metabolic-syndrome risk, and the symptoms that you are currently experiencing should begin to improve, as you take your first steps on the path to better health.

If having completed the metabolic syndrome checklist you have noticed that you have many of the symptoms of internal warming, you may be at risk of insulin resistance. If you are concerned, you should ask your doctor to check your glycosylated haemoglobin level, which is the best early indicator of risk. This test is also available as a home test kit (see page 326).

Now let's take a look at the key objective measures of metabolic syndrome, to sharpen up your own understanding of where you are along this slippery slope. Then I'll examine the evidence linking the symptoms you are experiencing.

Why being insulin resistant is so predictive of diabetes

It's almost impossible to develop type-2 diabetes without first becoming insulin resistant. Almost nine in ten people with diabetes, if tested, have insulin resistance.[8] To recap, insulin controls your blood sugar level, sending excess glucose in the blood to be stored as fat. So, if it's working, and you're eating too much sugar and carbs, you'll be gaining weight for sure, but your blood sugar level will be normal.

Gradually, the receptors for insulin become blunted through overuse and start to shut down, so you have to make more and more insulin. The more insulin you make, in response to eating carbohydrates or something sweet, the more insulin insensitive you become, so you have to make even more. Eventually, you are so insulin resistant you can't even bring your blood sugar level down. That's diabetes.

This progression is shown in the illustration opposite. (There is a fourth stage, shown on the right, which can happen in advanced diabetes (type-2) where the cells that make insulin in the pancreas stop working. In type-1 diabetes this happens because the body's immune system attacks the insulin-producing cells. In either of these scenarios insulin levels are low.)

The problem with insulin resistance is not only that you can't bring your blood sugar level down. Insulin resistance starves cells of glucose when they need it, and AGEs them (remember those advanced glycation end-products?). So, your brain goes foggy, your memory gets worse, your muscles feel tired, your arteries harden and your skin looks older with more 'age' spots and darkened areas. Insulin resistance attacks every cell in your body and is a fundamental cause of most Western 21st-century diseases.

The progression of glucose and insulin towards diabetes

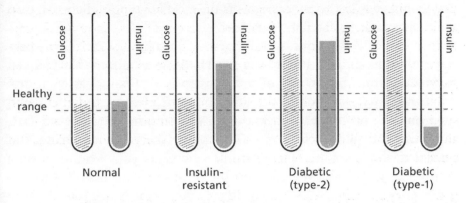

Normal   Insulin-resistant   Diabetic (type-2)   Diabetic (type-1)

Testing for insulin resistance

If you haven't developed diabetes but you are overweight or at high risk according to the metabolic syndrome questionnaire, the simplest way to know if you are insulin resistant is to have a blood insulin test after ingesting a measured amount of glucose, but this requires the cooperation of your doctor. If you can, I recommend having this done. It normally involves ingesting 75g of glucose, then measuring both your blood sugar and insulin levels after one and two hours. Your blood sugar should be less than 4.4mmol/l fasting and never rise above 6mmol/l to 6.6mmol/l after one to two hours. Your insulin should be less than 5mmol/l fasting and should never rise above 30mmol/l after one to two hours. This is an important test to have if you score high on the metabolic syndrome check above.

In the same way that glucose can vary minute to minute, however, so too can your insulin level. In the last chapter we learned that glycosylated haemoglobin is a better long-term indicator of your glucose level. In a similar way something called C-peptide is the best long-term indicator of your insulin level. If you are seeing a diabetes specialist or endocrinologist, the chances are that they will be monitoring this. Your level should be between 250 and 700pmol/l (25–70mmol/l). A high score shows that you are insulin resistant, producing more insulin because you have become relatively insensitive to it. If you score above 1200pmol/l (120mmol/l) then you have a high degree of insulin resistance. A score below 250pmol/l (25mmol/l) shows that either you are extremely healthy or you are following a low-GL diet, but if either of those is not the case you need to be screened for type-1 diabetes, using an antibody test. If you have a degree of destruction of insulin-producing cells in the pancreas, as is the case for type-1 diabetes, then your C-peptide level will be very low.

You can calculate your overall degree of insulin resistance by working out your 'HOMA Index' using a HOMA calculator that you can download from the website of the University of Oxford at www.dtu. ox.ac.uk/homacalculator/download.php. Your HOMA Index is based on a calculation made from knowing your fasting glucose and fasting specific insulin levels (you can use your C-peptide level instead of insulin if you know it). This formula calculates your level of insulin resistance (called HOMA-IR) and the health of your insulin-producing beta-cells (called HOMA-B). Ideally you want your HOMA-IR to be below 2. If your HOMA-IR is above 10 you are significantly insulin resistant. Your HOMA-B should be above 200. If your HOMA-B is low this means your pancreatic cells are not producing enough insulin and it may be wise to be screened for type-1 diabetes.

Testing your glycosylated haemoglobin

In Chapter 1, I mentioned the GLCheck for glycosylated haemoglobin. You may be able to get a glycosylated haemoglobin test through your doctor, but if not you can use this test. It tells you if you are starting to have blood sugar problems and I think it's well worth the investment – it's certainly much better than the glucose test that you'll get in a routine medical.

Here's how you do it:

1. You buy the kit (see Resources), which contains a device that pricks your finger (it doesn't hurt).

2. Put the lancet on your finger or thumb, press the purple part of the lancet down to pierce your skin. Massage your finger or thumb until there are large droplets of blood.

3. Hold your finger or thumb directly over the orange tube to drop the blood in. Keep massaging to produce a few droplets of blood until it reaches the orange line.

4. Immediately, place the orange tube inside the larger container tube. Put this and the used lancets in the prepaid envelope provided and return to the laboratory the same day. They will send you a result that looks like this:

Glycosylated haemoglobin (HbA1c) test results

Personal Details

Name:	Mr Example Results	Gender:	Male
DOB:	18 November 1978	Age:	32
Weight:	85kg	Height:	1.82metres

Body Mass Index (BMI) score: 25.6

Glycosylated haemoglobin level: 6.5% Normal range <5.5%

GLCheck result

Your overall GLCheck score is DARK AMBER

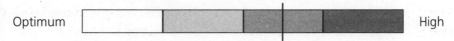

Optimum   High

As you look at the results chart, you want to be in the white area (with a HbA1c score below 5.5 per cent), not in the black (above 7 per cent). If you have a score in the dark grey range (6.1–6.9 per cent) you are at risk of developing diabetes or heart disease, and you probably already have a degree of insulin resistance and metabolic syndrome. If you are in the light grey range (5.5–6 per cent) you are out of danger, with mild dysglycemia, but with room for improvement in relation to your diet. (Note: your lab results will be in colour, ascending in risk from green, through amber to red.)

However, if your score is in the range of 5.5 to 6 per cent you have approximately doubled your risk of diabetes, compared to being in the range less than 5.5 per cent. If you score between 6 and 6.5 per cent you've quadrupled your risk. If you score above 6.5 per cent you have 16 times the risk.[10] A score above 7 per cent is indicative of diabetes, or certainly pre-diabetes. You are also likely to have similar increases in risk of a stroke or a cardiovascular problem.

Conversely, decreasing your score by 1 per cent gives you a 19 per cent reduction in the risk of cataract extractions, 16 per cent decreased risk of heart failure and a 43 per cent reduced risk of amputation or death caused by peripheral vascular disease.

There is growing evidence that glycosylated haemoglobin is perhaps the best early indicator of risk; for example, a three-year study screening people aged 45 to 64 at the Department of Veterans Affairs

Medical Center (VAMC) in the US found that those with a score greater than 5.6 up to 6 per cent doubled their risk of a diabetes diagnosis in the coming year, compared to those with a score below 5.5 per cent. Those with a score of 5.6 to 6 per cent who were also obese had four times the risk. Those with a score of 6.1 up to 6.9 per cent had seven times the risk of a diabetes diagnosis.[11]

Other studies have shown that, on its own, the glycosylated haemoglobin test is a highly sensitive test for either diagnosing or predicting the development of diabetes[12] and for predicting cardiovascular disease.[13]

Testing your blood pressure

One of the first signs of cardiovascular disease, which tends to run hand in hand with diabetes, is increased blood pressure. Imagine a hosepipe attached to a tap that turns on and off. When the tap is on the pressure is greatest, and when the tap is off the pressure is lowest. That's what blood pressure is all about. A blood pressure of 120/80 means that the maximum pressure when the heart has just beaten is 120 units, and the minimum pressure when the heart is in a lull is 80 units. Imagine if the hosepipe was metal rather than rubber. This would raise the pressure wouldn't it, because the metal is rigid whereas the rubber can expand? If the hosepipe was furred up, or if the fluid was thicker, these too would raise the pressure. So raised blood pressure is a reliable indicator that all is not right. Life insurance companies rely heavily on blood pressure to predict expected lifespan.

High blood pressure, also called hypertension, can be the result of any one of three main changes in the artery and is usually a combination of these:

Increased constriction The blood vessels contain a layer of muscle. If this muscle contracts too much the pressure increases. Smoking and stress can cause this kind of constriction as can too much salt (sodium), or not enough magnesium, calcium or potassium. This is because these minerals control the balance between muscles contracting and relaxing. Insulin also affects the musculature of the artery walls, increasing blood pressure.

Thicker blood If the blood is thicker, or stickier, this alone can cause small increases in blood pressure. The blood contains tiny plates, called platelets, which stick to each other. This ability to clot is what stops you from bleeding to death if you cut yourself. Too much clotting, however, and you increase the risk of producing life-threatening blood clots, especially if the arteries are already narrow due to atherosclerosis. Insulin doesn't clot the blood but it does affect the kidneys, keeping more water and salt in the bloodstream, hence more pressure.

Atherosclerosis This is a term that has come to mean a narrowing of a blood vessel due to damage, inflammation and thickening of the blood vessel wall. The blood vessel may also become less elastic, increasing the pressure. Too much blood glucose coats proteins in the arteries with sugar. These glycosylated proteins are hard, inflexible and unhealthy, and contribute to arterial damage.

Approximately one in four people in the UK have hypertension, whereas only half the population have a blood pressure in the optimal range (below 120/80).

Your ideal blood pressure

	Low Risk	Medium	High
Blood	90/60	126/80	136/86
pressure	to	to	or
	125/80	135/85	higher

A blood pressure measurement of 120/80 or less is ideal. A top figure (the systolic pressure) of more than 135, or a bottom figure (the diastolic pressure) of more than 85 indicates a potential problem. A blood pressure of 150/100 indicates a serious risk of heart disease. For example, a 55-year-old man with a blood pressure of 120/80, will, on average, live to the age of 78, while a 55-year-old man with a blood pressure of 150/100 is predicted to live to 72. High blood pressure is a silent killer. Only one in ten people with raised blood pressure are aware of it. After the age of 25 most people's blood pressure increases quite rapidly. So a yearly blood pressure check is always recommended. If you're healthy there's no reason why your blood pressure should increase with your age. Many primitive cultures show no such rise.

Testing your weight and your waist circumference

Your weight, or more specifically your body mass index (BMI) is also an indicator of diabetes risk. (Your BMI is calculated by dividing your weight by your height (squared), thus taking into account that taller people weigh more. You can work out your BMI by going to page 277, or using an online BMI calculator.) If you are in the 'obese' category, with a BMI above 30, your risk of diabetes is 70 times higher than someone in the 'ideal' BMI category. If you are in this category, it is imperative that you lose weight. It may literally be a matter of life or death, perhaps not now, but in the not too distant future. To put your mind at rest, though, many people lose a stone (14lbs/7kgs) a month on my low-GL diet, and I'll be explaining it in detail in Part 3, so your risk will come plummeting down along with your weight.

Your waist circumference is also highly predictive of metabolic syndrome and, consequently, diabetes. A high waist circumference, indicating that you have too much abdominal fat, puts you at high risk of type-2 diabetes, high blood pressure, high cholesterol and heart disease. It's another clear indicator that you need to lose weight for the sake of your health.

How to measure your waist correctly

Put one end of your tape measure midway between the top of your hip bone and the bottom of your rib cage (in line with your belly button), then wrap the tape all the way around your body until the ends meet. Make sure it's not too tight and that it is parallel with the floor. Don't hold your breath while measuring it!

A high-risk waist circumference is:

A man with waist measurement over 102cm (40in)

A woman with waist measurement over 89cm (35in)

Testing your cholesterol and triglyceride levels

If you are over 40 and live in the UK, you've most likely had your cholesterol level measured. It is important, however, to know not only your total cholesterol but also how much of it is in the form called HDL cholesterol (which is the 'good' kind) and LDL cholesterol (the 'bad' kind). Having a low HDL level is as important a risk factor as having a high total cholesterol level, because the HDL molecule helps to remove excess cholesterol from the arteries. Sugar directly raises the portion of cholesterol in the LDL form,[14] and this means that you have less cholesterol in the form of HDL, which is a problem for your body because it means you have more of the unhealthy cholesterol.

If your HDL is below 1.04mmol/l that's indicative of metabolic syndrome and a high risk of diabetes. Generally speaking, your cholesterol should be below 6, and ideally below 5, with at least a third in the form of HDL. So, if you have a cholesterol level of 6, but an HDL level of 3 (a ratio of 2 – meaning that half your cholesterol is the good guy) that's better than having a cholesterol level of 5 and an HDL level of 1 (a ratio of 5). This ratio of your total cholesterol divided by your HDL cholesterol is the most important figure. You want to get this down to 3 or less, meaning that at least a third of your total cholesterol is in the form of HDL.

Perhaps even more important is your level of blood fats, known as triglycerides. You don't want to have a level above 3.9mmol/l, although, according to one study in America, about a third of adults do, and the percentage is much higher among those who are both overweight and don't exercise.[15] Eating high-fat foods, such as red meat and dairy products, or high-sugar or a diet that is 'high GL' (meaning full of refined foods) especially if you have insulin resistance, raises your triglycerides, as does drinking too much alcohol (see Chapter 3 in this part for more on alcohol).

You may recall that the liver converts excess sugar into fat, and it is this that not only ends up stored in your body but also circulates in your blood as triglycerides. That's the biggest promoter of high triglycerides: eating too much sugar, or a high-GL diet. The fruit sugar fructose, particularly, raises triglycerides.[16] The second biggest promoter is a lack of omega fats. Increasing your intake of omega-3s can halve your triglyceride level.

Certain drugs, notably the contraceptive pill, steroid drugs (based on cortisone) and diuretics, given to lower blood pressure, can also increase triglycerides.

Triglycerides are normally tested as part of a routine medical and would be included in a standard medical screening. If you ask for a copy of your test results, this will be shown. If you've had your cholesterol measured, the chances are you will also have a result for your triglycerides.

How the two work together

The most predictive measure of all is your HDL to triglyceride ratio. This is because your triglycerides go higher in direct response to the excess fat you make from blood sugar spikes. If you remember, this happens because the liver converts the excess glucose from the blood that insulin couldn't cope with into fat. As blood sugar spikes increase, so the more LDL cholesterol and the less HDL cholesterol you have. This ratio is the most predictive of cardiovascular disease, and you want to get your ratio of triglycerides to HDL down to 3 or lower. For good health you want to have high HDL cholesterol and low triglycerides.

Other health problems linked to metabolic syndrome

As well as diabetes and heart disease, cancer, depression, memory loss, infertility, impotence and premature ageing are all linked to metabolic syndrome. These problems become more common in people with diabetes so, by reversing metabolic syndrome you can reverse your risk of these problems occurring and help to get rid of those you've already got. Research confirms the risks:

Cancer According to Dr Walter Willett, from the Harvard School of Public Health, being obese is associated with 14 per cent of cancer deaths in men and 20 per cent in women, compared with about 30 per cent each for smoking.[17] If you have gained weight with every decade since the age of 18 you've roughly doubled your risk of cancer.[18] Furthermore, postmenopausal women with high insulin levels have twice the risk of developing breast cancer.[19]

Eating foods with a high GL is linked to a higher risk of breast, colorectal, pancreatic, ovarian, thyroid, endometrial and gastric cancer. People with diabetes in particular have an 82 per cent increased risk of pancreatic cancer.[20] Conversely, low-GL diets are associated with a reduced risk of breast,[21] colorectal,[22] ovarian,[23] and endometrial cancers.[24]

Regularly eating sweet foods, including biscuits, ice cream, honey and chocolate, also increases the risk of breast cancer. Results from a study of more than 5,000 Italian women have shown that the effects may be significant: 'If real [if the results from a small study can be extrapolated to the larger population], the excess risk for frequent sweet consumption may account for 12 per cent of breast cancer cases' say the researchers.[25]

Depression People who are not depressed but who do have metabolic syndrome at baseline are twice as likely to suffer from depression seven years later, confirms research from Finland,[26] and children who have metabolic syndrome are much more likely to become depressed in adulthood.[27]

What is more, if you already suffer from depression, but you don't have metabolic syndrome, there's a very strong possibility that you are insulin resistant and that you are approaching metabolic syndrome. A big study by Harvard Medical School researchers found that women with depression were 17 per cent more likely to develop diabetes, while those taking antidepressants had a 25 per cent higher risk compared to those who weren't depressed.[28] Exactly the same finding was reported in a study of Chinese people, aged between 50 and 70.[29] And the studies continue to show links; for example, major depression predicts the onset of metabolic syndrome[30] and so does long-term depression.[31] Furthermore, depression and raised glycosylated haemoglobin tend to go hand in hand,[32] indeed a recent review article in a medical journal was headed 'Should depressive syndromes be reclassified as "metabolic syndrome type II?"'[33]

Eating sugar can improve your mood when you are feeling low, and this is part of its addictive nature, as I explain in Part 2, Chapter 1, but in Part 3 I'll show you how to break a sugar addiction.

Worsening memory Both metabolic syndrome and insulin resistance are strongly linked to worsening memory. Research shows that the more insulin resistance, the greater a person's risk of both Alzheimer's and dementia,[34] and that older women with metabolic syndrome are almost twice as likely to develop cognitive impairment over a four-year period.[35] As far as men are concerned, the fatter they become the worse their memory declines as they age.[36] Insulin resistance increases the risk of heart disease as well as dementia.[37]

Impotence and infertility Both metabolic syndrome and abdominal weight gain lead to reduced fertility, which is another far too common attribute of diabetes.[38] A worrying trend among adolescents is polycystic ovary syndrome (PCOS), which is strongly linked to insulin resistance and treated with the same kind of drugs as diabetes. Young women with PCOS have higher cholesterol and lower levels of HDL cholesterol and are more insulin resistant than their healthy peers.[39]

Vitamin D is associated with a reduced risk of metabolic syndrome,[40] and new research has found that a lack of it may contribute to infertility. Many people living in Europe and the northern hemisphere are deficient in this vitamin, which comes largely from the sun, but after supplementing with vitamin D, improvements were found in sufferers of PCOS.

Other vital nutrients, such as zinc, vitamin C and essential fats are vital for sperm production and function.[41]

Now you know that metabolic syndrome, and particularly insulin resistance, are the underlying drivers of so many common health problems – not only of diabetes. You also know what your risk is likely to be, and the tests you need to arrange if you haven't done so already.

It may be that you are already experiencing some of those common health problems. Yet, the simple truth is that it is so easy to turn this whole process around, undo the damage and reclaim your health, and that's what the next chapter explains.

3

How to Reverse Metabolic Syndrome and Diabetes

As we saw in the last chapter, type-2 diabetes and metabolic syndrome go hand in hand, but the good news is that they can be prevented. To make good health a possibility it is essential that you correct the problems that lead to metabolic syndrome, whether you have been diagnosed with diabetes or you scored high on my list of symptoms of metabolic syndrome – or even if you just wish to protect your health for the future. You can also reverse type-2 diabetes and metabolic syndrome to the point where you have stable blood sugar, with none of the signs of metabolic syndrome, and no need for drugs – even if you are in the advanced stages of the process.

Look at the case study below on Norwegian nurse Hannemor, whose story was published in the *Norwegian Journal of Medicine*.[42] Hannemor is one of many patients treated by Dr Fedon Lindberg, who have achieved perfect blood sugar control without the need for further medication.

Case Study: Hannemor

Hannemor started gaining weight in her thirties, from 60kg (9 stone 6lb/132lb) to 75kg (11 stone 11lb/165lb). She followed official nutritional recommendations and did not overeat but, year on year, she continued to gain weight. In 1992, at the age of 61, she was diagnosed with type-2 diabetes, hypertension and low thyroid – she weighed 120kg (18¾ stone/264lb). Her blood sugar was out of control and her glycosylated haemoglobin was 8.9 per cent. Hannemor was treated with a cocktail of drugs and ended up injecting 150 units of insulin a day. But, despite all this, her weight continued to increase, so she decided she had to do something different. She sought the advice of diabetes expert Dr Fedon Lindberg in Norway, who put her on a strict low-GL diet and exercise regime, together with nutritional supplements. To cut a long story short, today she needs no insulin, takes no medication, has a normal blood sugar and glycosylated haemoglobin (which is now an ideal 5.4 per cent), and her weight has stabilised below 80kg (12½ stone/176lb). Her total cholesterol:HDL ratio dropped from 5.4 to a healthy 1.7.

Is diabetes really reversible?

You might have been told by your medical practitioner that reversing type-2 diabetes isn't possible; that diet and lifestyle, together with medication, can keep diabetes under control but not reverse it. Yet, the truth is that if Hannemor was to go for a medical today she would not be diagnosed with diabetes. Remember also Kyra, whom we met in the Introduction. In six weeks her blood sugar became balanced and she was able to give up medication. So, why is there such a difference of opinion? The answer is that although most studies testing the effect of diet and lifestyle changes are steps in the right direction, they don't go far enough in applying the golden rules for reversing insulin resistance, the cornerstone of which is a strict low-GL diet (explained in Part 3), not a low-fat diet.

One example is a study that randomly assigned people with pre-diabetes to either a control group or a dietary advice group. After six years, 67.7 per cent of people in the control group had diabetes, compared with only 43.8 per cent in the advice group. This was a 33 per cent reduction.[43] In another study, 12 months of acting on dietary advice led to significant reductions in many diabetes-related factors, such as insulin resistance, blood glucose, triglycerides and cholesterol.[44] And in a further study looking at people with diabetes on medication, those in the diet group managed to drop their glycosylated haemoglobin score from an average of 8.9 per cent to 8.4 per cent. They also lost some weight and lowered their need for medication by 13 per cent. These are good developments but really they are only a start, because in this study the only significant change in the diet-intervention group was a reduction in the intake of saturated fat.[45]

Can it be prevented?

As far as prevention is concerned, two major trials (the Diabetes Prevention Study[46] from Finland and the Diabetes Prevention Program[47] from the US) have shown that intensive lifestyle intervention could reduce the progression from dysglycemia to diabetes by 58 per cent but, again, it still doesn't go far enough. Furthermore, we have to remember that in these studies not everybody would have complied with the advice given or followed it 100 per cent – if they had, it would have produced a much better result. But it's also important to be aiming for the right thing, because simply cutting calories and eating less fat and sugar won't achieve the results you need.

So, what *does* reverse the process of insulin resistance and metabolic syndrome that cause diabetes? There are ten golden rules.

The Ten Golden Rules of diabetes reversal

1 Eat a low-GL diet We have seen how a diet high in refined carbohydrates is one of the main factors behind weight gain and loss of blood sugar control. Such a diet is known as a high-glycemic load diet. Conversely, a low-glycemic load (low-GL) diet doesn't cause blood sugar spikes and will keep your blood sugar even. There are two ways to achieve a low glycemic load. One way is to eat no, or very few, carbohydrates, eating protein instead. The other way is to eat only those carbohydrates that have a low glycemic load – those are the foods that release their sugar content very slowly. Oats and berries are examples. The ideal is to combine these two strategies, eating relatively more protein and less carbohydrate, and by choosing low-GL carbohydrates. This is the diet I will be explaining to you in Part 3.

There are certain tricks to further stabilise your blood sugar, and these are also part of your Anti-diabetes Diet. One is to always combine carbohydrate foods with protein foods and foods which contain a small amount of healthy fats – for example, by having a few almonds or pumpkin seeds when you eat a piece of fruit such as an apple. Another is to eat little and often – five times a day – and never to skip breakfast. I'll explain exactly what you need to do in Parts 2 and 3.

The kind of protein you eat is also important, as I explain below. To make this easier for you I have included a collection of recipes that include all the healthy foods I recommend and you'll find those in Part 4.

2 Eat high levels of soluble fibres One of the reasons why it's good to have some low-GL carbohydrates is that many of these foods, such as oats and especially pulses such as lentils, beans and chickpeas, are naturally high in what are called soluble fibres. These not only have extraordinary effects on further stabilising your blood sugar levels but they also help to eliminate excess cholesterol and fat, so both cholesterol and triglyceride levels in the blood come down. I'm going to show you the evidence about some fibres that you can add to your food to turn your blood sugar balance into a gently undulating landscape instead of hills and mountain peaks.

3 Use the insulin helpers The above two principles mean that your body will need to make much less insulin, but how can you improve your sensitivity to insulin so that the insulin you make works better? This is what one drug, metformin, does – my favourite of those on offer. But the combination of the mineral chromium with a certain extract from cinnamon does it better, without side effects. I'll explain exactly how much you need to take, and when, to help reverse insulin resistance.

4 Increase omega-3 fats and monounsaturated fats; reduce omega-6 and saturated fats and avoid trans fats One of the key reasons why metabolic syndrome, insulin resistance and diabetes cause unpleasant symptoms and knock-on diseases is because they switch your whole system towards inflammation. This is part of the 'internal global warming' that I've been referring to. Inflammation is often experienced as pain, redness or swelling, but it can also be happening in your system, causing hidden problems, such as inflamed and blocked arteries, that eventually lead to a heart attack. Reducing inflammation is absolutely vital, because it helps you get out of the vicious cycle of metabolic syndrome. In the diagram opposite you can see all the factors that conspire to promote inflammation after a meal. Inflammation, you may remember, is another hallmark of metabolic syndrome or internal global warming, associated with your body producing more pain. Inflammation, in turn, promotes insulin insensitivity, feeding back into worsening diabetes.

The inflammation cycle

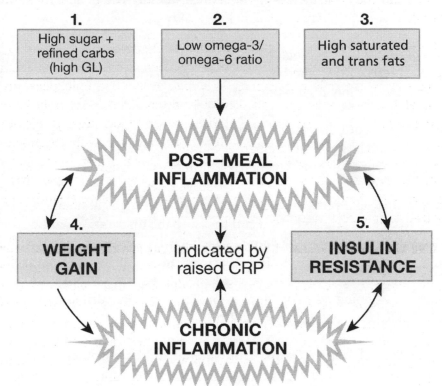

INFLAMMATION is promoted by:

1. High sugar + refined carbs (high GL)

2. Low omega-3/ omega-6 ratio

3. High saturated and trans fats

POST–MEAL INFLAMMATION

4. **WEIGHT GAIN**

Indicated by raised CRP

5. **INSULIN RESISTANCE**

CHRONIC INFLAMMATION

Inflammation after eating is promoted by the five factors indicated above. Obesity and insulin resistance tip your body into a state of permanent inflammation, promoting pain. This is indicated by a raised level of C-reactive protein (CRP) in the blood, which is also a good predictor of a lack of omega-3 fats in the diet.

Meat and dairy products such as cheese are high in saturated fats and tend to increase inflammation and make matters worse, so I encourage you to go for the many natural anti-inflammatory compounds found in food, ranging from spices like turmeric to fruits such as olives. Beans are high in plant sterols, which help to switch off inflammation and normalise cholesterol levels, but the most potent of all are the omega-3 fats found in oily fish. (The best vegetarian source of omega-3s are chia seeds. You might not have heard of these but they are genuine superfoods, full of good-quality protein, soluble fibres and antioxidants as well, see page 96.) You'll find the above healthy foods in many of the recipes in this book.

One of the best measures of inflammation in your system is something called C-reactive protein (CRP), which can be measured in the blood. (Ideally, I'd include it in the cluster of metabolic syndrome tests.) The ideal CRP score is below 1.69mg/l. Raised CRP is a hallmark of diabetes and is strongly associated with higher insulin levels and glycosylated haemoglobin.[48] Hannemor, whose story of diabetes reversal we heard at the beginning of this chapter, lowered her score from an incredibly high 9.0mg/l to just 0.4mg/l.

5 Increase your intake of antioxidants I'll show you which are the best antioxidants in Part 2, Chapter 5, but as a rough guide, foods with strong colours, such as blueberries, tomatoes, mustard and broccoli, have the most antioxidants, and these will help to reduce inflammation. Some, like red grapes, however, are also high in sugar, so you need to be a bit selective. You can measure the total antioxidant power of a food by its 'ORAC' rating, which I'll be explaining in detail in that chapter. (ORAC stands for oxygen radical absorption capacity – it's these oxygen radicals, or oxidants, that do the damage in your body.) I'm going to make sure you are eating and drinking at least 6,000 ORACs a day for good health.

6 Eat liver-friendly foods Antioxidants and certain foods, such as broccoli and red onions, are especially important because they help to support the liver's ability to work optimally. Although I haven't gone into detail, the liver has to work very hard converting excess glucose into fat, and a sluggish liver – or what's called fatty-liver disease – often lies behind the complications of diabetes. It's your liver, not your pancreas, that has a hard time if you have diabetes. You also want your liver's help to reverse the process – that is, burning fat instead of building it. I've included in your Anti-diabetes Diet foods that support liver function, such as the cruciferous vegetables, which include broccoli, cauliflower, cabbage, kale, Brussels sprouts, rocket, watercress and mustard.

You can actually measure your liver's ability to cope with processing the glucose by taking a simple blood test measuring two enzymes called AST and ALT. When your liver is making too much fat, these enzymes spill out into the blood, so your level will go up. If your doctor runs a liver check for you this is what he or she will measure. You can also do it for yourself using a home test kit called LiverCheck (see Resources). If your score is high you need to follow a liver-friendly diet and take certain supplements that support the liver's detoxification processes, since it is responsible for not only breaking down fat but getting rid of any toxins in the body.

I have written a book on exactly how to do this. It's called *The 9-Day Liver Detox*. If you want a rapid kick-start to improving your liver's ability to detoxify, this is the best way to do it (see also page 118). Many of the key principles are also imbedded in your Anti-diabetes Diet.

7 Take daily exercise This is a must if you have diabetes or insulin resistance. Exercise does so much more than burn calories. It actually lowers insulin; helps to stabilise your blood sugar level, and it helps you to burn fat and build muscle. Resistance exercise, such as using weights – which is the kind that helps build muscle – makes your body more sensitive to insulin. Also, simply moving after a meal, such as a ten-minute brisk walk, actually helps get glucose out of the blood into the cells that need it, such as the brain and muscle cells. I'll explain the best kinds of exercise for reversing diabetes, depending on your starting point, but you want to be doing about 20–30 minutes a day of exercise, even if it is just walking.

8 Reduce your stress and improve your sleep You might think that this is easy to say but not possible to do without winning the lottery, but the good news is that it is going to happen naturally when you follow my low-GL diet and take the supplements I recommend. This is because stress isn't just caused by things outside yourself that challenge you, it's also caused by changes in your blood sugar. If your cells are starved of sugar (in the case of advanced diabetes) or if your blood sugar level rebounds are too low, your body makes stress hormones called cortisol. The reason your body does this is to get you ready to hunt for food. It is simply reacting to the fact that your cells need sugar. You become more edgy, irritable, grumpy and hungry, craving carbs or sugar. That makes you react more stressfully. So, by stabilising your blood sugar level so that you never get blood sugar lows you'll naturally feel less stressed and you'll sleep better as a result. In Part 2, Chapter 8 I'll also be giving you simple ways to reduce the stress in your life to help keep your blood sugar and stress hormones in balance.

9 Change what and how you drink The biggest single increase in sugar consumption has come from drinks, many of which are loaded with high levels of fructose. These, and drinks with glucose, are the worst. If you have diabetes you have to be really careful about what you drink. Nothing is better for you than water or herb teas. A little tea and coffee is not a problem, but you need to be careful what you put in it and what you eat with it. Combining a coffee with a carbohydrate snack can send your blood sugar level three times as high, because there is something about this combination that almost halves insulin sensitivity.

Also, if you are in the habit of adding sugar and lots of milk, a latte perhaps, this becomes a deadly combination. Milk actually promotes high insulin levels, even though it is low in carbohydrate. If you must have coffee, drink it on its own, ideally black or with a dash of milk and unsweetened. Then wait 30 minutes before you eat anything. Lemon tea would be a much better choice, but ginger and cinnamon tea is best. I also drink red bush (rooibos) chai tea because red bush is high in antioxidants and the chai spices include ginger and cinnamon.

Many people use stimulant drinks as a pick-me-up, but when you get established on the low-GL diet, and are taking the supplements I recommend, your energy will increase big time.

Alcohol has a strange effect on blood sugar, sometimes sending it down and at other times making it soar up. It certainly doesn't help to stabilise blood sugar levels. It also promotes inflammation. I recommend that you have two weeks' abstinence when you first start the diet, then drink no more than a unit of alcohol (I'll explain what that means) a maximum of five days a week.

10 Take supplements twice a day, every day I know you've probably heard that if you eat a well-balanced diet you will get all the nutrients you need, but this really is completely untrue. Firstly, there are many nutrients you just cannot get enough of from eating food, and these include vitamins C, D and B_{12}. Vitamin D reverses insulin resistance and reduces your diabetes risk, as you'll discover in Part 2, Chapter 4. Much more important than this is the fact that in order to 'tip' your body back towards good health you need much larger amounts of nutrients than you'll need once you are healthy. Chromium is an example. The ideal intake for someone with diabetes is 600mcg a day – that's ten times what you need if you are healthy with no insulin resistance.

Vitamin C and the B vitamins are vital for turning sugar into energy rather than fat. Vitamins B_6, B_{12} and folic acid are vital for a process called methylation, which is essential for making fully functioning insulin, as well as vital neurotransmitters such as adrenalin and serotonin that keep you motivated and in a good mood. A lack of these B vitamins raises the level of homocysteine in your blood. Homocysteine is an amino acid found naturally in the blood. Our levels of it – or our 'H score' – tell us how well our bodies are performing the process of methylation, which is why your H score is a vital health statistic. A high score points to your need for more of these three B vitamins. Poor methylation, raised homocysteine and a consequent need for more B vitamins is the final piece of the equation in understanding how your body's metabolism goes haywire.

You can ask your doctor to test for your homocysteine level or it is easy to measure at home (see Resources). (In Germany homocysteine testing forms part of many medical screening tests.) You want to have a level below 7 or, if you are older than 70, below your age divided by ten. If your level is higher than this figure, then you are not getting sufficient B vitamins for your needs.

Metabolic 'global warming'

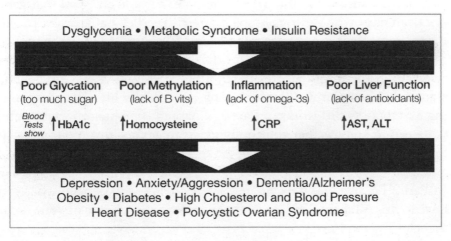

The fundamental contributors to metabolic overheating, the tests worth having, and the associated nutritional imbalances.

As you have seen, there are many factors that contribute to your metabolism overheating, leading to poor blood sugar control (dysglycemia or diabetes), insulin resistance and inflammation. These 'systemic' changes have a knock-on effect, increasing your chances of a wide range of common health problems. But they also go one layer deeper – they actually reprogramme your genes towards disease and premature ageing.

Be kind to your genes

What you eat directly changes your genes. Although you can't alter the genes you were born with, new research is showing that the foods you eat can affect which ones become active or, in technical terms, 'expressed'. That's possibly bad news. To make this clearer, a hundred years ago the Pima Indians – the original inhabitants of Arizona – were thin and fit, living on a high-carbohydrate diet, but the carbs were all natural, unprocessed plants, which were naturally high in fibre. No one ever had diabetes or obesity. Now, nearly all of their descendants are obese, and 80 per cent have diabetes by the time they are 30 years old![49] That's because they have turned from high-fibre carbs to refined carbs, sugar and saturated fat, and those, coupled with nutrient deficiencies, actually turn on the genes that promote diabetes.

In days of old, people whose metabolism was programmed to store carbohydrates as fat survived better when food was scarce. You could call this the 'survival of the fattest'. You are most likely from that gene pool, but now, with the trigger of a modern-day diet, nature is switching the extinction genes so that it will become 'the survival of the thinnest'!

The good news is that my Anti-diabetes Action Plan also does the opposite. It turns off diabetes-promoting genes and cranks up genetic signals that programme you for a long and healthy life. I'll be explaining exactly how this works in Part 2, Chapter 10. The important thing you need to know is that your body *wants* to get healthy. Your job is to create a set of circumstances that make anything else impossible.

In Part 2 I'll give you the evidence for each step and explain what you have to do. All these fundamental principles are included in your Anti-diabetes Diet in Part 3.

Although this approach is designed for those with type-2 diabetes, almost all the golden rules given above apply to those with type-1 diabetes. In the next chapter we explore why type-1 diabetes develops and what you can do to protect yourself. Unlike type-2 diabetes, type-1 is not completely reversible, although those with type-1 diabetes can massively reduce their need for insulin.

4

How to Prevent and Control Type-1 Diabetes

Type-1 diabetes, formerly known as insulin-dependent diabetes, is an autoimmune disease, whereby the immune system selectively attacks and destroys cells in the pancreas that produce insulin. As a result, a person with type-1 diabetes produces very little or no insulin, depending on how many insulin-producing cells have been destroyed. Without insulin, glucose levels rise but it doesn't get into the cells. This glucose starvation leads to cell-energy lows, experienced as extreme tiredness, dizziness and eventually collapsing. People with type-1 diabetes need to inject insulin at regular intervals. However, too much insulin is bad for you and too little is extremely dangerous. It's a balancing act that has to be controlled by the careful use of medication under the guidance of a medical practitioner.

The good news is that certain nutritional changes can decrease your likelihood of getting the disease and can help to alleviate it if you already have it. Research also shows that there are ways that mothers can help to protect their babies from developing the disease.

The nutritional strategy I have been describing that helps type-2 diabetes is also appropriate for people who have type-1, with certain changes that I explain in Part 3. Because my strategy is based on a low-GL diet, you will need less insulin, and the insulin you inject will also work better. According to diabetes expert Professor Charles Clarke, eating a low-GL diet can reduce insulin requirements by up to 40 per cent within two weeks.[50] If you follow my programme strictly there's a good chance that you can cut your insulin requirement from a half to a third of what it is at the moment, but you need to progress slowly, as I explain at the end of this chapter and in the Action Plan in Part 3.

Case Study: Fergus

Having been diagnosed with type-1 diabetes, Fergus followed the standard diabetic diet guidelines for 20 years, gradually gaining weight. He then switched to a low-GL diet: 'Very quickly I lost all my excess weight (4 stones), improved all my lipids, kidney function and retinopathy and saw my HbA1c return to a healthy non-diabetic range of between 4 and 5 per cent, where it has remained ever since. This was without reducing calorie intake, with a marked reduction in hunger and a 75 per cent reduction in insulin dose. I've been eating this way for 10 years now, have no diabetic complications and frankly I have never felt better.' He now runs a website (www.lowcarbdiabetes.co.uk) to help other diabetics.

Before we talk about how to reduce your need for insulin, I want to explain the underlying causes of type-1 diabetes, how you can help prevent it if you haven't got it, and how you can stop any further destruction of insulin-producing cells.

What causes type-1 diabetes?

The general conception is that type-1 diabetes is inherited and that there's nothing you can do to reduce your risk. This has led to a hunt for the gene or genes that makes people susceptible. Many of those with type-1 diabetes do have a variation of a particular set of genes, called the human leukocyte antigen genes, and these probably account for half of the cases of susceptibility to type-1 diabetes, but there are also many other genes potentially promoting susceptibility that have been discovered.[51] Some of these genes are shared in people who have rheumatoid arthritis or coeliac disease (a sensitivity to wheat gliadin).[52]

Inherited genes are only one side of the story. Genes can be switched on and off by environmental factors, and there's growing evidence that many aspects of our modern-day diet may be switching on these diabetes-promoting genes.

Just like type-2 diabetes, type-1 incidence is very much on the increase. A recent study in the *Lancet* medical journal predicts a doubling of new cases of type-1 diabetes in European children younger than five years between 2005 and 2020, and a 70 per cent increase in all those younger than 15 years.[53]

This surely means that something other than genes is driving the increased incidence of type-1 diabetes, since the genes we inherit haven't changed. Two main factors are thought to potentially trigger the body into producing antibodies that attack the pancreas. One is food allergies, the other is viral infections.

Protect your baby by avoiding food allergies

The food allergy link is thought to happen because the immune system can react against a food, producing antibodies that attack that it, but it may also mistakenly produce antibodies that attack the pancreatic cells instead. This is called cross-reaction. It has been proposed that the early introduction of foods other than breast milk, before the age of four months, might increase this risk. Early introduction of cow's milk, in animal studies, has been shown to increase the incidence of type-1 diabetes quite dramatically,[54] although human studies have not confirmed this.[55] It is known, however, that cow's milk proteins do end up in breast milk,[56] a factor not taken into account in these studies. With this in mind, it may be wise for breast-feeding mothers not to consume dairy products. In any event, it is a good idea not to introduce babies to any dairy products before the age of 12 months to minimise the possibility of developing an allergy to dairy, the most common food allergen. It takes several months for a baby's immune system and gut to form properly and no food is better than breast milk for at least the first six months. Other dairy products also raise insulin levels substantially.[57]

Coeliac disease and type-1 diabetes

Type-1 diabetics are much more likely to have coeliac disease, which is an allergy to a type of protein in wheat called gliadin. Almost half of all people with type-1 diabetes have ATG antibodies, which are a diagnostic marker of coeliac disease, and the majority have deposits of these antibodies in their intestines.[58] This suggests that the early introduction of wheat products might increase risk. Once again, this is a food well worth avoiding for the first 12 months of a baby's life.

The vast majority of people with coeliac react to the gliadin component of wheat, which is also present in rye and barley but is absent in oats. Gluten-free grains such as rice are also free from gliadin so are a much safer bet when weaning a baby.

Coeliac disease is far more common than most people think. Many medical textbooks say that it affects one in several thousand, however, a survey testing people for ATG antibodies found that it affects one in 111. Susceptibility to coeliac disease is, in part, genetically inherited – for example, if your mother, father, brother or sister has it, you have a one in eleven chance of having it too. If you have an autoimmune disease, your risk is even higher. A survey in Denmark found that one in eight children with type-1 diabetes also had coeliac disease.[59] Both conditions can result in being underweight: in the case of diabetes this is because cells are starved of sugar, and, in the case of coeliac disease, this is because it damages the gut making it difficult to absorb nutrients.

Testing for coeliac disease

Given the known link between food allergy and the destruction of insulin-producing cells, if you've never been tested it's worth doing it, especially if you have any digestive problems and/or a family history of coeliac disease. Ask your doctor first, but you can also use a home test kit called the Coeliac Test (see Resources) that gives you an instant result, much like a pregnancy test. It measures the presence of ATG and is a very reliable test.

In one study, not only did 100 per cent of those with coeliac disease test positive to ATG but the greater the degree of reactivity, the greater the level of damage to the gut mucosa. So, it not only tested whether or not the person was sensitive, but also the degree of sensitivity.

Other allergies

Whenever anyone who comes to me for help presents with an autoimmune disease I always recommend a proper IgG antibody food intolerance blood test to find out if they are producing antibodies against other foods, not just wheat and milk. (Most food allergies, often called food intolerances, involve IgG antibodies. Classic, immediate food allergies, such as a violent reaction to nuts, often involve the IgE antibody reaction. These can also be tested in a blood test – see Resources.) The theory is that if the immune system becomes hyper-alert against foods, it 'cross-reacts' against certain body tissues. So, the goal is to eliminate the food that you are allergic to and to lessen the immune system's belligerent attitude.

Immune reactions in the gut

There are more immune cells in the gut than anywhere else in the body for the simple reason that the gut is a major internal point of contact with the outside world. Here, the immune system checks out every-thing you eat to discover whether it is a friend or a foe. It could be that the early introduction, and high consumption, of wheat and dairy products – which are relatively new foods to homo sapiens – is trigger-ing autoimmune reactions in a substantial percentage of people who then go on to develop type-1 diabetes.

What's interesting is that 80 per cent of those with coeliac disease don't react to oats. This cereal is not only gliadin-free but also a rich source of beta-glucans, which are beneficial for the immune system. One of the prevalent theories as to why autoimmune diseases are on the increase is that we live in environments that are too clean and we don't have enough exposure early in life to bugs and bacteria. Most microbes have beta-glucans present in their cell walls and these stimu-late the immune system and help to build up normal, strong immunity. So, eating foods containing beta-glucans may help to lessen autoim-munity and improve general health.

Many foods that are known to be immune-enhancers – such as shii-take mushrooms and the herb Echinacea – are also rich sources of beta-glucans. I recommend eating more oats and shiitake mushrooms, but you can also get supplements of purified beta-glucans – choose those that contain (1–3) (1–6) beta-d-glucans, which have greater activity in the body than the (1–3) (1–4) beta-glucan form.

The role of nutrients in the fight against allergies

Another nutrient that seems to switch off a hyperactive immune system is glucosamine, famous for reducing inflammation in arthritis. In animal studies a form of this nutrient called N-acetylglucosamine was found to dampen down immune cells from attacking pancreatic tissue, as is found in type-1 diabetes.[60] Although we need human studies using people with type-1 diabetes to validate this, one other study did find that N-acetylglucosamine switched off autoimmune inflammatory bowel disease, possibly confirming the importance of this nutrient for further research. In my opinion, given that there are no down sides, it's worth trying for a couple of months and continuing if you find a benefit.

Another nutrient critical for healthy immunity is vitamin D. Made in the skin in the presence of sunlight, vitamin D is vital to general good health, but many of us are deficient in it, especially those of us living in the northern hemisphere, where it is a particular problem during the winter. Vitamin D deficiency has also been linked to a higher incidence of type-1 diabetes.[61] As well as coming from the sun, vitamin D is also rich in oily fish (see also page 49).

If you have type-1 diabetes but still have some insulin production, you might be able to prevent further cell destruction by avoiding foods that you are allergic to, and minimising wheat and milk products. Eating more oats and shiitake mushrooms for beta-glucans and oily fish for vitamin D will also be helpful, and you might also consider supplementing these nutrients, as well as glucosamine.

Viral infections

There's growing evidence that viruses in the gut, responsible for gastroenteritis, can also trigger type-1 diabetes.[62] This is, of course, another reason to keep your immune system strong and your digestive system healthy. If you do have digestive problems, supplementing a combination of probiotics, digestive enzymes and glutamine is a great place to start. It's also worth checking for food allergies, which further weaken the immune system.

Other factors

Another line of thought is that rapid growth in height and being over-weight lead to too much insulin being produced. (Rapid growth, by the way, is associated with very high dairy consumption.) Such an over-load on the insulin-producing cells may lead to their self-destruction.[63] A similar process is seen in advanced type-2 diabetes.

The importance of fat

One of the biggest promoters, or hinderers, of gut-associated immune reactivity is the balance of omega-3 to omega-6 fats in your diet. Omega-6 fats, although healthy in small amounts, need to be eaten in moderation. Most people eat too many omega-6 fats (found in convenience foods, fried foods, snacks and so on) and two few omega-3 fats. By increasing the proportional amount of omega-3s, your body can switch off your gut's over-reactivity.

Being overweight or insulin resistant also increases the gut's inflammatory potential. So, a low-GL diet really does help autoimmune diseases, because it helps you to lose weight or to maintain a healthy weight. A clear reason for this is that the damage caused by too high sugar levels, called glycosylation, affects proteins in such a way that they may start to misbehave, or can no longer be recognised as a friend but seen as a foe by the body's immune system. The more damaged proteins (AGEs) you have, the more your immune system is likely to react.

Fructose (fruit sugar) is particularly bad news, because the body finds it harder to burn than glucose. Although it could be described as more 'slow-releasing', and therefore better for us, evidence suggests that high-fructose diets, principally from fructose-sweetened fizzy drinks, are messing up the body's control functions. Small amounts are not so much of a problem because the body can metabolise some fructose, but once its limit is exceeded, fructose becomes a dangerous sugar, so I highly recommend you avoid all fructose. You will need to check the labels on drinks and foods as it appears in many foods. In Part 2, Chapter 7 I explain in more detail this very unhealthy sugar.

Go back to the Stone Age

Another successful diet approach to autoimmune diseases is a 'paleo' diet, or a Stone Age diet. Before we became peasant farmers, so to speak, humanity lived on lean meat, seafood, plants, fruit and nuts – we weren't yet eating grains or dairy products. Many people with autoimmune diseases report great improvements from eating an essentially grain- and dairy-free diet. The Stone Age diet is also naturally high in poly-unsaturated fats and has a good balance of omega-3 and omega-6 fats. It is also free from sugars, low in saturated fat and high in fibre and is, in many ways, similar to a low-GL diet.

There is another difference between modern living and paleo living: vitamin D exposure. Given that we were originally designed to be naked, outdoors and living a lot further south than many of us do, our intake of vitamin D has drastically declined.

As we saw earlier, vitamin D deficiency is linked to an increasing risk of type-1 diabetes and other autoimmune diseases.

Getting enough vitamin D

We need at least 30mcg of vitamin D a day. Eating oily fish and exposing your arms, face and legs for 30 minutes daily in summer might give you 15mcg, so it's best to supplement at least another 15mcg a day. Of course, it's important to be careful with babies and young children in the sun because their skin is so much more tender. Always cover them up after 20 minutes in moderate sun and use a high-factor sun-screen.

Minimising your risk

Putting all this together, for someone wanting to prevent type-1 diabetes from developing, or worsening, the right course of action would be to:

- Have more omega-3 fats in the diet (see Part 2, Chapter 4).

- Test for, and eliminate, food allergies – and also heal the gut with a combination of glutamine, probiotics and digestive enzymes, if testing shows multiple allergies.

- Follow a strict low-GL diet (see Part 3).

- Take a high-potency multivitamin–mineral that contains at least 15mcg of vitamin D.

- Supplement extra immune-boosting vitamin C (2g a day), and at least 15mg of zinc (see pages 122 and 124 for more about these nutrients).

- For mothers, breastfeed for the first six months (avoiding eating dairy produce during that time) and avoid giving your baby wheat and dairy products until they are one year old. (You can buy non-dairy follow-on milks.)

Start off slowly as you manage your blood sugar level

If you have type-1 diabetes – or are the parent of a child with it – the basic strategy for managing your blood sugar balance is essentially the same as for type-2 diabetes, with some important differences. If you go full steam ahead with an immediate low-GL diet, plus the recommended supplements such as chromium, your need for insulin may plummet and then the dose you are currently taking will become too much for you and will induce a hypo (low blood sugar level).

So, it is essential to go slowly. Exactly how to do this is explained in your Anti-diabetes Action Plan in Part 3, page 204.

5

The Truth about Diabetes Drugs

'Medicine might be winning the battle of glucose control, but is losing the war against diabetes. Because type-2 diabetes, which accounts for 90 per cent of diabetes, is largely rooted in reversible social and lifestyle factors, a medical approach alone is unlikely to be the solution. A strong, integrated, and imaginative response is required, in which the limits of drug treatment are recognised.'

These are not my words but those of an editorial in a special edition of the *Lancet* medical journal in 2010.[64] It goes on to say 'the fact that type-2 diabetes, a largely preventable disorder, has reached epidemic proportion is a public health humiliation'.

The treatment of diabetes, say the guidelines, should be done as a partnership: you and your doctor collaborate on what fits your needs best. It's a fine idea but it can be tricky if you are relying on drugs to keep your blood sugar under control, because to make sensible decisions you need to have good information and with drugs that can be hard to come by. Doctors should now be more aware of the potential problems with drugs for diabetes. In this chapter I will describe the drugs on offer to help you to make an informed choice so that you will have more knowledge when discussing with your practitioner the best steps to take.

Metformin and biguanides

The chances are, if you have type-2 diabetes, that you will have been prescribed metformin. It is what's called a 'biguanide' and has been around for about 30 years – it is still the most widely used drug. Metformin works to lower your levels of blood sugar by increasing insulin sensitivity in the muscles so that they take up more glucose. It also increases sensitivity in the liver, which means that that organ doesn't release so much glucose. It doesn't cause weight gain – which other treatments do – and may even result in some weight loss. There is some evidence that those on metformin have a reduced incidence of cancer.[65] Whether this is a beneficial effect of the drug or a result of lowering blood sugar isn't yet clear. It's the best of the bunch by far, but it is even more effective if you are following a diabetes-friendly diet and lifestyle.

When you start using metformin, it sometimes causes gastrointestinal symptoms such as mild nausea, cramps and vomiting, and soft or loose stools, although a new, slow-release formulation minimises the likelihood of these side effects. Some people tolerate it well although others don't.

The problems with metformin

Metformin has a black-box warning (the most serious kind) in the US because of a very small risk of a potentially fatal condition known as lactic acidosis. Furthermore, metformin is processed in the kidneys, so it shouldn't be used if you have serious kidney problems. That said, it's probably one of the better diabetic drugs in relation to side effects.

Perhaps the most serious side effect of metformin, however, is that it knocks out vitamin B_{12} levels in the body, especially in those who suffer from gastrointestinal symptoms from taking metformin. This is likely to allow your homocysteine level to rise, which is strongly associated with increasing the risk of heart attack. I introduced you briefly to homocysteine in Chapter 3 – a high level of this amino acid in the blood is associated with an increased risk of strokes, cardiovascular disease, osteoporosis, depression and age-related memory loss. This effect on vitamin B_{12} was first reported in 2004,[66] but most doctors aren't aware of it or acting accordingly. This is probably more likely to be an issue for you if you have experienced digestive symptoms with the drug.

A trial, published in the *British Medical Journal* in 2009 confirms this. A dosage of 850mg of metformin was given to 196 of the study's participants and a placebo to the other 194 people three times daily for more than four years.[67] People who had taken the metformin were found to have a 19 per cent reduction in their vitamin B_{12} levels, compared with those who had taken the placebo, who had almost no change in their levels during the study. In addition, the reduction of levels of vitamin B_{12} by metformin was not temporary but persisted and became more apparent over time. There was also a significant rise in the number of people with seriously deficient levels of vitamin B_{12} from 3 patients to 19 over the period of the study if they had been taking metformin. The equivalent number for the placebo group rose from four patients to five. Compared with people taking a placebo, people taking metformin also had a 5 per cent increase in homocysteine, but their folate levels were the same. Homocysteine levels increased especially in individuals in whom vitamin B_{12} levels decreased – showing that the decrease in vitamin B_{12} levels were functionally meaningful. The authors say: 'Our study shows that it is reasonable to assume harm will eventually occur in some patients with metformin-induced low vitamin B_{12} levels.'

The authors conclude: 'Our data provide a strong case for routine assessment of vitamin B_{12} levels during long term treatment with metformin.' However, although current guidelines indicate that metformin is a cornerstone in the treatment of type-2 diabetes, no recommendations are made on the detection and prevention of vitamin B_{12} deficiency during treatment.

What you can do

I suggest that if you are on metformin you check your homocysteine level. If it is raised, you need to supplement more vitamin B_{12} – ideally in combination with the other homocysteine-lowering B vitamins: B_6 and folic acid. The recommended daily allowance (RDA) for this vitamin is far too low. A basic level of B_{12} to supplement for everybody is 10mcg a day. A good multivitamin needs to provide this, but if your B vitamin levels are low, or your homocysteine level is high, you'll need more like 500mcg to correct the deficiency.

Vitamin B_{12} is increasingly poorly absorbed as you age, and deficiency is known to increase the rate of brain shrinkage, and hence the risk of accelerating memory loss and Alzheimer's. According to a survey by researchers at the University of Oxford, two in five people over the age of 61 in the UK have insufficient B_{12} levels to stop accelerated brain shrinkage.[68] The chances are you'll be lacking B_{12} if you are over 60 and on metformin – and even more likely if you are taking a proton pump inhibitor (medication such as Nexium for indigestion), as this stops you making stomach acid, which is vital for the absorption of B_{12}. Under these circumstances your doctor really should test your homocysteine and B_{12} levels. If they won't, you can test your homocysteine level yourself with a home test kit (see Resources). Your homocysteine level should be below 7. Above 9 correlates with accelerated brain shrinkage and increased risk of heart disease and stroke.

The natural alternatives to metformin

The best alternative to metformin is to follow my Anti-diabetes Action Plan, including the recommended low-GL diet, as well as taking chromium and other supplements, and to take at least 20 minutes' daily exercise.

I'll look at the effectiveness of natural alternatives shortly, but first I want to look at the other drugs that are prescribed for diabetes.

Sulfonylurea drugs are bad news

Amaryl, Euglucon and Diamicron are what are known as sulfonylurea drugs. These drugs stimulate cells in the pancreas (called beta cells) to produce more insulin. Most people with type-2 diabetes produce too much insulin – the problem is that the insulin that's produced doesn't function properly. It makes little sense, therefore, to stimulate the pancreas to produce even more in order to accommodate the very same poor dietary choices that lead to the development of diabetes in the first place. When you get your diet right, these drugs often become unnecessary and should be the first to go.

What you can do

The most common side effect with sulfonylureas is an excess of insulin, causing too much glucose to be taken out of the blood. This can lead to a potentially serious drop in glucose supplies to the brain, known as a 'hypo' – blacking out because your blood sugar level drops too much. Watch out if you've suddenly improved your diet, as this side effect may become more common as your need for the drug becomes less: for example, within six weeks of following my low-GL diet, and taking chromium, one patient's blood sugar level normalised and she started experiencing hypos when she took her Amaryl. Her doctor then stopped the drug. Advise your doctor that you are starting on the diet and that you expect to see your blood sugar level drop so that he or she can be prepared to adjust your medication.

Sulfonylureas can also cause gastrointestinal problems including nausea, vomiting and diarrhoea, or constipation and weight gain. The weight gain can be significant, triggered by rising insulin levels in people who typically have dangerously high levels to begin with. There is also evidence that these drugs can damage the pancreas into early failure, so control of sugar, although quick, is brief. Not surprisingly, I feel sulfonylureas are bad news and should be avoided.

Why you should be suspicious of new drugs

There is a simple financial fact you need to be aware of regarding drugs. Pharmaceutical companies can only make money on patented drugs for which they effectively have a monopoly and hence can charge a high price and fund their marketing campaigns. Once a patent runs out, usually after 15 years, anyone can produce the drug, so the price and profit comes right down. The patent for metformin, for example, has run out and it is therefore much less expensive than other drugs.

An example is Avandia (rosiglitazone), one of a new family of diabetes drugs called glitazones (also known as thiazolidinediones) that were licensed over a decade ago to treat diabetes. Avandia works by increasing your body's sensitivity to insulin. This sounds like a good thing to do, and it's very effective at bringing blood sugar levels down – but at a cost. Well-known side effects include significant weight gain, fluid retention, a raised risk of heart failure and a link with osteoporosis.

What you may not have been warned about is the growing evidence that Avandia could increase your risk of a heart attack even though the first warning bells were sounded four years ago.[69] The evidence for harm continued to grow but so too did the prescriptions. By 2009 around 500,000 prescriptions a year were written for the drug in the UK.[70]

By July 2010 both the American drug regulator, the Food and Drug Administration (FDA), and the European one, the European Medicines Agency (EMA), considered taking it off the market and strengthening the warnings about it. The EMA did neither.

Behind the scenes, a fight was on to keep the drug on the market. A major plank in Glaxo Smith Kline's (GSK's) evidence was a big trial that reported no increase in the risk of heart disease among nearly 4,500 patients taking Avandia. It was called Record, and it began in 2002/3; the results were published in 2009.[71]

Dr Thomas Marciniak, a scientist working for the FDA, described it as 'seriously flawed'. He reported that his detailed examination of only a small percentage of all the cases had found a dozen instances where patients taking Avandia appeared to suffer serious heart problems that were not counted in the total of adverse events. One patient, for example, was hospitalised after a severe stroke. But the study record doesn't list them as having a cardiovascular problem. In reply GSK said that it stood by the Record study and that five further studies had all concluded that Avandia was safe.[72]

This reassuring picture was challenged further by the most high-profile and persistent critic of Avandia, cardiologist Dr Steven Nissen of the Cleveland Clinic in Ohio. He had carried out the study in 2007 which first set alarm bells ringing, with its conclusion that Avandia raised the risk of heart attack or stroke by 40 per cent.

At the hearing, he presented new data which estimated the number of people who would have to take Avandia for one of them to be harmed. 'Even if you accept the favourable Record data, you would still get one extra heart attack for every 52 people treated with Avandia,' he said.[73] Dr Nissen has since published a meta-analysis of all trials which makes the risks associated with Avandia very clear.[74]

The Avandia story is still relevant

Avandia is now banned (although still occasionally prescribed). During the years between Dr Nissen's original paper and the 2010 hearings the official advice was that the 'benefits outweighed the risks' for Avandia; however, many diabetes clinicians didn't agree. 'We have had serious doubts about the safety of Avandia for a number of years,' says Dr Ralf Abraham who heads a private clinic, the London Diabetes and Lipid Centre.

It was only following a headline article in the *Daily Mail*, a *Panorama* TV documentary, and a strong article in the *British Medical Journal* that the EMA took action, effectively banning all marketing of Avandia in September 2010.[75]

The fierce disagreements over the safety data of Avandia is a prime example of why making informed decisions about drugs can be tricky. Furthermore, the EMA is charged with protecting you from the dangers of drugs, yet they are mainly funded by the pharmaceutical industry. As the editor of the *British Medical Journal* aptly said, 'Even the most loyal Manchester United fan wouldn't expect Alex Ferguson to be the referee for a match.'

Yet, back in 2007 a lead editorial in the *New England Journal of Medicine* said, 'Insofar as the findings of Nissen and Wolskire present a valid estimate of the risk of cardiovascular events, rosiglitazone represents a major failure of the drug-use and drug-approval processes.'[76]

Why it's best to be wary of new drugs

The fact that a harmful drug was licensed in the first place, and then took three years to come off the market from the point of clear evidence of harm, should make you suspicious of any new drugs.

It's not just Avandia that has been under scrutiny recently. There are some new kids on the block that work in a completely different way from existing drugs for diabetes and promise to avoid the problems of weight gain and raised risk of heart problems that come with glitazones. It is possible that the companies involved are being totally straightforward about the potential risks but, even so, rarer or serious side effects are unlikely to appear until they have been on the market for several years.

Some of these new drugs are designed to replace the sulfonylurea drugs, including Amaryl, Euglucon and Diamicron discussed above, whose patents are about to, or have, expired.

The new drugs all target GLP-1, a peptide that is released in the gut when you eat. GLP-1 normally acts to trigger the release of insulin from the beta cells in the pancreas so by manipulating its level, these drugs affect how excess sugar is cleared away from the blood. These drugs are a more sophisticated version of the old sulfonylurea drugs (described on page 54), which also stimulate the beta cells to produce insulin.

Sulfonylureas produce the same boost to insulin release regardless of how much you have eaten. However, the new drugs are sensitive to your meal size. This means that the amount of GLP-1 produced and the amount of insulin released is appropriate to your food intake. As you now know, making more insulin isn't such a good idea because excess insulin is, itself, harmful. Another benefit is fewer of the hypos that are a major drawback of the older drugs.

In general, the new drugs increase the amount of GLP-1 that's produced at meal times to compensate for the loss of insulin sensitivity and overcome the decline in production that often occurs in people with diabetes. One approach is to make the GLP-1 produced stay active for longer by blocking an enzyme called DPP-4 whose job it is to clear away GLP-1.

Drugs that do this include Januvia (sitagliptin) and Galvus (vildagliptin), which are widely regarded as a big improvement, not least because rather than causing you to put on weight, as the glitazones Actos and Avandia do, they can cause weight to drop off. There are more unpleasant side effects, however, including more vomiting, stomach ache and diarrhoea, than you get with more traditional drugs.

There is also a more serious concern because the job of the blocked enzyme DPP-4 isn't just to clear away GLP-1, it cleans up a number of other bodily processes that you don't want to go on for too long (such as inflammation), and targets cells that are turning cancerous. There have been some early reports of raised risk of inflammatory problems in patients with rheumatoid arthritis and of cancers, particularly melanoma, prostate and lung.[77]

Another approach to raising GLP-1 is by making a synthetic version of it. Two drugs that do this are Victoza (liraglutide) and Byetta (exenatide), which have to be injected. Both of these drugs stay in the body for much longer than the natural version. They are arousing a lot of interest because they can also produce considerable weight loss, but both can also cause nausea which, in the case of Victoza, affected nearly half of the patients using it in the trials. The drug is also being tested for possible cancer links.

What you can do

If you are offered a new drug, apart from finding out about the side effects, you should ask your medical practitioner if the new drug is more effective than the older ones. Although established drugs are less profitable, and hence not marketed aggressively to doctors by the pharmaceutical companies, at least they've been around for a long time.

There is certainly a good case for comparing new drugs, not against placebo but against the best available treatment; for example, a major review on the effectiveness of diabetes drugs concludes:

'*Compared with newer, more expensive agents (thiazolidinediones, alpha-glucosidase inhibitors, and meglitinides), older agents (second-generation sulfonylureas and metformin) have similar or superior effects on glycemic control, lipids, and other intermediate end points. Large, long-term comparative studies are needed to determine the comparative effects of oral diabetes agents on hard clinical end points.*'[78]

Those 'hard ... end points' mentioned above mean whether or not you suffer less or survive for longer.

Aggressive drug treatment is not the answer

It is not just new drugs and their possible long-term side effects that people with diabetes have to be aware of. Some doctors are rethinking the way high-risk diabetes patients are treated. Conventional wisdom says it should be as aggressively as possible to bring down their markers for heart disease.

A recent trial known as Accord, however, found that people with diabetes who had a high risk of heart disease, because they had high blood pressure, high blood sugar and high cholesterol, actually had more deaths from heart attacks when they were intensively treated with higher doses of drugs, including statins, than those who received regular amounts.[79]

In fact it's not really clear why diabetes causes heart disease. People with diabetes are certainly at a greater risk but their level of risk doesn't seem to be related to the usual symptoms. 'Very little of the additional risk is explained by obesity, blood pressure, lipids [fats in the blood] or kidney problems', says Dr Nadeem Sawar of Cambridge University, discussing his recent study.[80] So the drugs may not be doing much for those who need help.

Consider the natural alternatives

When you view diabetes and its associated complications as part of a process of 'internal global warming' and metabolic syndrome, as I've been explaining in this part, it becomes obvious that changing your body's ecology through nutrition and lifestyle changes has to be the best way forward, rather than taking a cocktail of drugs with their attendant side effects to lower the indicator of risk, be it high glucose, cholesterol or blood pressure.

The dangers of insulin and insulin-promoting drugs

By now you are well aware that the last thing you want is very high insulin levels. If you have type-1 diabetes, on the other hand, you need insulin

continued

injections to get glucose from the blood into your cells – the last thing you want is no insulin, because that can induce a diabetic coma. The good news is that following my Anti-diabetes Action Plan can dramatically reduce your need for insulin and help you to balance your blood sugar levels, making you feel better and more energised.

In the case of type-2 diabetes, you should never have got to the point where you needed or were given insulin. Of course, this does happen because people don't want to change their diet, or can't break free from their sugar addiction. But, provided you are committed to change, there is every reason why you should be able to come off insulin (unless your pancreatic cells are irreversibly damaged) and every reason to do so.

In Chapter 1, I explained how excess insulin promotes fat storage and stops you breaking down fat, increases your cholesterol and triglyceride levels, and increases your risk of heart disease. It causes the kidneys to retain both water and salt, which increase your blood pressure, but it also increases cancer risk. In a Danish study, insulin users had a 50 per cent higher risk of cancer[81] and in a Canadian study the greater a person's use of insulin the greater their risk of cancer. In this study, metformin users had a lower risk compared to those taking sulfonylurea drugs, which, as we've seen, stimulate insulin production.[82]

The healthy alternative

So, just how effective is a healthy diet plus exercise in preventing or treating diabetes in the longer term? Trials on lifestyle are much harder to do than trials on pills, but a good attempt was made by researchers at George Washington University in Washington DC, who published their findings in 2005.

The team selected volunteers who had signs of glucose intolerance and were therefore at high risk of developing diabetes, then split them into three groups. One received placebos, the next 850mg of metformin twice a day, and the third began to make lifestyle changes designed to lower their weight by 7 per cent, including 2½ hours of exercise a week (20 minutes a day). At the end of three years, among those who made the lifestyle changes, 41 per cent were no longer glucose intolerant. Among those who took metformin, 17 per cent more were no longer glucose intolerant, compared to those on placebo. So the lifestyle change was more than twice as effective.[83]

The comparative costs of drugs v. lifestyle changes

Despite the prevailing medical view, the dietary approach is likely to be more cost-effective. Based on the data from a massive diabetes-prevention programme launched in the US in 2002, Dr William Herman, professor of internal medicine at the University of Michigan School of Medicine, built a computer simulation to estimate the cost-effectiveness of changing one's lifestyle versus taking diabetes drugs.[84] His study showed that taking metformin as a preventative might delay the onset of diabetes by three years, while changes in diet and exercise delays it by 11 years. His team estimated that the drug would cost $29,000 per year of healthy life saved, while the diet and exercise regime would cost $8,800. 'The bottom line,' says Herman, 'is that lifestyle intervention is more cost-effective than a pill.'

Another landmark study, which also found diet and exercise to be twice as effective as metformin in preventing at-risk patients from developing diabetes, estimated that the non-drug approach was also very cost-effective.[85] In this study, published in 2002, one case of diabetes was prevented in every seven people treated for three years.

Eat your oats and supplement chromium

Oats, or specifically oat bran, contain a powerful anti-diabetes nutrient. It's called beta-glucan. Diabetic patients given oatmeal or foods rich in oat bran experienced much lower rises in blood sugar compared to those who were given white rice or bread. In fact, it's been known for nearly a decade that having 10 per cent of your diet as beta-glucans can halve the blood sugar peak of a meal.[86]

This level of effect is as great as you'll get from taking metformin (at a fraction of the price). Practically, that means eating half oat flakes, half oat bran, cold or hot as porridge, with a low-GL fruit such as berries, pears or apples, and snacking on oatcakes (rough oatcakes have the most beta-glucans). With over 1,000 studies on beta-glucans, the evidence really is overwhelming. (Oats have a relatively low GL, too, as I explained in Chapter 3.)

Chromium works better than metformin, but without any side effects. It also improves insulin sensitivity, kicks in faster, and lowers blood sugar levels more effectively. It is cheap, since nutrients can't be patented, and has plenty of good-quality 'double-blind' trials to prove its efficacy. A systematic review in the top diabetes journal *Diabetes Care* in 2007 concludes: 'Among participants with type-2 diabetes, chromium supplementation improved glycosylated haemo-globin levels and fasting glucose. Chromium supplementation significantly improved glycemia among patients with diabetes.'[87] I'll tell you exactly how much chromium to take in Part 2, Chapter 6.

Work with your doctor

Your doctor is aware of the diabetes epidemic and should have the same goals that you have in mind to control diabetes and its associated complications. He or she should also be keen for you to do this as much as possible through diet and lifestyle, rather than drugs, especially those that have quite serious side effects.

In about a third of cases patients' and doctors' goals are not the same. A study of patients with diabetes who had high blood pressure found that while both patients and doctors agreed that bringing down hypertension is important, twice as many doctors as patients rated it as the most important goal. What patients considered more important was reducing pain and depression – subjective problems that doctors all too often put on the back burner.[88]

If you are on medication, firstly it is important not to change it without consulting your doctor. But you may also want to tell him or her that you are pursuing an aggressive low-GL diet strategy and, if successful in lowering your blood sugar and glycosylated haemoglobin (your HbA1c), discuss at what point would your doctor reduce your medication, if this is your goal? Some patients find it difficult to approach their doctor but I strongly recommend you do this.

Are you taking a sulfonylurea?

If you are on a drug such as a sulfonylurea, as mentioned above, it is important that you and your doctor know that once the low-GL diet effect kicks in this drug may become dangerous for you to take, with the possibility of causing a hypo (a blood sugar low, initially making you dizzy). You may ask that, in the event that taking the drug causes a hypo, should you stop the drug or lower the dose?

In any event, the more you can work with your doctor, and keep him or her informed of what you are doing, the better. Keeping a diary of key changes and your blood sugar levels, as I will explain in Part 3, will help this collaboration.

PART TWO

Ten Ways to Prevent or Reverse Diabetes

There are ten principles that you need to understand to become a master of your blood sugar control. Nine of them are essential to undo the damage caused by diabetes and metabolic syndrome, and the final one, which is optional, takes my Anti-diabetes Action Plan one step further to reprogramme your genes for good health. Applying these principles is the fastest way to reverse diabetes, and the surest way to prevent it.

1

Follow The Holford Low-GL Diet – the Gold Standard for Stable Blood Sugar

In Part 1, I explained how diabetes develops, and that your number-one aim is to eat in such a way that keeps both your blood glucose level as stable as possible and your need for insulin low. The question is how do you do it?

The most accurate measure of the total effect a food or a meal has on your blood glucose level is called its glycemic load (or GL). This is based on what is called the glycemic index (GI). Carbohydrate foods that release their sugar content in the body more slowly have a low GI. The GL is calculated using the GI and a portion size, so that you can see at a glance what food is best to eat and what portion to have. I'll be explaining this in detail later in this chapter and giving you a list of these values later in the book.

Why GLs are important for you

Becoming aware of the GL of what you eat and knowing how to lower the GL of a meal is a much more effective way of reversing diabetes than simply eating less sugar or less carbohydrates – or eating foods with a low-glycemic index (GI) score. The GL of your diet is the most predictive measure of your risk of diabetes, says a recent European study of over 37,000 people;[1] it predicts your glycosylated haemoglobin level very accurately, says another;[2] and, according to a recent review in a top diabetes journal, it is the one aspect of a person's diet that most predicts their risk of metabolic diseases associated with metabolic syndrome[3] (see pages 15–17 for an explanation of metabolic syndrome and its implications). A major review of 11 good-quality studies in 2009 concluded that a low-GL diet works for diabetes, lowering glycosylated haemoglobin without causing hypos (blood sugar dips).[4] It's the bee's knees as far as mastering your blood sugar balance is concerned; below is just a selection of the many studies that have found that low-GL diets are superior to high-carbohydrate, low-fat diets in controlling and treating type-2 diabetes.

The evidence in studies

Study 1 One group of people followed a low-GL diet while another group followed a conventional low-fat, low-calorie diet (Canada's Food Guide to Healthy Eating). After six months those following the low-GL diet had not only lost more weight but they also had greater improvements in the 'good' HDL cholesterol (up), 'bad' LDL cholesterol (down), triglycerides (down) and fasting glucose (down a lot) compared to those on the conventional low-fat, low-calorie diet, who actually had an increase in fasting glucose. These health gains were sustained or improved upon after 12 months. The researchers concluded that 'implementation of a low-GL diet is associated with substantial and sustained improvements in abdominal obesity, cholesterol and blood sugar control'.
    S. A. LaHaye, et al., *Canadian Journal of Cardiology*, 2005; 21(6):489–94

Study 2 Researchers at the Harvard School of Public Health monitored the health of 42,000 middle-aged men for six years and found that those who ate a high-GL diet were one and a half times more likely to develop diabetes than those who ate a low-GL diet. This positive association between GL and risk of diabetes was after taking into account other factors such as age, BMI, smoking, physical activity, family history of diabetes, alcohol consumption, cereal fibre, and total energy intake.
    J. Salmeron, et al., *Diabetes Care*, 1997; 20(4):545–50

Study 3
In a separate study, researchers at the Harvard School of Public Health also monitored the health of 65,000 middle-aged women for six years and found that those who ate a high-GL diet were also one and a half times more likely to develop diabetes than those who ate a low-GL diet.
    J. Salmeron, et al., *Journal of the American Medical Association*, 1997; 277(6):472–7

continued

Study 4 Fifteen volunteers followed a low-GL diet for 12 weeks while 15 others followed a conventional low-fat, low-calorie diet. Both diets contained identical numbers of calories. The volunteers then switched diets for a further 12 weeks. Fasting insulin concentrations were significantly lower in the low-GL group. Lower fasting insulin is associated with decreased risk of obesity, diabetes and heart disease.

M. Slabber, et al., *American Journal of Clinical Nutrition*, 1994; 60(1):48–53

Study 5 This study of 85,059 women found that low-carbohydrate diets are better than low-fat diets in preventing diabetes. The study followed the women over 20 years and found that women who ate less carbohydrate and got most of their fat and protein from vegetable sources were at less risk of developing diabetes. This is the equivalent of my low-GL diet and is yet more evidence that this is the best choice for preventing diabetes.

T. Halton, et al., *American Journal of Clinical Nutrition*, 2008 Feb: 87(2):339–46

If you'd like to see the evidence of more studies showing just how effective low-GL diets are for preventing and reversing diabetes, go to www.holforddiet.com/evidence

Now, not all so-called 'low-GL' diets are the same in their effect. A similar analogy would be to say that not all 'low-calorie' diets have the same effect. One might be 500 calories, another 1,000 calories. The calories might also come from different classes of food; some low-calorie diets, for example, are strictly no fat.

The Mediterranean diet – a big step in the right direction

A Mediterranean diet is a relatively low-GL diet despite the inclusion of pasta, because it is based on more wholefoods. Although the general diet is very good, however, it is not as effective as my strict low-GL diet for reversing diabetes or achieving weight loss.

One critical feature of the traditional Mediterranean way of living in days of old was the large amount of exercise it included. Many people walked on average seven miles a day as part of their work and regular routine, and this combination of diet and exercise brought positive health benefits. Today, diets have changed, and with the convenience of modern transportation the population is generally less active. In fact, Greece now has a higher percentage of obese men than the US! Having said that, there are many good qualities in a Mediterranean-style diet that are echoed in my Anti-diabetes Diet: more fish, less meat and dairy; more beans, nuts and seeds; plenty of fresh vegetables; wholefoods and wholegrains. Olives are also excellent, with virtually no GL. As far as prevention is concerned, this way of eating is very good.

Strict adherence to a Mediterranean diet has been shown to cut diabetes risk by 83 per cent; this was the conclusion of a Spanish study of 13,000 people followed over four years and published in the *British Medical Journal*.[5] This kind of diet, while good for general health, is not enough for the rapid reversal of diabetes – a modified Mediterranean diet, however, containing less carbs (and hence a lower GL) does the trick.

This was demonstrated in a recent trial by researchers at Tel Aviv University's Meir Medical Centre in Israel, which compared three diets for diabetes: the kind of diet recommended by the American Diabetes Association (55 per cent of calories as carbs, 30 per cent as fat, 20 per cent as protein), with a Mediterranean-style diet (containing 55 per cent of calories as *low-GL* carbs, 30 per cent as fat, 20 per cent protein) and a low-GL Mediterranean diet (with only 35 per cent of calories as low-GL carbs, 45 per cent fat and 20 per cent protein).[6]

This third low-GL Mediterranean diet had the best results in many respects – participants experienced more weight loss, a bigger decrease in glycosylated haemoglobin and glucose levels, a bigger drop in triglycerides and LDL cholesterol, and a bigger increase in HDL cholesterol. This kind of diet is closer to my low-GL diet, which contains a little more protein and a bit less fat, and is stricter in controlling not only the amount of GL but also the spacing of the glycemic load from food over the day.

The four principles of the low-GL diet

Foods are measured in ⅁, and I'll be giving you full details as well as a list of foods with their GL values later in the book. You will get the best results if you eat and drink no more than 45 ⅁ in carbohydrate a day, spread out evenly throughout the day and always eaten with protein foods. This is just about the lowest you can go without ever feeling hungry. (If you are more than 1.8m (6ft) tall and exercise a lot you'll need more. I'll explain how to personalise your GL requirements on page 232). To achieve this there are only four principles you need to adhere to:

1 Eat 45 ⓖ a day You'll be learning exactly what the GL of a food is. Some foods have such a high GL score that you would only be able to eat the smallest amount of them; for example, a whole 300g (10½oz) punnet of strawberries is 5 ⓖ but so is just 10 raisins! (You'll begin the diet on 40 ⓖ a day, increasing to 45 ⓖ after two weeks.)

2 Graze rather than gorge, eating less food, more often. Divide the ⓖ throughout the day as follows:

10 ⓖ for breakfast
5 ⓖ for a mid-morning snack
10 ⓖ for lunch
5 ⓖ for a mid-afternoon snack
10 ⓖ for dinner
5 ⓖ for drinks or desserts (optional and also not to be used during the first two weeks, when you will begin your diet on 40 ⓖ per day)

You'll soon know exactly what a 5-GL snack or a 10-GL main meal means, and there are plenty of example menus and recipes in this book. In Part 3 I'll personalise this for you depending on your current blood sugar levels.

3 Eat fewer carbs, but more protein You can achieve a low-GL diet in one of two ways: the first is by eating no, or less, carbohydrate, since only carbohydrates raise blood sugar levels; for example, you could just eat meat. The trouble here is that your body needs glucose, but just not too much. Also, eating very high amounts of animal protein, especially from red meat, is bad for your kidneys and your bones and is associated with an increased colon cancer risk. It's an extreme. Perhaps it's a useful direction to go in the short-term but not a good long-term diet. That's the Atkins-type diet direction.

Another way is simply to eat carbohydrate foods that release their sugar content more slowly. These, as we have just seen, are called low-GI foods – for example, wholemeal brown bread instead of refined white. This is a step in the right direction, giving you a better 'quality' of carbohydrate foods, although you can still go overboard. In other words, you need to not only eat brown rather than white but also eat less carbohydrate overall.

The GL score of a food already factors this in, so when you eat 45 🌀 a day you have automatically eaten both a lesser quantity of carbs and a better quality of them as far as your blood sugar is concerned. But you do also need to consciously eat a little more protein and healthy fats.

4 Only eat carbs with protein You don't just need to eat more protein and healthy fat overall but you also need to eat it whenever you eat carbohydrate, because this helps to release the carbohydrate slowly. So, egg and sugar-free beans is in, whereas jam on toast is out. If you have an apple, you must have, for example, some nuts or seeds. The reason for this is that even if a food has a particular GL score, eating it with protein lowers the GL of the meal. The GL score for strawberries, for example, was initially worked out by feeding volunteers strawberries on their own and measuring what effect it had on their blood sugar level. But when you eat strawberries with yoghurt, for example, the protein takes longer to digest, so the sugars in the strawberries are also released more slowly, further lowering the GL of the meal.

Anything that slows down the release of sugars in foods lowers the GL. The combination of proteins with healthy fats will also help lower the GL score of your meal. In the next chapter I'm going to tell you about some amazing fibres that, if you add a teaspoonful to your meal, will automatically lower the GL.

Now that you know the 'rules' you could jump straight to Part 3 and get on with the diet if you like, but it's a good idea to understand why these rules exist and why eating my low-GL diet is the ultimate way to control your blood sugar.

What determines GL?

How a food is processed, prepared or cooked is a key element in the GL value of a food and therefore what it will do to your blood sugar.

In the illustration opposite you can see how blood sugar levels, followed by insulin, rise and fall after eating spaghetti. As the blood glucose level rises, the body produces insulin, and down it comes again.

Glycemic response to spaghetti

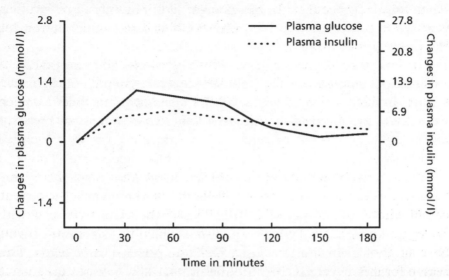

Within 40 minutes of eating spaghetti, blood sugar levels are at a maximum. The body releases insulin to help get the glucose out of the blood and into body cells. Two hours later both blood glucose and insulin levels have returned to normal.

Glycemic response to bread

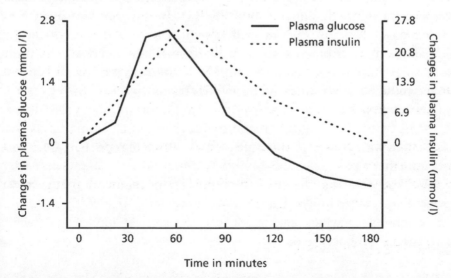

Within 40 minutes of eating bread, blood sugar levels are almost double those seen with spaghetti. The body produces more than three times as much insulin to bring blood glucose levels under control. The body over-reacts and blood glucose goes too low, leading to strong cravings for something sweet or a stimulant such as caffeine, peaking three hours later.

The second illustration on page 71 shows what happens when you eat white bread. Notice that the blood sugar level not only peaks twice as high when compared with the pasta but it also dips much lower. It's the peaks that damage your arteries, making them less responsive to insulin, and the troughs that leave you tired, sleepy and craving carbohydrates or stimulants. Again, you can see a massive increase in insulin release. In fact, compared with levels for spaghetti, four times as much insulin was produced in the first two hours after eating that bread! If you are already insulin resistant you'll produce even more to achieve your body's required result – bringing your blood glucose level down.

What's fascinating is that this particular bread and spaghetti were made from the same type of flour, using the same amount.[7] So the only difference is in the processing. Bread rises when you feed yeast with sugar, and it is then baked for some time, which turns complex sugars into simpler sugars. Pasta is just wheat and perhaps some egg. (Pasta with egg has a lower GL because the protein slow-releases the carbs.) It contains no yeast or sugar and it isn't cooked for so long.

It's obvious that this small difference in preparation makes a big difference in blood sugar response, and hence in how much weight you put on. That's why I recommend that you eat very little bread, but you certainly don't need to give up pasta, especially if it's wholewheat as opposed to refined. You can buy low-GL pastas too. However, how much pasta you can tolerate will depend on your degree of insulin resistance. If your blood sugar is way off, you may need to omit pasta and other starchy foods until you are able to bring it down. Then you may gradually reintroduce such low-GL foods.

Harking back to Rule 4, above, it's also important how you eat your low-GL carbs. I'm going to recommend that you eat some fat as well as protein with your carbohydrate because this will reduce its GL score even further.

We'll be looking at the kinds of combinations that work best to lower your blood sugar in a while. But, for now, let's stick to the GL scenario, exploring which carbohydrates you can eat lots of and which you should probably avoid.

The glycemic index (GI) explained

It was the discovery that even quite similar foods could have very different effects on blood sugar that led to classifying foods as slow- or fast-releasing carbohydrates. The fast-releasing foods include white bread, which as we saw above act rather like rocket fuel, releasing their glucose in a sudden burst. They give a quick shot of energy with a rapid burnout. Slow-releasing carbohydrates, such as wholewheat spaghetti, supply steadier energy over a longer period of time, and thus help in balancing blood sugar levels.

But how do you know what is fast and what is slow releasing? This is where the GI – the glycemic index – comes in. The GI is a scale that compares the levels to which different foods raise your blood sugar with the effect of pure glucose (see illustration below). It is also key in determining a food's GL.

Measuring the glycemic index of a food

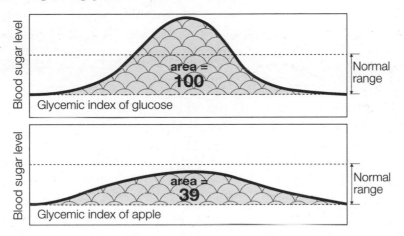

To discover a food's GI, a portion that provides 50g (1¾oz) of carbohydrate is eaten, and the effect on the person's blood sugar over a three-hour period is compared to the effect of eating 50g (1¾oz) of the 'reference' food, which is glucose. Glucose is the fastest-releasing carbohydrate, because it requires no digestion.

In the illustration above, the curve created by eating 50g (1¾oz) of glucose is given a value of 100. If another food raises the blood sugar level significantly, and for some time, the area under the curve made by glucose is bigger. Conversely, if a food hardly raises blood glucose levels at all, and only for a short time, the area under the curve is smaller. The amount of food tested obviously affects how high the blood sugar level will go.

Overleaf you can see the GI scores for a variety of foods. As a general rule, a high GI score indicates the ones to avoid; a low GI score, the ones to eat.

The glycemic index of common foods

Sugars	GI
Maltose	105
Glucose	100
Honey	55
High-fructose corn syrup	50–70
Sucrose (sugar)	68
Lactose	46
Fructose (pure fruit sugar)	19
Xylitol	8

Fruit	
Dates	103
Watermelon	72
Pineapple	59
Melon	65
Raisins	64
Kiwi fruit	53
Banana	52
Grapes	46
Orange	42
Strawberries	40
Raspberries	40
Plum	39
Apple	38
Pear	38
Grapefruit	25
Cherries	22

Grains and grain products	
French baguette	95
White rice	72
Bagel	72
Wholemeal bread	71
White bread	70
Crumpet	69
Ryvita	64
Pastry	59

Basmati rice	58
Wholegrain rye bread	58
Brown basmati long-grain rice	47
Brown rice	55
Instant noodles	47
Wholegrain wheat bread	46
White spaghetti	40
Wholemeal spaghetti	37
Barley	26

Cereals	
Puffed rice	82
Cornflakes	81
Shredded wheat	75
Weetabix	70
Kellogg's Special K	69
Porridge oats	58
Muesli	55
Kellogg's All-Bran	42

Pulses	
Baked beans	48
Chickpeas	42
Black-eyed beans	42
Haricot beans	38
Butter beans	36
Lentils	29
Kidney beans	28
Soya beans	14

Dairy products/substitutes	
Ice cream	61
Yoghurt	36
Skimmed milk	32
Whole milk	27

Vegetables	
Parsnips (cooked)	97

Potato (baked)	85	Jelly beans	80
French fries	75	Fanta	68
Beetroot (cooked)	64	Squash (diluted)	66
Sweet potato	61	Corn chips	63
Potato (new, boiled)	57	Muesli bar	61
Sweetcorn	54	Potato crisps	54
Peas	48	Orange juice	50
Carrot	47	Mars Bar	49
		Chocolate bar	49
Snacks and drinks		Apple juice	40
Lucozade	95	Peanuts	14

Carbohydrates are not all the same

So much for the GI, but what's the inside story on what makes one food fast-releasing and another slow? There are two main factors.

The first is how 'complex' the carbohydrate is. The illustration below is a diagram of the chemical structure of glucose, regular white sugar and oats. You don't need to be a scientist to see that oats are more complex than sugar and that sugar is more complex than glucose. All it means is that there's more to them.

Oats are more complex than glucose

Oats need digesting into single glucose units, which takes time and slows down the release of its sugars. This sugar, which is a molecule of glucose and fructose, is slower in turn than a glucose molecule, which needs no digesting and directly enters the bloodstream.

Since the body can use only glucose for fuel, the sugar pictured – sucrose – has to be chopped into two to release the glucose. When you eat sugar, an enzyme released in the gut does this job for you and, before long, the glucose is whizzing around your bloodstream.

The carbohydrate in oats, however, needs a lot of digesting into smaller and smaller units in the digestive tract before the glucose is released into the blood. This takes longer, so you don't get such a massive and immediate blood sugar rise.

Cooking some foods affects the release rate by 'pre-digesting' the carbs they contain. That's why the more you cook a carbohydrate food the faster releasing it becomes. Take potatoes, for example. A baked potato, with a GI score of 85, is worse than a boiled potato, which has a GI of 57. Oats, however, are an exception. There's little difference between porridge and oat flakes eaten cold. This is largely because the cooking time is very short – you are really rehydrating the oats rather than cooking them.

Another factor that slows down the release of carbohydrate in food is fibre. Fibre is an indigestible carbohydrate and, generally, the more fibre a food contains the slower is the breakdown of carbohydrate. This is doubly true for foods that contain soluble fibre such as oats. (We'll be looking at fibre in more depth in Chapter 3 of this part.)

Why sugars are different too

There's one more important thing you need to know. Not all simple sugars raise your blood sugar level. In the illustration opposite you can see the chemical structure of lactose (milk sugar), sucrose (white sugar), maltose (grain sugar or malt) and high-fructose corn syrup (a sweetener that is added to many drinks). The body can only use glucose for energy. So, once the glucose is removed from lactose you're left with galactose, and once the glucose is removed from sucrose you're left with fructose.

What happens to fructose and galactose (shown in grey in the diagram)? The answer is that they go to your liver, where they can be converted into glucose or fat. But this takes time, so they're classed as slow-releasing. If you flood your already overworked liver with too much fructose, however, it sets up a chain reaction that pushes you towards metabolic syndrome. (This, unfortunately, is what's happening in most people's bodies since the beverage industry switched to high-fructose corn syrup as its preferred sweetener.) So, fructose is better than glucose, but only in small quantities, and if eaten with fibre as nature intended (see also The Problems with Fructose on page 79). Fructose is the sugar found in fruit, so eating small amounts of whole fruit, which combines both fibre and natural fruit sugar, is healthy.

Most high-fructose corn syrup is actually 55 per cent fructose and 45 per cent glucose. That's basically exactly what sugar is. As far as your body is concerned, there's no difference.

Lactose versus sucrose versus maltose versus high-fructose corn syrup

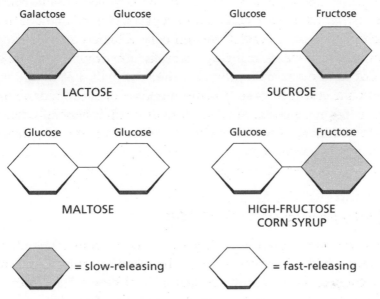

Galactose and fructose (shown in grey) are slow-releasing sugars whereas glucose is fast. Hence, lactose (milk sugar) and sucrose (white sugar) are more slow-releasing than maltose, a grain sugar (malt) which is quickly digested into two glucose molecules. High-fructose corn syrup, used in many sweetened drinks and foods, is very similar in chemistry and effect to sucrose.

Now look at the GI score of glucose, sucrose and fructose on page 74. As you would expect, glucose is ranked as the fastest-releasing carbo-hydrate (100), because it requires no digestion. (Although the GI of maltose is higher (105), it is made up of two glucose molecules, so it must be digested.) Fructose is the slowest (19), and sucrose – a com-bination of glucose and fructose – is in the middle (68). You'll also notice that maltose is just as fast as glucose, and honey isn't far off, at

55. Malt, the sugar, is naturally present in grains and artificially added to things such as cereals and breads – as malted wheat, for example. As you can see from the illustration, malt is just two glucose molecules; it needs virtually no digestion. Most honey is basically glucose (also called dextrose, or grape sugar, because it's also found in grapes), especially commercial honey, which is heated to clean out impurities and to make it easier to pack into jars.

The sugars in dairy products

You'd expect things such as ice cream to be high GI, but it isn't that high. It scores 61. This is because lactose is quite slow-releasing. (Be aware, though, that poor-quality ice creams have added glucose.) Milk or yoghurt score lower still (27–36). Dairy products are actually a little bit misleading as far as diabetes is concerned. Yes, they are relatively low GI, but drinking milk promotes the release of insulin and insulin-like growth factor (IGF-1). This is not good news if you are already insulin-resistant. Hence, you'll find my recipes use fewer dairy products. Furthermore, if you are allergic to dairy products, which many people unknowingly are, they are bad news.

Fruits and their sugars

Looking at fruits, even these can be fast or slow-releasing. Not all contain mainly fructose. Dates, for example, contain mainly glucose and bananas are high in starch (long chains of glucose), while most other fruits and berries are mainly fructose. Even better than fructose is a natural sugar called xylose, which is particularly high in cherries, berries and plums. This is the reason why plums have a low GI score. Xylitol, which is made from xylose, looks and tastes just like white sugar, but has less than half the GI score of fructose and a ninth of the GI score of sugar – it is highly preferable to any artificial sweetener. So, nine teaspoons of xylitol has the same effect on your blood sugar as one teaspoon of regular sugar, and it tastes just as good. I use only xylitol as a sweetener, in moderation, and never use sugar.

Be aware that if you have too much xylose or xylitol you will get loose bowels. That's why prunes (which are dried plums) help to keep you regular. Unsweetened prunes, dried cherries or berries are the only dried fruits I recommend and, even then, only in moderation.

Another advantage of using xylitol is that it is very tooth friendly. A study published in the *Archives of Pediatric and Adolescent Medicine* in July 2009 gave young children aged 9 to 15 months a xylitol syrup two or three times a day, versus placebo, over a ten-month period. The incidence of tooth decay had more than halved:

'Our results suggest that exposure to xylitol (8g per day) in a twice-daily topical oral syrup during primary tooth eruption could prevent up to 70 percent of decayed teeth ... Dividing the 8g into three doses did not increase the effectiveness of the treatment. These results provide evidence that xylitol is effective for the prevention of decay in primary teeth of toddlers.'

Xylitol has been shown to effectively prevent tooth decay by acting as an antibacterial agent against organisms that cause cavities. Bacteria that feed off xylitol become unable to stick to teeth and cause rotting.

The problems with fructose

As we have seen, although fructose may appear to be better for you because it is lower GI, be careful. Our ancestors consumed very little, but they ate lots of fibre, by eating whole fruits, for example, thus slow releasing the natural fructose. In contrast, we consume loads of fructose without the fibre, because it's added to foods and drinks as sugar and high-fructose corn syrup, which is half fructose and half glucose.

If you have a big serving of fructose – in a soft drink, for example – it doesn't cause an increase in blood glucose, doesn't raise your insulin level and consequently doesn't trigger the appetite-suppressing hormones, ghrelin and leptin, so you don't feel satisfied, and you keep drinking. Fructose in the blood causes damage (glycation) resulting in lots of AGEs (see page 8), and is metabolised in the liver, producing more fat and promoting metabolic syndrome.[8] A study on college students gave them either a measured amount of glucose or fructose. Ten times more fat was generated from the fructose than from the glucose.[9] Fructose turns into fat, stored as triglycerides.[10] So, even though it is technically low GI it's not good news for you and is going to make you fatter. You are better off staying away from foods or drinks sweetened with fructose and choosing either unsweetened foods or drinks or those that contain a small amount of xylose or xylitol. (See also Chapter 7 in this part for healthier drink options.)

It's the *GL* that counts

Although the GI score of a food is very useful, there's one problem. Look at the list on page 75 again and compare carrots with chocolate, or watermelon with French fries. You're probably wondering why they have such similar scores – and aren't carrots supposed to be good for you? You'd be absolutely right. Apart from the vitamins and other important nutrients they contain, a carrot or a slice of watermelon contains comparatively little carbohydrate. In fact, you'd have to eat two large carrots to get the same amount of carbohydrate, and the same effect on your weight, as four pieces of chocolate. The chances are you'll eat a lot more than four pieces of chocolate and fewer than two carrots. This kind of inconsistency is why knowing the GI alone is a bit misleading.

This is where the GL comes in – it's the best way to tell what a food will do to your blood sugar level and how much weight you'll gain from it. It's a simple calculation, taking into account both the amount of carbohydrate in a food (the quantity) and its GI score (the quality).

To find a food's GL, you multiply its GI score by the amount of carbohydrate it contains (I give the formula in Appendix 3). The result will tell you exactly what a given serving of a food does to your blood sugar, so it's more practical when you plan what to eat. But you don't need to work this out yourself because I've already done this for literally hundreds of foods. You can find my GL index in Appendix 4.

To illustrate the GL values more clearly, the chart below shows a list of high- and low-GL foods. The GL score for each of the quantities is 10 ⑤ – so, you can see that two entire punnets of strawberries (weighing 600g/1lb 5oz) have the same GL score as just two dates.

Common foods scoring 10 ⑤

Low-GL foods	High-GL foods
4 small cans tomato juice	1 small can cranberry juice drink
2 slices wholegrain rye bread	1 slice white bread
2 large punnets of strawberries	2 dates
1 large bowl of peanuts	1 packet of crisps
1 carton of orange juice	1 glass of Lucozade
3 bowls of porridge (sugar-free)	1 bowl of cornflakes

As the golden rule of my low-GL diet is to eat no more than 40 ⒼⓁ a day when you first start, it's obvious that if you choose high-GL foods you won't be eating much. You could lose weight this way, but that's not what I want you to do.

It's infinitely more satisfying for you to eat low-GL carbohydrates. You'll be able to eat more, experiment with the recipes more and generally enjoy your food (remember how that feels?). Let me make this real for you by showing you a typical day in your Anti-diabetes Diet versus a typical diet. ⒼⓁ are shown for each food.

The Holford Low-GL Diet versus the average diet

Holford daily diet	ⒼⓁ	Average daily diet	ⒼⓁ
Breakfast		**Breakfast**	
A bowl of porridge (30g/1oz)	2	A bowl of cornflakes	21
½ grated apple	3	Banana	12
1 tbsp seeds	0	Milk	2
Small tub of yoghurt	2	Total ⒼⓁ for breakfast	35
Some dairy or soya milk	2		
Total ⒼⓁ for breakfast	9		
Morning snack		**Morning snack**	
Punnet of strawberries		Mars Bar	26
plus a few almonds	1		
Lunch		**Lunch**	
Substantial tuna salad		Tuna salad baguette	15
3 oatcakes	11		
Afternoon snack		**Afternoon snack**	
Pear plus a small handful		Packet of crisps	11
of peanuts	4		
Dinner		**Dinner**	
Tomato soup, salmon,		Pizza with Parmesan cheese	
sweetcorn and green beans	12	and tomato sauce, plus salad	23
'Good day' total ⒼⓁ	37	'Bad day' total ⒼⓁ	110

Take a good look at the food in the column on the left on page 81. Imagine you ate that breakfast, rather than the one on the right. It would definitely be more filling, wouldn't it? But it's not just that: by eating it, you'd have cut your blood sugar spike by a third! The great news about eating the GL way is that you can actually eat more food and lose more weight and never feel hungry! And it's all delicious.

Let's see what that means in real terms. All the meals below have identical GL scores, and identical effects on your blood sugar.

For breakfast you could have:

either	*or*
Scrambled egg on rye toast	Fruit and yoghurt smoothie

As a snack you could have:

either	*or*
Hummus with crudités	Oatcakes with peanut butter

For lunch or dinner you could have:

either	*or*
Trout with Puy lentils and roasted tomatoes	Chicken fajitas with salsa and salad

It doesn't look much like hard work, does it? And this is a mere taster. I'm going to give you many mouth-watering recipes and menus ranging from the simple to the elegant, all designed to keep you going at 40 ⑭ a day. In addition to the recipes in this book, if you want to widen your repertoire of meals there are also three books of recipes available: *The Low-GL Diet Bible*, *The Low-GL Diet Cookbook* and *Food GLorious Food*, containing low-GL recipes from around the world. Between the recipes and your own 'freestyle' choices using the complete GL food chart in Appendix 4, you'll soon learn which carbohydrates to go for, while your body unlearns how to store glucose as fat.

Super fibre

As I pointed out previously, fibre slows down the release of carbohydrate – it therefore helps to lower the GL of foods. Both the amount and the kind of fibre is important and in Chapter 3 of this part I'll

explain how to increase the fibre content of a meal – for
adding a teaspoon of oatbran to your cereal – and lower its G.

The other factor that makes a difference is the amount of prot   you
eat with each meal.

The power of protein

As I have explained, combining protein-rich foods with low-GL carbohydrates helps to stabilise your blood sugar, reducing the need for
insulin and also burning fat. Remember how high insulin is bad news
(discussed earlier on page 9)? There's another hormone, glucagon,
which raises rather than lowers blood sugar. It is good news as far as
fatburning is concerned because it helps to turn fat back into glucose
when your blood sugar level is too low.

Protein foods tend to trigger a small and equal release of both insulin
and glucagon – which happens to be the ideal. Carbohydrates, especially fast-releasing carbohydrates such as cakes and sweets, trigger a
substantial release of insulin with little or no glucagon response. Eating
fat has little direct effect on either insulin or glucagon. Eating a bit
more protein with low-GL carbs produces a small release of insulin,
together with glucagon. Long term, this is the most ideal. I'll be talking
about the right kind of fats to eat in Chapter 4 of this part. The relative
effects of each combination are shown in the chart below. The foods
with the greatest number of + signs have the greatest effect on your
insulin and glucagon levels, so those with the fewest + signs will be
better for your blood sugar and therefore your health and weight loss:

Effects of protein, carbohydrate and fat on insulin and glucagon

Food eaten	Insulin level	Glucagon level
Carbohydrate only	+++++	No change
Protein only	++	++
Fat only	No change	No change
Carbohydrate and fat	++++	No change
Protein and fat	++	++
High protein and low-GL carbohydrate	++	+
High-GL carbohydrate and low protein	++++++++	+
Low-GL carbohydrate and medium protein	+++	++

From this research, you can see that the best three combinations are either protein only, protein and fat, or low-GL carbohydrates and medium protein. The trouble with a high-protein and fat diet is that it isn't good for your health. You can get away with it for a couple of months, but it's not a good long-term regime. It's also very restrictive. That's why the best all-round diet for consistent and easily maintained weight loss and blood sugar control, with the lowest boredom factor, is to eat low-GL carbohydrates, plus protein. It's great for your health and equally effective for your overall weight as a high-protein diet, although it's more effective for fat loss and it's better for you in the long run.

How much protein should you eat?

Very high-protein diets have proved effective in weight control, partly because they adversely affect the body's ability to turn food into fat and also because you eat less on them. But a lot of the weight loss is water. This is partly because when you starve the body of glucose it breaks down stores of glucose called glycogen, which is stored with water. The other reason is that, when you eat too much protein without enough carbohydrates, compounds called ketones are produced. These are toxic, and the body tries hard to get rid of them in the urine, and this contributes to the fluid weight loss. But any pounds of water lost will come back.

Although we all need something in the region of 40g (1½oz) of protein a day, eating above 80g (2¾oz) a day over the long term may increase your risk of developing osteoporosis. Because protein is acidic it can deplete the bones of calcium, which is drawn out from the bones in an attempt to maintain the body's acid–alkali balance. Too much protein also stresses the kidneys. If the protein source is red meat, this may increase the risk of colon cancer, while high dairy consumption may increase the risk of prostate cancer. Also, if a person chooses meat as their main source of protein, their diet will inevitably become higher in saturated fat, which, as I'll explain later in Part 2, is not good news. It might not be that red meat, per se, is bad for you, it's just that wild animals would normally be exceedingly fit and lean, with around 5 per cent of their body mass as fat, whereas most animals we eat are unfit, like us, and have around 20 per cent of their body weight as fat. Even if you cut off the fat, the so-called lean meat is still marbled with too much if it.

The acid test

One of the reasons why combining protein with carbohydrate works is because protein, being made of amino acids, makes the digestive environment more acidic, and this slows down the digestion of carbohydrates. They need a more alkaline environment lower down in the small intestine, although the stomach's environment is more acid. So, food stays longer in the stomach, making you feel fuller for longer.

If you increase the acid level by adding lemon juice (citric acid) or vinegar (acetic acid) you get a similar effect. In a study on people with type-1 diabetes, adding two tablespoons of vinegar to a meal lowered the glycemic load by 20 per cent, measured by plotting the rise and fall in blood sugar levels after the meal.[11] The vinegar meant fewer high blood sugar spikes. In another study, this time using people with type-2 diabetes, the effect of adding vinegar to either a high-GL meal or a low-GL meal was investigated. Once again, the added vinegar substantially lowered the GL, and slightly lowered insulin levels, in those eating a high-GL meal but not in those eating a low-GL meal.[12] So, there is probably a limit to how much additional benefit you can get by adding vinegar. But, for example, if you ever eat chips, which I don't recommend, at least make sure you have lots of vinegar!

This may be the basis for the old wives' tale about cider vinegar being good for you. In practical terms this might mean eating a salad with a vinegary salad dressing or drinking a shot of cider vinegar plus water with a meal or adding balsamic vinegar for flavour to a meal. Adding lemon juice or vinegar also reduces the formation of AGEs when food is cooked.[13]

The best ratio for burning fat

On a short-term basis, such as 30 days up to three months, increasing your protein intake to between 60g (2⅛oz) and 75g (2¾oz) a day and focusing on fish, chicken and vegetarian sources does help to restore blood sugar control[14] and boost fatburning. For this reason, your Antidiabetes Diet provides a greater proportion of calories from protein than the average diet – 25–30 per cent over a norm of 17 per cent – to control blood sugar balance and reduce insulin resistance. After 30 days – or once you've reached your goal, if less than that period – you need only to maintain your weight and blood sugar balance over the long term, so the ideal amount of protein would be 20–25 per cent of calories.

Fortunately, you won't have to mess about with calorie counting, as this isn't that kind of diet. Exactly what all this means in terms of the food you eat is explained simply and clearly in Part 3. I'll tell you exactly what to do. For now, though, check out the table below showing estimates of the ideal balance of proteins, carbs and fats.

The perfect balance

	Protein	Carbohydrate	Fat
Average diet	17%	48%	35%
Anti-diabetes Diet	25–30%	40–50%	25–30%
(first 30 days up to 3 months)			
Low-GL maintenance diet	20–25%	50%	25–30%

Because we all need to eat some protein, some carbohydrates and the right kind of fats, the best combination is to eat low-GL carbohydrate foods that are also rich in protein. Beans and lentils are an example. People who live in countries whose diets contain these are consistently thinner and healthier, with a very low risk of diabetes.

The easiest and healthiest way to achieve this perfect balance is to eat the equivalent of 60g (2⅛oz) of protein (that's the weight of protein, not the weight of the food) and 120g (4¼oz) of low-GL carbohydrate in a day, and to divide it evenly between each meal; that is, 20g (¾oz) of protein and roughly 40g (1½oz) of carbohydrate, at breakfast, lunch and dinner. (To clarify, 25g (1oz) of meat or fish has 7g (⅛oz) of protein; a 175g (6oz) can of tuna has 40g (1½oz) of protein; 1 large egg has 6g (⅛oz) of protein.) You needn't worry too much about the maths though, the recipes will do this for you. (Details on the quantity and quality of fats to be eaten are given in Chapter 4 of this part.) Roughly two-thirds of your carbohydrates need to come from vegetables and low-GL fruits, and one-third from things such as grains and more 'starchy' vegetables.

The simplest way to visualise your meals, as far as lunch and dinner are concerned, is to eat any one of the protein-rich foods shown opposite, with an equivalent-sized serving of any carbohydrate-rich food, plus two servings of vegetables.

If you have quite advanced diabetes, you may need to increase the protein to a third of the plate, reducing the carbohydrate portion even more until your blood sugar balance starts to even out.

You will probably be eating more protein-rich foods in relation to carbohydrate-rich foods than you are used to, as well as more fresh

The perfect plate for main meals

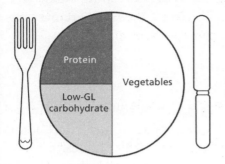

NORMAL BLOOD SUGAR CONTROL

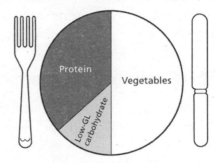

RAPID BLOOD SUGAR CONTROL

fruit and veg. The amount of carbohydrate or protein provided by non-starchy vegetables (broccoli, kale, cabbage, peas, spinach, carrots, and so on) is small, so these can be eaten relatively freely on your Anti-diabetes Diet. Aim, too, for two pieces of low-GL fruit a day. Here are a few examples of food combinations:

Fatburning food combinations

Protein	Carbohydrate	Vegetables
Poached salmon	on brown basmati rice	with a green salad
Marinated tofu	on wholewheat pasta	with steam-fried vegetables
Grilled chicken breast	with boiled new potatoes	with steamed runner beans
Cottage cheese	on oatcakes/rye bread	with broccoli and tomato salad

(You'll be able to work out more combinations using the comprehensive list of foods is given in Appendix 4.)

The anti-diabetes snacks are also great protein–carb combinations. Eating a few almonds or pumpkin seeds, which are high in healthy fats and protein, at the same time as some low-GL fruit can further slow the effect of fruit sugar on your blood sugar. And remember, fruits such as apples and strawberries have a low-GL, so those are better choices than some other fruits (again, you'll find a full list in Appendix 4).

For breakfast, you can achieve the correct balance and amount of protein and low-GL carbohydrate by, for example, eating a cup of oat flakes with some seeds, some berries and either skimmed milk or soya milk.

Above all, don't worry about having to calculate all this – the low-down in Part 3 and the menus and recipes in Part 4 make it remarkably easy.

Have you lost your 'appestat'?

Another sign of the internal health issues that show your body is affected by the modern Western diet is losing your appetite control. Part of this is a natural reaction to blood sugar dips. One of the hottest areas of research is related to leptin, nick-named the 'appetite hormone'. The purpose of leptin is to suppress your appetite when you are satisfied. Paradoxically, overweight people tend to have more circulating leptin than non-overweight people but the result is that they become increasingly 'leptin resistant' and no longer respond to the hormone's attempt to curb their appetite, hence the body keeps producing more. It's as if their body's 'appestat' has stopped working so they keep eating. Does this sound like you?

Leptin resistance is very much like becoming insulin resistant. In fact, leptin and insulin resistance are closely related, indicating your metabolism has gone out of sync. This scenario is often also accompanied by adrenalin resistance, which makes you more tired and in need of stimulants. The critical question is, what makes you become leptin resistant and hence unable to stop eating soon enough? And how do you regain your sensitivity to leptin?

Leptin is made in certain kinds of fat cells called white adipose tissue (nicknamed WAT); this is the stuff that accumulates around your belly. The more fat you make, the more leptin you produce, and, if working properly, this should curb your appetite. Furthermore, research has found that high levels of leptin increases the desire for alcohol, which can further exacerbate the problem, as it leads to loss of appetite control and merely adds more weight around the middle.

High levels of stress also contribute to making you more leptin resistant, as does a lack of exercise, according to one study.[15] There's also accumulating evidence that eating a high-GL, high-carbohydrate, grain-based diet may be a major reason why we become resistant to leptin, and research also shows that a high intake of fructose increases leptin resistance.[16]

My low-GL diet is designed to lower leptin resistance as well as insulin resistance. Including daily exercise will bring greater improvements, as exercise not only improves insulin resistance[17] but it is also a great stress reliever.[18]

Case Study: Adrian

You may remember meeting Adrian, the chef from South Africa, in the Introduction. He was diagnosed with diabetes when his glucose level was checked and found to be 19.8 (a normal level is 5)! He just couldn't stop eating, but after two months on my diet he felt satisfied and could even leave food on the plate because he was full. His health has also benefited in other ways:

'I no longer get any gout at all – even when I eat the foods I had to avoid before. I've lost 38kg [6 stone/84lb] in six months and ten inches [25cm] off my belly. I'm meant to take metformin every day, but most of the time I forget to take it. After a month on the diet my blood sugar was stable – never above 6.

Are you a sugar addict?

Sugar is literally addictive. Sugar actually stimulates the same areas of the brain that are involved in nicotine and other drug addictions. According to addiction expert Dr Simon Thornley, a registrar with the Auckland Regional Public Health Service, 'Drug addicts have to keep taking larger amounts of some chemical, they find it difficult to stop, they keep on doing it despite negative consequences and they feel bad if they do stop. People do all those things around refined carbohydrates.'[19] In tests with animals you only need to give them a drink of water with 10 per cent of the calories coming from sugar and they will start craving sugar. This is a lot less than many people are drinking in sweetened drinks.

A recent study found that overweight people who are already feeling the need to have carbohydrate snacks daily behave like addicts. 'The idea that carbohydrates can be addictive is an old one but until recently it was out of favour,' says leading researcher Bonnie Spring, professor of preventative medicine at the University of Illinois, Chicago. 'But the evidence has been building for the fact high blood sugar levels affect brain circuits involved in addiction.'[20]

In one study, Professor Spring gave a group of overweight women two drinks that appeared and tasted identical, but one only contained sugary carbohydrates, such as dextrose and rice syrup, while the other had some protein added. They were then asked to think about something sad for sufficient time to make them feel slightly low, then asked to drink again. Most of them, when asked, greatly preferred the pure carb drink and said that it cheered them up. Experiments like these are regularly used to test if a drug is addictive. Professor Spring said:

'The way these women behaved in response to the pure carbohydrate drink was similar to patterns we see in addicts … Addicts become tolerant of a drug so they need more of it and we saw that with the women. How big a part addiction plays in the obesity crisis isn't clear yet.'

If you think you've got hooked on sugar, and crave it often, especially when you feel low, then you'll be pleased to hear that the combination of my low-GL diet plus the supplements recommended in Part 3 will rapidly reduce your cravings for sweet foods, literally in around five days. So this diet does not entail a battle of will, fighting your desires. Your desire for sweet food will fall away.

The best time to eat

Obviously it is best to eat when you are hungry, not when you are bored or upset but equally important, you don't want to wait so long that your blood sugar level is on the floor so that you then can't stop eating.

Your blood sugar level is at its lowest when you wake up, so it is important to eat a breakfast containing plenty of protein, such as eggs for example. If you do go for a grain cereal such as oats, make sure you have a tablespoonful of ground seeds and a protein-based milk such as soya milk. This helps to reduce your appetite later on.

Finish eating dinner at least two hours before you go to sleep. It is very important to eat a low-GL dinner, with sufficient protein. Having beans, lentils or chickpeas as your 7-GL carb portion really helps to keep your blood sugar level stable. This will actually lower the GL of your breakfast the next day.

Never eat after dinner. That means no snacks or drinks other than water or non-sweetened herb teas. Aim for eleven hours without eating between dinner and breakfast. Research has found that night eating promotes obesity.[21] Do make sure you get enough sleep, because research has found that a lack of sleep also messes up your appetite hormones.[22] Chapter 8 in this part shows you how to get a good night's sleep.

What about low-calorie diets

Just after the first edition of this book went to print, a small trial by Professor Roy Taylor from Newcastle University, published in the journal *Diabetologia*, showed reversal of type-2 diabetes by giving people a very low-calorie (600kcal) diet for eight weeks.

I believe this is the effect of eating what is essentially a very low-GL diet. By cutting food intake so drastically, the body not only burns fat but also doesn't need to produce so much insulin. These may be the two conditions that bring insulin-producing cells back to life. Eating between 500 and 800 calories can switch genes away from diabetes although, interestingly, animal studies indicate that you don't have to do this every day but every other day, for one month, to turn genetic expression away from diabetes (see Chapter 10, pages 174 and 178 for more details).

If you decide to try this strategy, please make sure you tell your doctor what you intend to do as it will affect your need for medication. In this study all volunteers were withdrawn from medication prior to the study. I'd appreciate your feedback too, at www.patrickholford.com/diabetes.

Summary

- You need to be on a strict low-GL diet.
- Eat and drink a maximum of 45 ⑩ a day (40 ⑩ for the first two weeks), made up of 10-GL main meals and 5-GL snacks.
- Combine protein with carbohydrate.
- Have three meals and two low-GL snacks a day, always starting your day with a substantial low-GL breakfast.

2

Eat the Eight Key Food Groups that Keep Your Blood Sugar Level in Check

Some simple changes to what you put in your supermarket trolley can have a profound effect on your ability to control your blood sugar, your appetite and also your cardiovascular health. If you aren't already eating the following foods on a regular basis, you really need to. As well as explaining why they are important, I'll give you plenty of simple recipes and ideas to introduce them into your diet on a regular basis.

1 Oats rule

As we have seen, oats are a superb food choice for keeping your blood sugar level even. You can eat them as oat flakes (cold) or soak and cook them to make porridge. You can also make delicious oat pancakes (see the recipe on page 244). Oatcakes are the best 'bread' choice, for example, with your scrambled or boiled egg, or as a snack during the day with a high-protein spread such as hummus. Nowadays you can also find oat bakes (so much better than crisps) and oat biscuits, but do check that they say low-GI or GL on the box. The Nairn's brand is particularly GL conscious.

The best oat choices are those highest in the soluble fibre called beta-glucans. This is found in oat bran, the rougher outer layer of the grain. So, it's best to choose 'rough' oatcakes rather than 'fine'. You can lower the GL of your breakfast further by adding a spoonful of oat bran. This simple act makes a big difference to the GL of the meal. Since oat bran is highly absorbent, if you add it to cereal, it is best to leave the cereal to soak for a few minutes before eating, and put in more liquid than you normally would.

You want to eat as much beta-glucans as you can to help balance your blood sugar. Not only does the presence of beta-glucans in food slow-release the carbohydrates you eat but it also helps to lower cholesterol. An example of this is a study, conducted by Dr Allan Geliebter of the New York Obesity Research Center at St Luke's-Roosevelt Hospital.[23] In that study, Dr Geliebter gave volunteers either an oatmeal breakfast, high in beta-glucans, or a sugared cornflakes breakfast, containing equal calories. Those who had the oat-based breakfast consumed 30 per cent fewer calories at lunch, compared with those who ate sugared cornflakes for breakfast.

According to Dr Geliebter, 'The effect may be due primarily to a delay in gastric emptying, the time it takes for oatmeal to leave the stomach and enter the blood as glucose and other nutrients. The slower the stomach empties the longer food stays in the stomach and the longer people feel full and satisfied.'

The best foods for beta-glucans[24] are shown below, giving the percentage of beta-glucans per food:

Celery	20% of dry weight
Carrot	20% of dry weight
Radish	20% of dry weight
Oats	up to 7.5% (e.g. Nairn's rough oatcake, which is 88% oatmeal, would contain up to 6.6% beta-glucans)
Pearl barley	4% (e.g. ¼ cup pearl barley contains 2.5g beta-glucans soluble fibre)
Soya bean	0.8% of dry weight
Shiitake mushrooms	0.4% of dry weight

2 Choose rye or barley instead of wheat

The whole rye grain is also excellent in terms of GL. Rye bran, in one study, lowered glycemic load better than oat bran.[25] In practical terms this means a wholegrain rye bread, in moderation, would be a good choice for breakfast or a snack, together with a protein-rich food. The best choice of all would be the slow-cooked German-style breads called pumpernickel, sonnenbrot or volkenbrot. Bear in mind that some use wheat as well, so it's best to go for those breads that are wheat-free (they're now widely available in supermarkets).

You can also find whole rye sourdough bread, which is good. These breads will be more dense and heavier than regular wheat bread – this is a good sign, but make sure you have thinner slices. One thin slice will be 5 Ⓖ; 10 Ⓖ for two thin slices.

Rye also changes genetic expression (see Chapter 10 later in this part) away from insulin resistance, reversing the indicators of metabolic syndrome.[26] So, if you really want to go for it, stay away from wheat as much as possible, choosing oats and rye.

Healthy barley

Barley is another good grain to use, better than wheat. A study conducted by Dr Joseph Keenan, MD, of the University of Minnesota Medical School in Minneapolis, showed that eating barley makes you feel less hungry.[27] Dr Keenan fed a group of overweight people who also had high cholesterol the same diet, but either with barley muffins, high in barley bran and beta-glucans, or wheat muffins. The groups who ate the barley muffins felt significantly fuller and more satisfied throughout the study than those who ate the wheat muffins. 'We attribute the improvement in satiety almost entirely to the beta-glucan. Foods rich in beta-glucan stay in the stomach for a longer period of time compared to foods low in this fibre. That leads to a feeling of fullness, or satiety,' said Dr Keenan. Those eating the barley muffins lost, on average, 225g (8oz) per week whereas those who ate the wheat gained 225g (8oz) per week. Also, those who consumed the beta-glucan-rich muffins had significantly reduced total cholesterol (11 per cent) and the 'bad' LDL cholesterol (12 per cent), while high-density lipoprotein cholesterol levels remained unchanged. 'This is a very significant result,' said Dr Keenan. 'Such reductions are estimated to produce a 20 per cent reduction in the risk of developing heart disease.'

You can buy wholegrain pearl barley, which boils like brown rice. It is also full of beta-glucans and soluble fibres and has a good flavour – quite chewy. Chewing is good because it means you take a little longer to eat your meal.

Pasta tends to be a lower GL than bread anyway but a variety of pastas is now available made from rye, quinoa and chickpeas. You'll find these more often in health-food stores. These are a good choice, and you may also find Dreamfields pasta, which is especially low GL.

3 Eat more beans, lentils and chickpeas

This food group, known as pulses, is a staple in countries with low diabetes incidence, but we just don't eat enough of these highly nutritious foods in countries with a typical Western diet. Other than beans on toast, most people don't eat enough pulses (beans on toast is not a bad choice if you pick sugar-free beans – Whole Earth, sweetened with apple juice, are the best tasting). Pulses are all relatively high in protein, making them lower GL.

If, for example, you chose a serving of beans or lentils as your 7 GL carbohydrate portion in a main meal, you'd be achieving your low-GL goals easily:

130g (4¾oz) of cooked chickpeas is 7ⓖⓛ
150g (5½oz) of red kidney beans is 7 ⓖⓛ
175g (6oz) of butter beans is 7ⓖⓛ
210g (7¼oz) of lentils is 7ⓖⓛ
260g (9½oz) of borlotti beans is 7ⓖⓛ

Including a serving of lentils, or beans, for dinner actually has a knock-on effect on breakfast, quite substantially reducing the blood sugar spikes of breakfast the next day. This was proven in a study that fed people different kinds of evening meals, then different kinds of breakfast, while measuring their blood sugar levels after the meals. The lower the glycemic load of the evening meal, the flatter the increase in blood sugar was after breakfast the next day. A dinner containing roughly a 130g (4¾oz) serving of cooked lentils was the best.

In Part 4 there are lots of recipes using beans, lentils and chickpeas. One of my favourites is Chestnut and Butterbean Soup (see page 250). You can make this in less than 5 minutes and it is absolutely delicious either as one of your snacks or as part of a main meal, perhaps with some oatcakes and a salad.

4 Discover quinoa – the secret of the Incas

Quinoa has been grown in South America for 5,000 years and has a long-standing reputation as a source of strength for those working at high altitudes. Called the 'mother grain' because of its sustaining properties, it contains protein of a better quality than that of meat.

Although known as a grain, quinoa is technically a seed. Like other seeds, it is rich in essential fats, vitamins and minerals, providing almost four times as much calcium as wheat, plus extra iron, B vitamins and vitamin E. Quinoa is also low in fat: the majority of its oil is polyunsaturated, providing essential fatty acids. Quinoa is also one of the highest protein sources in the vegetable kingdom, with 16 per cent of its calories as protein (soya has the most, at 38 per cent protein, and some other beans are also higher). As such, quinoa is about as close to a perfect food as you can get.

Quinoa can be found in many supermarkets these days, as well as health-food stores, and can be used as an alternative to rice. To cook it, rinse well, then add two parts water to one of quinoa and boil for 15 minutes. It is also gluten-free and is a much lower GL than rice. A 7-GL serving of cooked quinoa is 130g (4¾oz). The GL comes down even more if you serve it with protein, such as some fish or maybe tofu for a vegetarian option. Sesame Quinoa and Quinoa Taboulleh are two great recipes that can be served with a grilled tuna steak or tofu.

5 Eat chia, flax, pumpkin seeds, walnuts or almonds most days

You might not have heard of chia seeds but I've been aware of them for some time as the richest source of omega-3 fats from the vegetable kingdom, and a staple food for thousands of years going back to the Aztecs and beyond. It's just that you couldn't get chia seeds in the UK and many other countries until recently.

The first record of chia's consumption by humans is in 3500 BC, and by 1500 BC it had become a cash crop in Mexico. Aztec rulers received chia seeds as an annual tribute from conquered nations, and the seeds were offered to the gods during religious ceremonies. But chia dropped out of the Meso-American diet and culture after it was banned by the Catholic Spanish conquistadores, because it had been worshipped by the locals. Instead, agriculture was forced towards growing foods that Europeans were accustomed to.

Now, chia is making something of a comeback – and rightly so. Along with the South American grain quinoa, chia is a highly nutritious food that should become a daily part of our diet, going a long way to restoring our essential fat intake back towards more omega-3 than omega-6.

Like flax seeds (also called linseed), chia is very high in soluble fibres, as well as omega-3 fats and protein, all of which are good news as far as reversing metabolic syndrome and diabetes are concerned. Chia has more than double the soluble-fibre content of oats but, of course, you wouldn't eat the same quantity. Added to oats, for example in porridge, it is a great way to greatly increase your soluble fibre intake. The three reasons I prefer chia to flax are, firstly, it is nutritionally superior; secondly, it tastes better; and thirdly, it stores and remains fresh for longer. This is because it's naturally high in antioxidants. In a study giving people with diabetes 37g (1¼oz) of chia a day, which is about two heaped tablespoons, versus wheat bran, which was used as a placebo, those eating chia had a decrease in their glycosylated haemoglobin and their blood pressure.[28]

Like flax, chia is a very good source of protein – about 20 per cent, which is much higher than grains, including even quinoa. Rice is only 7 per cent protein, while oats are pretty much the best grain with 17 per cent protein. Chia, however, is richer in antioxidants and soluble fibre than flax – and it is also nutritionally superior in the following ways:

- Chia oil is 64 per cent alpha linolenic acid (omega-3) and 19 per cent linoleic acid (omega-6), compared to flax, which is 58 per cent omega-3 and 15 per cent omega-6.

- Chia provides 631mg of calcium and 466mg of magnesium per 100g (3½oz), whereas flax contains 199mg of calcium and 362mg of magnesium.

- Chia is also very low in sodium – 19mg versus 34mg per 100g (3½oz) in flax.

I have a 15g (½oz) serving every day (a tablespoon), which gives me 100mg of calcium and 70mg of magnesium, a really decent amount for maintaining good health and also ideal if you have diabetes. A 15g (½oz) serving also has an antioxidant rating of 1,335 ORAC points (which I mentioned in Part 1, Chapter 3 and discuss further on page 119). This represents more than a fifth of your daily target of 6,000 ORAC points. Having a quarter of a cup of berries is another 1,000, as is four walnuts or pecan nuts. So, all three with breakfast is more than half your ideal daily antioxidant intake.

Taste-wise, chia has a much nicer, slightly nuttier flavour than flax and tastes good on its own, added to cereal, bread or cakes and in salads or soups. Many health-food stores stock it. (See Resources for details on other suppliers.) Chia seeds are tiny, like sesame, so need grinding before consuming to release all the goodness, or they can be soaked for ten minutes. You can also buy ground chia seeds. Much like oat bran, they absorb a lot of water, so if you add them to cereals, shakes or soups they will bulk up, much like the oats in porridge. This makes you feel fuller.

The other healthy seeds and nuts

Flax seeds are also a great source of omega-3, soluble fibres and protein. Much like chia they are best either ground or soaked for ten minutes. Aim for a tablespoon of these seeds once a day.

The next best seeds are pumpkin seeds. These are 21 per cent protein, and reasonably high in omega-3. An advantage of pumpkin seeds is that they are very high in magnesium, which you'll see is also vital for blood sugar control. Pumpkin seeds are large enough and soft enough to be eaten whole, either on cereal, or as a snack, perhaps with a piece of fruit. If you are 'on the road' it's a good idea to have a supply so that when your blood sugar dips you can have a carbohydrate food, plus some pumpkin seeds. Aim for a tablespoonful.

Other good nuts for helping to reverse metabolic syndrome and reduce cardiovascular risk are walnuts and almonds. Walnuts have been shown to improve circulation in those with diabetes,[29] and generally to help reduce indicators of cardiovascular risk. Whether you choose chia, flax or pumpkin seeds, or nuts, you really want to be having a tablespoon of seeds, or a small handful of nuts, every day, either in your food, for example on breakfast, or as part of a low-GL snack. My Four Seed Mix (see page 187) is a simple way to get a good balance of these seeds.

You can also get almond butter and pumpkin-seed butter, which are better for you than regular butter or margarine. Peanuts and peanut butter (sugar-free) are also an excellent source of protein but won't provide the other benefits of omega-3 fats and soluble fibres.

6 Choose squashes

I'm not talking about squash drinks here, but the vegetable family, which includes courgettes, marrows, pumpkin, butternut squashes and many other varieties of winter squash. These are a very low-GL vegetable so a great choice for your 7 GL carbohydrate portion for a main meal.

Recent research reveals that an extract from pumpkin promotes the regeneration of damaged pancreatic cells in type-1 diabetic rats, boosting levels of insulin-producing beta cells and insulin in the blood.[30]

A group, led by Tao Xia of the East China Normal University, found that diabetic rats fed the extract had lower insulin levels and less destruction of insulin-producing cells. Xia says: 'pumpkin extract is potentially a very good product for pre-diabetic persons, as well as those who have already developed diabetes'. He adds that although insulin injections will probably always be necessary for these patients, pumpkin extract could drastically reduce the amount of insulin they need to take.

The protective effect of pumpkin is thought to be due to both anti-oxidants and D-chiro-inositol, a molecule that affects insulin activity. It's a bit early to say the same effects will occur in people with diabetes but, given that squashes have a very low GL as well, I encourage you to make them a regular part of your diet. Try Roast Squash and Sweet Potatoes with Shallots (page 269) or Spicy Pumpkin and Tofu Soup (page 255).

7 Enjoy berries, cherries and plums

As you saw in Chapter 1 earlier in this part, the principal sugar in most berries, cherries and plums is xylose, making these fruits especially slow-releasing. The bluer the berries the better, so blackcurrants, blackberries, blueberries and cooked black elderberry are all super-foods. In a recent study, blueberries were put to the test on a group of overweight, insulin-resistant volunteers deemed at high risk of diabetes. They were given a blueberry smoothie every day for six weeks, or an identical-looking and tasting fake smoothie. Those getting the real thing had a 22 per cent increase in their insulin sensitivity.[31]

The Montmorency cherry is exceptionally high in antioxidants (see Part 2, Chapter 5) and Montmorency cherry extract (called Cherry Active), as a cordial, is the only fruit drink I recommend. Since the predominant sugar in cherries is xylose, this drink is relatively low in GL (even so, be careful not to have more than a shot a day), whereas grape juice contains pure glucose.

Plums, when in season, are a great fruit snack, together with some protein such as a few almonds or pumpkin seeds. Try my Plum Amaretti Slices on page 275. Prunes are dried plums and three or four on cereal is an alternative fruit, but make sure they haven't been soaked in sugar.

The next best fruits are apples and pears, but the kind of apple or pear you choose makes a difference. The harder and less sweet conference pears, for example, have the lowest GL.

8 Take a spoonful of cinnamon

A spoonful of cinnamon a day really does help keep diabetes at bay. Cinnamon is a safe and inexpensive aromatic spice, which has been used for many years in traditional herbal medicine for the treatment of type-2 diabetes. The active ingredient in cinnamon, MCHP, mimics the action of the hormone insulin, which removes excess sugar from the bloodstream. Cinnamon also appears to reduce blood cholesterol and fat levels[32] and decrease blood pressure.[33] I certainly recommend you make a daily teaspoon of cinnamon part of your reverse-diabetes programme.

While we no doubt have much to learn about cinnamon, animal studies have found that there is a positive effect on blood sugar levels when treated with cinnamon. A study in 2005 found that following a high-sugar meal, cinnamon reduced blood sugar and increased insulin levels for up to 30 minutes.[34]

Another animal study found that after just two weeks of cinnamon administration, there were positive effects on fat levels and blood sugar levels, and after six weeks insulin levels and 'good' HDL cholesterol had also increased.[35]

There have also been positive findings in human studies. A research group found that when people who are in the early stages of diabetes development rather than just at higher risk were given a cinnamon extract called Cinnulin for 12 weeks, there were improvements in several features of metabolic syndrome (blood sugar levels, blood pressure and body fat percentage).[36] A follow-on study found that the cinnamon extract also improves antioxidant status, thus potentially giving protection from arterial damage caused by oxidants.[37]

Another recent study in people with diabetes found similar results. Thirty-nine patients were given cinnamon extract for four months and showed a substantial reduction in post-meal blood sugar levels and a 10 per cent reduction in fasting blood sugar levels. Interestingly, people with diabetes with the poorest blood glucose control showed the biggest improvements with cinnamon.[38]

How much cinnamon do you need?

Once again, studies are showing us the most effective levels of cinnamon to take. In one study, in 2003, researchers gave three groups of people with diabetes 1g, 3g or 6g (a heaped teaspoon) of cinnamon per day. All responded to the cinnamon within weeks, with blood sugar levels 20 per cent lower on average than those of a control group. Some of the volunteers taking cinnamon even achieved normal blood sugar levels. Tellingly, blood sugar started creeping up again after they stopped taking cinnamon. The biggest improvements were seen with the highest dosage.

A more recent Scandinavian study in which volunteers were given rice pudding, with or without cinnamon, found that those given 3g of cinnamon produce less insulin after the meal. In an earlier study the researchers also found that cinnamon may slow down gastric emptying. This would have the effect of slow-releasing the carbohydrates in a meal. This effect was seen with 6g of cinnamon, not 3g. A teaspoon is roughly 3g. A heaped teaspoon is closer to 6g.

I recommend you take 1 teaspoon (3g) per day, and see also page 132 for more about supplementing with cinnamon extract. Try my Apple and Cinnamon Compote (page 240) or Scots Porridge with Cinnamon and Apple (page 245) for two ways to cook with cinnamon.

Summary

To control your blood sugar, regulate your appetite and improve your general health:

- Eat your oats (and shiitake mushrooms and barley) for their beta-glucans.
- Vary your grains – don't always eat wheat, but opt for rye or barley.
- Eat pulses (beans, lentils and chickpeas) regularly.
- Make the super-grain quinoa a regular part of your diet.
- Snack on a small handful of chia seeds, walnuts or almonds every other day to help improve your cardiovascular health.
- Include squashes and pumpkins for their pancreas-promoting power.
- Pick deep-coloured blueberries, blackberries, blackcurrants, cherries and plums, or apples and pears, which are all naturally lower in sugar.
- Sprinkle a spoonful of cinnamon onto your cereal each morning or add to your soups and bakes to subtly spice them up.

3

Increase the Soluble Fibre In Your Diet

We've all heard about the importance of fibre, which was first put on the map back in the 1970s when doctors Denis Burkitt and Hugh Trowell (aptly named) travelled the world collecting stool samples. They found that those countries where the stools were loosely formed (which you would expect from people whose bowels moved regularly) had small hospitals, but those with a harder stool (in other words a more constipated population) had large hospitals with many patients. Doctors Burkitt and Trowell identified an indigestible type of carbohydrate in food, now called fibre, which effectively bulks up faecal matter leading to regular and healthy bowel movements, and their conclusion was that those who ate a diet which included more fibre and therefore had looser, more frequent stools also enjoyed better health.

The basics of fibre explained

The fibre in grains, which comes from the outer husk, is called bran. Vegetables also contain fibres, but some of these break down on cooking and are at their best eaten raw or lightly cooked. Fruits also contain fibre, which helps to slow-release the fructose contained in them but, as we saw in Chapter 1 of this part, fructose in large quantities acts more like a poison than a nutrient. All these fibres slow down the release of sugars in food and lower the amount of insulin you need to produce. Our ancestors ate in excess of 100g (3½oz) of fibre a day. In the 21st century we consume less than 10g (¼oz).

Foods that are high in fibre will naturally have a low-GL score, so I recommend you increase them in your diet. These include:

- Whole grains and their bran (some foods have added wheat or oat bran)

- Beans and lentils

- Nuts and seeds (especially chia and flax seeds)

- Raw and lightly cooked (steamed) vegetables

- The skins of fruits (there is virtually no fibre in the juice)

In your Anti-diabetes Diet you don't have to think about the above foods so much because I'll be giving you recipes made from low-GL foods that are naturally high in fibre.

The benefits of soluble fibres

Since the 1970s a whole world of different kinds of fibres has been discovered and studied, with wide-ranging effects, including controlling blood sugar, eliminating excess cholesterol, improving many aspects of digestion and boosting the immune system. Particularly significant was the discovery of 'soluble' fibres, which dissolve and become gel-like, absorbing lots of water, unlike wheat bran, for example, which absorbs very little. (Adding wheat bran to foods is not recommended as it acts as an irritant rather than providing moisture and softness.)

The best-known example is oat fibre or bran, which is rich in the fibre beta-glucans. When added to or cooked with water, beta-glucans becomes viscous giving porridge it's soft consistency. This soluble fibre helps to coat foods and the digestive tract in a way that slows down the release of sugars from food, effectively lowering the GL. It also attaches to cholesterol in the gut and helps to eliminate it. Generally speaking the more viscous, that is the more water-absorbing, the better. This also makes you feel fuller so you naturally eat less.

Other examples of foods that are exceptionally high in soluble fibres to help stabilise your blood sugar level are barley and chia seeds. As we saw in the previous chapter, these are some of my top anti-diabetes foods. You'll find a number of recipes in Part 4 using these foods.

Other common soluble fibres in foods include pectin, which is particularly high in citrus fruit and apples, and algin in seaweed.

The less well-known fibres

There are other food sources that you are unlikely to eat, such as konjac fibre, which is a potato-like tuber found in Japan, psyllium husks, guar gum and xanthan gum. In Japan you can buy dishes made with konjac fibre, but they're not on the menu in the West. These ingredients are often used as thickeners in foods and can also be used to create 'super-fibres' that you can buy as powders or capsules or in special shake mixes – all are designed to help stabilise your blood sugar levels. These are well worth knowing about, because taking a capsule before a meal, or a spoonful dissolved in water, makes a massive difference to the GL of the meal you are about to eat.

The super-fibres that halve blood sugar spikes

Some fibres are particularly useful for people suffering with diabetes or wishing to reduce their risk. These are my super-fibres:

Glucomannan

One of my favourite fibres, widely used in Asia but not in the UK, is glucomannan, the soluble fibre in konjac. Glucomannan absorbs 50 times more water than wheat bran, bulking up the food you eat and making you feel fuller for longer. Because of its highly absorbent properties, it is very important to take it with a lot of water. Its absorbent properties mean two things: firstly, it helps to eliminate cholesterol by binding to it in the digestive tract; and secondly – and this is the real gold of glucomannan – it has the ability to lower the glycemic load of a meal, and hence help to balance your blood sugar.

A study in Thailand found that giving 1g of glucomannan before meals significantly lowered the GL, and the need for insulin, in people with type-2 diabetes.[39] Other studies have shown that glucomannan lowers cholesterol[40] and also stabilises blood sugar,[41] which is associated with improving insulin sensitivity.

It's also a brilliant aid for healthy weight loss. Two studies, one in Japan[42] and one in the US,[43] reported an additional 450g (1lb) in weight loss a week when patients took 3g of glucommanan a day. At the Institute for Optimum Nutrition, we decided to put glucomannan to the test by giving 3g a day to ten overweight people over a three-month period.[44] None made any apparent change to their diet or exercise regime. Nine completed the trial, with an average weight loss of 3kg (6.6lb) each. A review of all studies to date, in 2005, concluded, 'At doses of 2–4 g per day, glucomannan was well-tolerated and resulted in significant weight loss in overweight and obese individuals.'[45]

You need about 3g, or a level teaspoonful, for this kind of effect. This would be the equivalent to three capsules, perhaps two or three times a day, before main meals. Be aware that, thanks to a quirk in a food law (the Emulsifiers & Stabilisers Act), pure glucomannan is not allowed to be sold in the UK; however, konjac root extract is. Konjac extract contains about 60 per cent glucomannan, so a daily intake of 5g would be equivalent to 3g of glucomannan, hence you'll need five capsules or a heaped teaspoon before meals (see Resources).

PGX – the king of all fibres

There is something even better than glucomannan. The most exceptional results have been demonstrated for a special type of fibre called PGX. It is the most highly water-absorbing fibre, created by reacting glucomannan with other plant fibres (alginate, from seaweed, and xanthan gum). PGX is a powder and is also available in capsules. Taking a heaped teaspoonful (5g) in a glass of water two or three times a day before meals reduces the appetite and substantially reduces the GL of the meal you are about to eat.[46]

Professor Jenny Brand-Miller, from the University of Sydney, has been very instrumental in promoting the value of low-GL eating. In a study she found that taking 5g of PGX powder with water before, with or immediately after breakfast cut the GL of the meal by around a quarter.[47]

You can see this effect in the first graph overleaf. You should be aiming to avoid blood sugar spikes, which means less glucose damage and less need for your body to produce insulin. As you can see, a teaspoonful of PGX does this very effectively. In addition, taking 5g with the evening meal has a knock-on effect of lowering the GL of breakfast the following day by up to a quarter.

You may recall that in Chapter 1 of this part I explained how the GI of a food is worked out by comparing the blood sugar curve created by glucose versus the food you want to test. In the second graph overleaf you can see the average curve created by glucose, in some healthy volunteers, compared to giving the volunteers both glucose and 5g of PGX. As you can see, adding the PGX effectively lowers the GI or GL of the

The effects of PGX

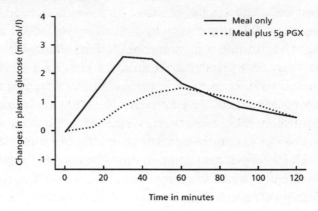

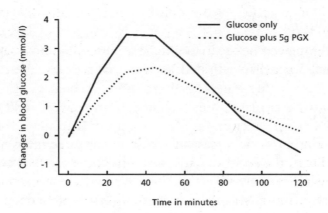

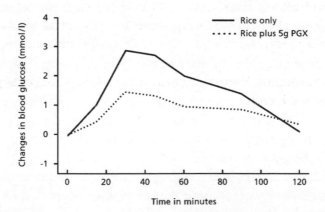

Used with the permission of the authors, J. Brand-Miller and A. Jenkins, adapted from J. Brand-Miller, et al., *European Journal of Clinical Nutrition*, 2010 Oct, advance online publication; A. L. Jenkins, et al., *Journal of the American College of Nutrition*, 2010 Oct; 29(2):92–8; and A. L. Jenkins, et al., *Nutrition Journal*, 2010; 9:58.

glucose.[48] The GL-lowering effect is even greater when added to a meal; for example, if you have a teaspoon of PGX with a meal containing a serving of rice (see the third graph) you dramatically stabilise the blood sugar spike of the meal, turning it from a mountain into a rolling hill.[49] This is almost the equivalent to halving the GL of the meal.

PGX has been shown to be very effective for losing weight. In one study, overweight volunteers lost, on average, 13lbs (6kg), and 12cm (4½in) off their waist in a 14-week trial, while their total cholesterol dropped by almost 20 per cent, with the 'bad' LDL cholesterol dropping by a fifth. PGX has also been shown to reduce the amount of food you want to eat in the accompanying meal.[50]

In a study on diabetic rats, PGX fibre was added to their meal and it was found to significantly reduce insulin resistance, cholesterol levels and damage to kidneys, and it also resulted in more healthy cells in the pancreas than in those animals not given PGX.[51] All of these are clear signs of reducing metabolic syndrome and reversing the usual pattern of 'internal global warming' that is the hallmark of diabetes.

You can use PGX to prevent or reverse diabetes

Faced with the kind of evidence outlined above, I strongly advise you to take a heaped teaspoonful of PGX, in water, before each main meal, as well as following my low-GL diet. That's why this supplemental fibre is one part of my basic building blocks for the prevention and reversal of diabetes. Ideally, you want to have your super-fibre drink up to 15 minutes before a main meal to help bulk up the food you are about to eat with much more water and fibre, thus lowering the GL of the meal. I have included this in your supplement programme in Part 3, Chapter 4.

If PGX is not available, then glucomannan, or konjac fibre, is your next best choice (see Resources).

Summary

Increase the soluble fibre in your diet for a lower GL option and to help stabilise your blood sugar levels:

- Eat wholegrains (like oats and barley), beans and lentils, which are rich in soluble fibres.
- Eat a small handful of chia or flax seeds every day.
- Include raw or lightly steamed vegetables in your daily diet.
- Eat whole, unpeeled fresh fruit to benefit from the fibre in their skins.
- Take a heaped teaspoon of PGX, in water, before each main meal, or take 3g glucomannan, or 5g (five capsules or a heaped teaspoonful) of konjac fibre before meals. (See Part 3, Chapter 4 for your supplement programme.)

4

Eat the Fats that Heal and Avoid the Fats that Kill

One of the biggest misconceptions about diabetes is that you should reduce your fat intake to lower your risk. This widespread fallacy stems from two misconceptions.

The first is that obesity causes diabetes. It is certainly associated with it, but that doesn't prove it is the cause. I believe we will find that it is the fundamental loss of blood sugar balance plus insulin resistance that is driving both weight gain and diabetes.

The second misconception is that if being overweight is the cause then you should eat less fat because fat has more calories per gram than carbohydrate or protein. Countless people with diabetes are put on low-fat diets, but most low-fat foods are high in carbohydrate. Hence, the result is a high-GL diet, which is the last thing you want if you have diabetes. These kinds of high-carbohydrate, not low-fat, diets are also a major promoter of heart disease.

Of course, this doesn't mean you should be aiming to eat high-fat foods such as dairy and red meat. Before I talk about the fats that are healthy to eat, I want to explain more about the research that has shown that focusing on high fat in the diet has overlooked the effects of a high-carbohydrate diet on people's health.

Higher fat, low-GL diets reduce diabetes risk

A study from Harvard Medical School followed over 85,000 nurses over a 20-year period to examine the diet drivers for diabetes.[52] Over that time 4,670 of the women developed diabetes. The researchers had kept measurements of their overall diets and worked out where each participant fell on a scale from eating a high-fat diet to a high-carbohydrate diet. According to the author of the study, Dr Thomas Halton, 'This study showed that a low-fat diet didn't really prevent type-2 diabetes in our cohort when compared to a low-carb diet. I was also surprised that total carbohydrate consumption was associated with type-2 diabetes, and that the relative risk of the glycemic load was so high.' They had found that it isn't cutting fat that reduces your risk but lowering the glycemic load. In this study a higher GL more than doubled the risk of developing diabetes.

According to Halton, 'The one diet that did seem to show a protective effect was a vegetable-based, low-carb diet which consisted of higher amounts of vegetable fat and vegetable protein, and lower amounts of carbohydrate.' This is a pretty good description of my low-GL diet, and the one you'll be following in Parts 3 and 4. It includes good fats (more on these in a minute) and plenty of vegetable-based protein.

High-GL, not high-fat diets, cause heart disease

Since the 1970s almost all medical advice has been that you must reduce fat in the diet to reduce your risk of heart disease as well as obesity and diabetes. But is fat really the killer? If you look at the evidence it really isn't that strong. In 2010, a large meta-analysis of studies, published in the *American Journal of Clinical Nutrition*, involving 21 studies and 350,000 patients, sent shock waves through the conventional medical and dietetic establishment. 'There is no significant evidence for concluding that dietary saturated fat is associated with an increased risk of coronary heart disease or cardiovascular disease,'[53] it reported.

What's more, the authors point out that replacing saturated fat in the diet with more carbohydrates, especially refined carbs, makes all the risk factors for heart disease and diabetes worse. 'This is striking,' says Dr Dariush Mozaffarian of Harvard, 'because it is what we have been doing for years.' Mozaffarian's own research suggests that polyunsaturated omega-6 vegetable oils like soya may reduce heart attack risk.

Part of the case against saturated fat is that it increases total cholesterol levels; however, this idea is 'based in large measure on extrapolations, which are not supported by the data,' says Meir Stampfer, professor of nutrition and epidemiology at Harvard School of Public Health. The point is that although it does raise levels of 'bad' LDL cholesterol, it also increases 'good' HDL cholesterol, higher levels of which are protective.

Two years ago, Stampfer was co-author on a study, published in the *New England Journal of Medicine*,[54] which found that the group on a low-carbohydrate diet who ate the most saturated fat ended up with the healthiest ratio of HDL to LDL and lost twice as much weight as those on a classic low-fat diet. Many other studies have found the same thing. In Canada a comparison between those on a low-GL diet and those following the conventional low-fat diet guidelines of Canada's Food Guide for Healthy Eating found that those on the low-fat diet had a substantial increase in fasting glucose, whereas those on the low-GL diet had a substantial decrease plus very positive improvement in cholesterol, with LDL 'bad' cholesterol going down, HDL 'good' cholesterol going up, and triglycerides going down.[55]

Sugar, not fat, is the real health problem

As we saw in Chapter 1 of this part, the real villain as far as both diabetes and heart disease is concerned is sugar and starch, not fat, or more specifically a high-GL diet. 'The authorities have been very slow in acknowledging the problem with carbohydrates,' says diabetes expert Professor Charles Clarke, Fellow of the Royal College of Surgeons of Edinburgh.

'The official advice for losing weight, controlling diabetes and reducing the risk of heart disease is to eat what is known as a "healthy balanced diet". This means keep your fat intake low but make sure you get a good amount of carbohydrates like pasta, bread and potatoes. Unfortunately that allows you to consume a lot of high-glycemic foods. In fact it's perfectly possible to follow a "healthy balanced diet" and consume the equivalent of 60 teaspoons of sugar a day, which is not good.'

Although high-fat diets do raise cholesterol, as Professor Stampfer points out, 'total cholesterol is not a great predictor of risk'. In the study he published in the *New England Journal of Medicine*, those with the lowest carb intake, eating high fat, lost twice as much weight as those eating a low-fat diet, which is good news as far as diabetes is concerned.[56]

There are many studies now that clearly show that eating too much sugar and refined carbohydrates, or too many carbs in total, best indicated by the GL of your diet, is a much more important health factor, and predictor of weight gain, cardiovascular risk and diabetes, than intake of fat.[57]

Low-fat, low-cholesterol diets are bad for you

One of the biggest myths in nutrition is that eating cholesterol-rich foods raises your blood cholesterol levels. It doesn't. You can have six free range or organic eggs every week and it won't make any difference to your blood cholesterol levels.

The body makes lots of cholesterol, mainly in the liver, as the vital starting material for all fat-based hormones, such as cortisol, testosterone, oestrogen and progesterone. If you take a statin drug, which stops the liver being able to make cholesterol, the liver will suck as much cholesterol as it can out of circulation to make these essential hormones. So your blood cholesterol level decreases. When you are under constant stress, the reason your cholesterol level rises is because the body is struggling to make more cortisol, so it increases its production of cholesterol. When you eat too much sugar, and a high-GL diet, or drink too much alcohol, the liver makes LDL cholesterol (the bad guy) in the process of turning the excess sugar into fat (triglycerides). So, the real cause of high LDL cholesterol and high triglycerides is a combination of high stress, and a high sugar or alcohol intake.

Low-fat diets affect testosterone levels

People put on low-fat, low-cholesterol diets, especially if also low in protein (such as a poorly designed vegan diet), often suffer with decreases in vital hormone levels. One of these is testosterone.[58] Testosterone levels are often low in people with diabetes, and testosterone deficiency is also a risk factor for developing metabolic syndrome. Testosterone deficiency is associated with a wide range of symptoms in middle-aged men, not dissimilar to menopausal symptoms and known as the andropause. These include weight gain, loss of enthusiasm, constant tiredness, decreased sex drive and, sometimes, impotence. There is also a link between heart disease and low testosterone.

Correcting testosterone deficiency can make a big difference to helping you reverse diabetes and metabolic syndrome. If you are working with a nutritional therapist or a switched-on doctor, they can test you, but don't only rely on blood tests – symptoms are also very important.

You can find out more about this subject in Dr Malcolm Carruther's book *The Testosterone Revolution* (see Recommended Reading).

Omega-3 fats are positively good for you – saturated fats are bad

There are good reasons to increase your intake of the right kind of fats. A diet high in omega-3 fats, found in cold-water oily fish, as well as certain seeds, notably chia, flax and pumpkin, helps reduce your risk of diabetes and heart disease, and also lowers triglycerides and improves insulin sensitivity. A particular kind of omega-3 fat, called EPA, which is abundant in fish oil, is a very strong natural anti-inflammatory agent, which helps to undo much of the damage caused by glycation (see Part 1, Chapter 1). The other main kind of omega-3, called DHA, is linked to improving insulin sensitivity in muscles.[59] You'll find that supplements of omega-3 fish oils contain both EPA and DHA.

The highest consumers of omega-3-rich fish are the Alaskans, Inuit and the Japanese, all of whom have a lower risk of metabolic syndrome and insulin resistance.[60] Eating a Mediterranean-style diet, which emphasises fish over meat, also means you get more omega-3s – a two-year study in Italy found that when patients with metabolic syndrome followed this kind of diet it reduced inflammation and improved insulin sensitivity.[61] On the other hand, a diet high in saturated fat, which is higher in meat and dairy products than fish, promotes insulin resistance, when combined with a high glycemic carbohydrate diet.[62] As I explained in Chapter 1 of this part, my Anti-diabetes Diet goes further than a Mediterranean diet although it shares many of its attributes.

Omega-3s also raise the level of a hormone, called adiponectin, which helps to burn sugar rather than storing it as fat. Having a high level of this hormone is associated with a reduced risk of diabetes.[63]

Having a high intake of omega-3s also reduces your risk of heart disease because they regulate inflammation, improve blood flow, reduce the stickiness of the blood and decrease blood pressure.[64]

Studies giving fish oils to people with diabetes, however, haven't always come up trumps. Almost all show a reduction in triglycerides (blood fats) but not all show an improvement in glucose control. I think the real benefit of including omega-3s in your diet is because they help to reduce the risk of many of the health problems associated with diabetes, and also because if you eat more fish, but less meat and dairy products, you are likely to reduce your intake of saturated fat. You'll find some great recipes for fish in Part 4 – try Sardines on Toast (page 254) or Pesto-crusted Salmon (page 262).

Eat a small handful of nuts or seeds every day

Omega-3 fats are also found in cold-climate nuts and seeds. The richest source is called the chia seed, which I mentioned in Chapter 3 of this part, and I recommend you eat them every day as suggested. One of the best nuts for omega-3s are walnuts, which I also discussed in that chapter. Walnut and Three-bean Salad (page 256) and Carrot and Walnut Cake (page 273) are two great walnut recipes.

Vitamin D cuts diabetes risk

Another essential fat found in oily fish is vitamin D. As explained in Part 1, Chapter 4, most of the vitamin D in our bodies comes from the action of sunlight on the skin. In the winter, if you live in the northern or far southern hemispheres, however, your body won't make enough.

A lack of vitamin D is known to increase the risk of other autoimmune diseases, so it's perhaps no surprise to find that children with type-1 diabetes have lower vitamin D levels than those without.[65] A lack of vitamin D is also associated with an increased risk of type-2 diabetes and metabolic syndrome.[66] But does supplementing more vitamin D help if you've already got diabetes? One small trial involving only ten people with diabetes found that it both improved insulin production and lessened insulin resistance,[67] and there are more studies underway.

We all need 30mcg of vitamin D a day. If you eat oily fish three times a week and six eggs a week, and if you spend 30 minutes outdoors each day exposing at least your face and arms you'll probably achieve half this quantity. Therefore, it is well worth supplementing at least 15mcg a day, and possibly more in winter.

Summary

Both for helping reverse diabetes and its associated complications and for general health, I recommend that you:

- Cut back on red meat and processed foods, but watch out for 'low-fat' foods, because most replace the fat with sugar. Stick to low-GL food choices. Replace meat with poultry and fish/shellfish, eggs, nuts and seeds.
- Have oily fish (salmon, mackerel, herring, kippers, trout, sardines or fresh tuna) three times a week.
- Eat a small handful of chia, flax, pumpkin seeds or walnuts every day, as recommended in Chapter 3 of this part.
- Eat six free-range eggs a week – this won't raise your cholesterol level.
- Supplement extra EPA and DHA in an omega-3 fish oil supplement and make sure your multivitamin provides 15mcg (600iu) of vitamin D (I give more details on supplementing in Part 3, Chapter 4).

5

Increase Your Intake of Antioxidants and Liver-friendly Foods

One hallmark of diabetes, insulin resistance and metabolic syndrome is increased inflammation and oxidation. Inflammation causes pain, redness and swelling, and oxidation, much like glycation, causes damage, as I will explain. This includes damage to insulin receptors, arteries and the liver. Fortunately, you can reverse much of this damage and switch your body's metabolism away from inflammation by increasing your intake of antioxidants and liver-friendly foods and nutrients.

Before I explain how you do this, and which foods and nutrients are most important, it is going to help to have a good understanding of how your liver and antioxidants work to keep you healthy.

Oxidants and the anti-ageing antioxidants

Think of oxidants as exhaust fumes generated from turning food into energy. Every day we generate trillions of oxidants simply as a by-product of eating. This 'pollution' damages all cells, because every single day all our cells are making energy from glucose. You can see the visible effects of oxidation in ageing skin which has lost elasticity, and in ageing eyes which have lost the ability to focus close and far, but the same process is going on throughout your body.

Anything burned, whether it's bacon or car exhaust fumes, creates these harmful by-products. A single puff of cigarette smoke contains a trillion oxidants. These literally age you by damaging your cells. The average cell has millions of tiny 'scars' caused by oxidation. As a consequence, your body and brain gradually work less and less well and look less and less youthful. But you can dramatically slow down, and even reverse, this trend if you've been on the ageing fast-train, by increasing your intake of anti-ageing antioxidant nutrients and minimising your exposure to, and internal generation of, oxidants.

How your liver keeps you healthy

Antioxidants are extremely important for liver function, and your liver is the hub as far as sugar metabolism is concerned. Your liver is responsible for turning glucose into fat, and turning fructose or alcohol into fat or energy. Most of the hallmarks of metabolic syndrome are linked to liver function. The liver makes uric acid as a by-product of sugar metabolism, raising blood pressure as a result. It makes LDL cholesterol and triglycerides and does its best to protect sugars from AGEing (creating damaged advanced glycation end-products). The more sugar and its by-products you can 'mop up' in the liver before they do damage the better.

How the liver detoxifies

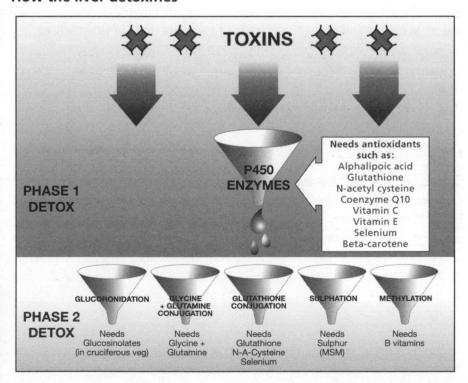

Contrary to popular belief your liver is the organ that suffers most in diabetes, not your pancreas. According to Dr Jacqueline Paltis in the *Sugar Control Bible*, Johns Hopkins University found that in 5,000 diabetics autopsied only 2 per cent had a degenerated pancreas, whereas 98 per cent had damaged livers.

As you can see from the illustration on the previous page, the liver needs a wide range of nutrients to detoxify your body. The first phase of liver detoxification, which is required to detoxify both sugar and alcohol, depends largely on antioxidant nutrients.

The second phase depends on other nutrients such as glucosinolates (found in cruciferous vegetables such as cabbage, cauliflower, kale, broccoli and Brussels sprouts); glycine (found in root vegetables); glutamine (found in tomatoes); glutathione and sulphur (present in onions and garlic, as well as eggs); and B vitamins (found abundantly in nuts, seeds, beans and greens).

Glutamine is an interesting amino acid which can be used as fuel by some cells, notably in the gut and the brain, and it can also reduce sugar cravings. It has been shown to help lessen insulin resistance and improve the function of the insulin-producing beta-cells in the pancreas.[68]

All these essential foods are included in your Anti-diabetes Diet, and I'll be talking about the importance of each nutrient in this chapter.

Cleanse your liver

If you have concerns about your liver's ability to detoxify you can go one step further and follow my Liver Detox Diet, explained fully in my book *The 9-Day Liver Detox* (it comes complete with shopping lists, recipes and daily menus). During those nine days you also take a supplement pack called the 9-Day Detox Pack (see Resources) that gives you all the essential liver-friendly nutrients listed in this chapter and helpful herbs, plus a daily sachet of 5g of glutamine powder. This is the fast track to optimising liver function – the equivalent to sending your liver to a health spa for nine days.

Essential help from antioxidants

Although there are many different kinds of antioxidants in foods, the main players, which work as a team to disarm harmful oxidants, are shown below.

Antioxidants are team players

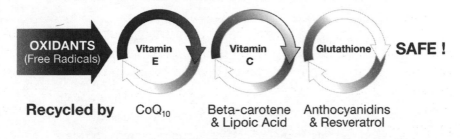

There are two ways you can increase your intake of antioxidant nutrients, thereby reversing the signs of internal global warming, and that is to eat them or supplement them. I recommend both. The reason for supplementation is that (a) you can guarantee the level of your intake, which you cannot do with food because it varies so much; and (b) there is proven value in taking larger amounts of specific nutrients than you can reasonably obtain from food for reversing disease processes. (More on this in a minute.) Also, in the case of diabetes, if you pee a lot you are literally losing nutrients and therefore need supplements to replace them.

Firstly, how do you increase your antioxidant intake from food?

You can measure your food's antioxidant power

Not all fruit and veg packs the same anti-ageing punch. The way to know the antioxidant power of a food is to measure its ORAC (oxygen radical absorbency capacity) potential. This is an objective measure of how good a food is at dealing with the oxidant 'exhaust fumes' of life. A consistent finding among populations that remain healthy into their hundreds is the consumption of at least 6,000 ORACs a day, but what does this mean for *your* daily diet?

6,000 ORACs a day keeps ageing away

The chart below shows the ORAC scores of 20 different foods that you can incorporate easily into your daily diet. Each serving given below contains approximately 2,000 units. Just choose at least three of these daily to hit your anti-ageing score of 6,000.

Foods with high ORAC scores

1	⅓ tsp ground cinnamon	11	7 walnut halves
2	½ tsp dried oregano	12	8 pecan halves
3	½ tsp ground turmeric	13	¼ cup pistachio nuts
4	1 heaped tsp mustard	14	½ cup cooked lentils
5	⅕ cup blueberries	15	1 cup cooked kidney beans
6	½ pear, grapefruit or plum	16	⅓ medium avocado
7	½ cup blackcurrants, berries, raspberries or strawberries	17	½ cup sliced red cabbage
8	½ cup cherries or a shot of Cherry Active concentrate	18	2 cups of brocolli florets
		19	1 medium artichoke or 8 spears of asparagus
9	An orange or apple	20	⅓ medium glass (150ml/5fl oz/
10	4 pieces of dark chocolate (70% cocoa solids)		¼ pint) red wine

Source: Oxygen Radical Absorbance Capacity of Selected Foods – 2007, US Department of Agriculture
Note: 1 cup = 250ml (9fl oz)

How to increase your antioxidant intake from food

Generally speaking, those foods that have the most colour and flavour also have the highest antioxidant levels. The reds, yellows and oranges of tomatoes and carrots, for example, are caused by the presence of the antioxidant beta-carotene. Artichoke has the highest rating of all the vegetables, whereas other vegetables, such as peas and spinach are lower in units, so aim for five to ten servings daily of a range of fruits and vegetables to keep your intake high. Try my Artichoke and Red Pepper Tortilla (page 249).

Fruits that have the highest levels are those with the deepest colour, such as blueberries, raspberries and strawberries. These are particularly rich in powerful antioxidants called anthocyanidins, which I'll be explaining about later in this chapter. One cup of blueberries will provide 9,697 ORAC units – you would need to eat 11 bananas to get the same benefit!

The cherry on the top

One of the simplest and easiest ways to achieve 6,000 ORACs is to have a daily shot of a Montmorency cherry concentrate, called Cherry Active, diluted with water. This measures 8,260 on the ORAC scale, which is the equivalent of around 23 portions of regular fruit and vegetables! Other juices, such as pomegranate and acai (made from berries of the South American acai palm tree, a relative of blueberries that are rich in flavonoids and anthocyanidins) claim high ORAC scores, but Cherry Active tops the lot. This is the only fruit juice I would recommend, since the predominant sugar in cherries is xylose which, you may remember, is very low in carbs. But, even so, don't have more than one shot, which is the equivalent of 5 ⓖⓛ. That's your daily drink quota.

Not just any 'five a day'

The number of portions of fruit and vegetables you need per day really does depend on your choices, as you can see in the menus for two days below. Both days have five portions selected, but Day 2's selection is 8,000 ORACs more than that for Day 1.

Comparative ORACs for two days' food choices

DAY 1		DAY 2	
Fruit/vegetable portion	**ORAC**	**Fruit/vegetable portion**	**ORAC**
⅛ large cantaloupe melon	315	½ pear	2,617
1 kiwi fruit	802	½ cup strawberries	2,683
1 medium carrot, raw	406	½ avocado	2,899
½ cup green peas, frozen	432	1 cup broccoli florets, raw	1,226
1 cup spinach, raw	455	4 spears asparagus, boiled	986
Total score	**2,410**	**Total score**	**10,411**

Antioxidant nutrients in supplement form

The following nutrients help to reverse your risk of diabetes or to reduce your risk if you have metabolic syndrome:

Vitamin C is extremely important to supplement and to eat, if you have diabetes. And having a high level of vitamin C in your blood, consistent with that achieved by supplementation and eating a diet high in fruits and vegetables, reduces your risk of diabetes by 62 per cent. That's the conclusion of a study of over 21,000 people over a 12-year period, published in the *Archives of Internal Medicine*.[69] Those with the highest amounts of vitamin C in their blood plasma were 62 per cent less likely to develop diabetes, compared to those with the lowest amounts. To reach the optimal level of vitamin C in your blood for diabetes reduction you will need to supplement 1,000mg a day and eat lots of fruit and vegetables. I take 2g a day for general good health.

One study in India gave people with diabetes either 500mg or 1,000mg of vitamin C. Only those taking the higher amount had a significant decrease in both their blood sugar levels and glycosylated haemoglobin, as well as triglycerides and cholesterol.[70]

Although most people think of oranges and other citrus fruits as being the highest sources of vitamin C, there's actually more in greens such as broccoli. A review of six studies, published in the *British Medical Journal*, found that an intake equivalent to 100g (3½oz) a day – roughly a serving – of dark green leafy vegetables, such as broccoli, spinach, cabbage and cauliflower, cut diabetes risk by 14 per cent.[71] These foods also help your liver to detoxify, because they are high in glucosinolates. For a tasty meal, try Oriental Green Beans and Broccoli (page 269).

A high intake (2g) of vitamin C a day also protects the eyes, which are prone to damage from the accumulation of slowly processed sorbitol, a consequence of diabetes. Taking a daily dose of vitamin C halves the amount of sorbitol the body produces.[72]

Vitamin E on its own, although good for you, doesn't appear to reduce diabetes risk, but when taken with vitamin C it helps to keep the arteries[73] and kidneys[74] healthy in those with diabetes. One trial gave people with diabetes vitamins C and E plus chromium, as well as counselling in behaviour modification, which included a low-fat diet, exercise and giving up smoking. The incidence of cardiovascular problems halved, compared to those receiving conventional medical treatment.[75] It's worth supplementing 100mg of vitamin E, so look for a multivitamin that provides this, along with vitamin C and chromium.

Co-enzyme Q$_{10}$ recycles spent vitamin E to return it to its active anti-oxidant form. Supplementing CoQ$_{10}$ helps to lower blood pressure and glycosylated haemoglobin.[76] CoQ$_{10}$ also plays an important role in energy production. I take 10mg every day to maintain good health, but if you have advanced diabetes, nine times this amount – 90mg – can help to speed up your recovery. This is especially helpful if you have cardiovascular disease, and essential if you are taking statins because these cholesterol-lowering drugs knock out CoQ$_{10}$.[77] Cholesterol-lowering drugs stop the production of CoQ$_{10}$ (produced further along the same pathway as cholesterol production), which is important for energy production.

Alpha lipoic acid is a vital antioxidant that helps vitamin C to work efficiently, recycling it back to antioxidant status once it's disarmed a harmful oxidant. But it does much more than that. Glycation and oxidation damage tissue such as the arteries, kidneys, nerves and eyes, as well as insulin-producing cells and insulin receptors, making you more insulin resistant. When your blood sugar levels are high it increases both glycation and oxidation.[78] Alpha lipoic acid protects you from that damage and it is important for people with type-1 or type-2 diabetes to minimise the damage caused by sugar.

A study in Greece gave diabetic patients supplements of alpha lipoic acid for four weeks and found that it increases insulin sensitivity.[79] Many studies have shown that it protects against nerve damage,[80] and another has found that it improves circulation in diabetics.[81] In many European countries high doses of alpha-lipoic acid (600–1,200mg) are given intravenously to treat neuropathy, the nerve damage that leads to loss of feeling in extremities and, ultimately, amputations.[82] It's well worth supplementing. I take 10mg a day as part of my supplement regime for maintaining good health, but the level recommended if you have diabetes is 100–200mg a day.

Glutathione is the body's most important antioxidant, but people with diabetes don't make enough of it. Supplementing glutathione – or the amino acids from which it is formed – N-acetyl cysteine (NAC) and glycine – helps to restore normal levels, thereby reducing inflammation.[83] I supplement 50mg of glutathione every day, but if you have advanced diabetes, you will need ten times this amount: 500mg of either glutathione or NAC to help to speed up your recovery. The combination of NAC and lipoic acid is very effective at raising glutathione levels, whey protein, rich in these amino acids, also helps boost glutathione.

Resveratrol and anthocyanidins are the purple colours in berries and red grapes. Anthocyanidins reactivate glutathione, so if you take these two together you get a much more substantial antioxidant effect. Resveratrol is concentrated in red grapes, and hence good-quality red wine. In both animal trials and two human trials involving ten older people with pre-diabetes and 19 people with diabetes, resveratrol improves insulin resistance and lowers glucose levels after a meal.[84] Resveratrol has some interesting effects on switching genes away from metabolic syndrome, as I'll explain later in this part in Chapter 10.

Zinc is a vital antioxidant mineral, but also, together with magnesium, it is essential for insulin production and function. Both these minerals help to turn sugar into energy, and help insulin to work properly.[85] Not surprisingly, a study reports that women with the highest zinc intake have a 10 per cent lower risk of developing diabetes.[86] Zinc is found richly in nuts and seeds, as well as seafood. I recommend supplementing at least 10mg a day, as well as eating these foods on a daily basis.

Magnesium levels tend to be low in people with diabetes, and the lower the magnesium the higher the insulin levels.[87] A 14-year study tracking over 75,000 people found that the lower a person's magnesium level the higher was their risk of diabetes.[88]

Magnesium is found in nuts, seeds, lentils, beans and green leafy vegetables, and it is perhaps the most commonly deficient mineral in the modern diet. The RDA in the UK is set at 300mg a day, but should be 500mg, especially if you have diabetes. The average person achieves only 270mg from their diet. If you eat a good diet containing those foods listed above you may achieve 350mg, but that leaves a shortfall of 150mg from the ideal total daily intake of 500mg. This is what I recommend everyone should supplement on a daily basis in a high-strength multivitamin–mineral. If you have diabetes, you might benefit from double this supplemental amount: 300mg a day.

In one study, diabetics with low magnesium were given magnesium or a placebo for 16 weeks. At the end of that period only those taking the magnesium had lower blood sugar levels, insulin levels and glycosylated haemoglobin, which dropped from an average of 10 per cent to an average of 8 per cent.[89] According to diabetes expert Dr Fedon Lindberg, 'Almost every diabetic patient I see needs extra magnesium.'

Milk thistle, containing the active nutrient silymarin, is particularly helpful for diabetes. It's worth supplementing even if you don't have any liver-related issues because it makes you more sensitive to insulin. There have been three good studies giving people with diabetes milk thistle supplements, and every one has shown a significant reduction in glucose and in glycosylated haemoglobin.[90] These studies gave the equivalent of 500–600mg of milk thistle a day; for example, 250mg twice a day. I recommend you start with 200mg twice a day of a milk thistle extract standardised to give at least 70 per cent silymarin (see Resources).

Gymnema sylvestre is an ancient Indian herb called *gurmar*, which means 'the sugar destroyer'. It's renowned for reducing cravings for sweet foods, so it is potentially useful if you are a sugar addict. There have been two good studies showing that both blood glucose levels and glycosylated haemoglobin levels decrease with daily supplements of 400mg a day, usually taking 200mg twice a day, standardised to contain at least 24 per cent gymnemic acid, which is the active ingredient.[91]

In Part 3 I'll explain how to build these important nutrients and herbs into your daily supplement programme. Often, a good place to start is an antioxidant complex containing vitamins C and E, alpha lipoic acid and glutathione or n-acetyl cysteine.

The B vitamins and homocysteine

In Part 1, Chapter 3 I mentioned a process call methylation, and you may also have noticed it in the illustration on metabolic syndrome (see page 41). If your body is not efficient at methylation your blood level of the amino acid homocysteine goes up and, as I explained earlier, this is strongly associated with a number of health risks. A raised homocysteine level means that you need more of the homocysteine-lowering B vitamins. The main ones are vitamins B_6, B_{12} and folic acid, although B_2 and B_3 (niacin) are also involved. You'll receive a good dosage of these B vitamins in a decent high-strength multivitamin–mineral which, in Part 3, Chapter 4, I will be recommending you take every day. However, for a raised homocysteine level you will need to supplement more.

If your homocysteine level is slightly high (above 7 mmol/l), high (above 9 mmol/l) or very high (above 15 mmol/l), you'll need more than a multivitamin can supply. Having a high homocysteine level is a risk factor for diabetes, but there isn't much evidence to date that taking high-dose B vitamins then reverses your risk.

Nevertheless, it is not a good idea to have a high homocysteine level, so my recommendation is to supplement a homocysteine-lowering formula if your level is raised. But do note that there are some studies that show potentially harmful effects from very high doses of B vitamins if you have kidney disease.[92] There's a catch-22 situation here in that people with kidney disease do often have high homocysteine levels. If this applies to you, my recommendation is to work with a nutritionally oriented doctor or nutritional therapist.

B vitamins and cholesterol

Many people with diabetes have high cholesterol, so it is worth knowing that high doses of vitamin B_3 (niacin) is the most effective agent for both lowering cholesterol and raising HDL (the 'good' cholesterol). You can buy it over the counter, but it is also available on prescription as a drug called Niaspan or Tredaptive. Pure niacin, usually taken as 500mg twice a day with food, will make you blush for about 30 minutes. There are some non-blushing forms of niacin available that mitigate this side effect but they may not be as effective at lowering cholesterol. There had been some concerns that high-dose niacin could trigger low blood sugar, especially during a blush; however, this has been specifically researched and ruled out.[93] Even so, I recommend caution.

Given that your liver has to detoxify sugar, fat and every other toxin you consume, and that your body generates trillions of oxidants, ensuring you have an optimal supply of all these liver-friendly and antioxidant nutrients helps to undo the damage caused by diabetes and metabolic syndrome.

Summary

To reduce your inflammatory status and support the liver in its essential metabolic processes:

- Eat a 'food rainbow' every day – choose red, yellow, orange and green fruit and vegetables, berries, tomatoes, carrots and cabbage to ensure the widest range of antioxidants.
- Drink one shot of diluted Cherry Active each day for a huge antioxidant boost.
- Supplements of liver-supportive antioxidants, herbs and vitamins can be included as part of your daily supplement programme. You'll find more on this in Part 3, Chapter 4.

6

Take Chromium – The Mineral that Makes Insulin Work Better

The most important aim for both weight and diabetes control is to keep insulin levels naturally low, but, as you've seen, we often become increasingly insulin insensitive or resistant. That's where the essential mineral chromium makes all the difference. For insulin to work properly it has to attach to an insulin receptor. Chromium not only increases the number of insulin receptors present but it also helps insulin bind more strongly to its receptor – thereby improving its overall effectiveness. The result is improved glucose transport into muscle, fat and liver tissue, and therefore better glucose control. The further you are along the road to diabetes the more you need to make sure you are really hearing the insulin message.

What about chromium from food?

Although chromium is naturally present in foods such as beer, whole grains, cheese, liver and meat, the typical intake in a Western diet is much lower than the recommended daily requirement of 50–200mcg per day. The average intake is thought to be in the region of 28–35mcg. One reason for this low consumption is that white flour, which is the most frequently eaten type, has 98 per cent of its chromium removed. Also, typical Western diets, which are high in sweetened and refined foods, such as white bread, cakes, sweets and biscuits, increase chromium losses because it is used up by the body to process the sugar. So, every time you binge on something sweet you are losing your body's stores of chromium.

You need high doses of chromium for diabetes repair

Although eating unrefined food – a cornerstone of my low-GL diet – should give you at least 30mcg of chromium, and taking an optimum multivitamin–mineral should provide at least another 30mcg (totalling 60mcg), that's not enough to undo the damage. It's good enough for maintenance but not for repair. What you need, if you have diabetes, is 600mcg a day – ten times this amount.

The evidence for chromium reversing diabetes

Not only is low chromium status associated with an increased prevalence of type-2 diabetes but there's also lots of good-quality research showing that chromium helps to restore blood sugar balance in people with diabetes better and faster than the most commonly prescribed anti-diabetes drug, metformin.

A 2007 review of over 40 randomised controlled trials found that giving chromium to people with type-2 diabetes improves their fasting blood sugar levels and also decreases glycosylated haemoglobin levels (another measure of poor sugar control). In the words of the reviewers, 'Among participants with type-2 diabetes, chromium supplementation improved glycosylated haemoglobin levels and fasting glucose. Chromium supplementation significantly improved glycemia among patients with diabetes.'[94]

This study, published in the highly respectable journal *Diabetes Care*, found that the best effects were seen with chromium picolinate (which is much better absorbed than cheaper forms of inorganic chromium, such as chromium chloride) in doses of 400–1,000mcg per day. Despite being more than eight times the current RDA in the UK, there are no known side effects at levels of up to 100 times greater than this.

A landmark study in 1997 looked at 120 Chinese patients with type-2 diabetes, 60 of whom were given 200mcg chromium per day and 60 of whom were given 1,000mcg per day. After just two months, significant improvements were seen in glucose control, in both groups. After four months, there was almost a 30 per cent reduction in glucose levels in the higher dosage group.[95]

The effect of chromium on blood sugar and insulin resistance

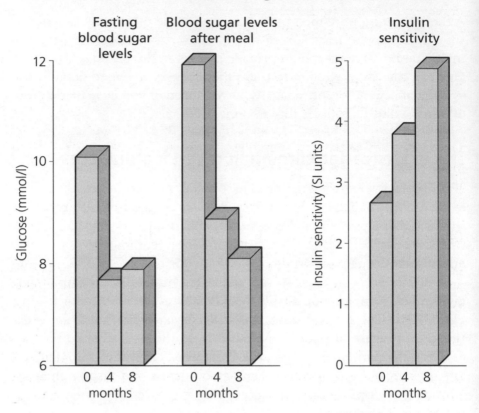

Length of time taking chromium supplements

As you can see from the illustration, after four months of taking chromium there was a significant drop in blood sugar levels recorded during fasting and after meals, and increased insulin sensitivity. After eight months the insulin sensitivity continued to improve significantly.

There are other studies confirming that chromium is effective and safe to supplement. One larger study in 1999 followed over 800 people with diabetes who were taking insulin or anti-hyperglycemic drugs.[96] The patients were given 500mcg of chromium per day for nine months, and after just one month, fasting and post-meal glucose levels had significantly fallen. At the end of the nine months, 90 per cent of patients reported a decrease in fatigue, thirst and the need for frequent urination.

More recently, a double-blind placebo-controlled study randomly assigned 42 overweight adult women who experienced carbohydrate cravings to receive chromium or placebo for eight weeks. Chromium, when compared to placebo, reduced food intake, hunger levels and fat cravings, and decreased their body weight.[97]

That's just about everything you could ever hope for.

Chromium gives you quick results

In many studies, the benefits of taking chromium are seen within a month, so you don't have to wait long.[98] In my experience, if you also take cinnamon extract (more on this shortly) and follow a low-GL diet, you'll experience a considerable improvement in blood sugar control in a matter of days, not weeks.

Chromium as an alternative to diabetic drugs

As we have seen, conventional anti-diabetes drugs, such as metformin and sulfonylurea, as well as glitazones, frequently cause side effects such as nausea, cramps and vomiting. They can also lead to weight gain and elevated blood pressure, leading to a need for weight-loss drugs in addition to anti-hyperglycemic medication.

Of greater concern is the evidence of glitazones increasing heart disease risk and metformin promoting vitamin B_{12} deficiency. This in turn elevates homocysteine levels, a major risk factor for stroke and cardiovascular disease.

Chromium has no known side effects up to 10,000mcg a day, according to the UK's Committee on Toxicity[99] – that's 20 times the therapeutic level. Therefore, this natural substance is surely much more desirable as a way of helping to stabilise blood sugar, thus reducing the symptoms of diabetes.

In fact, chromium has been shown to dramatically decrease the need for medication in many people with diabetes, and in some cases to eliminate the need for drugs completely.[100]

Which type of chromium is best?

There is some debate about the best form of chromium. Is it chromium picolinate, or chromium polynicotinate (chromium polynicotinate contains vitamin B_3 which works in synergy with chromium)? Both appear to be effective and better than another cheaper form, chromium chloride.

How much chromium should you take?

The majority of studies showing improvements in glucose control have used quantities of over 400mcg of chromium per day, although in two studies improvements in insulin sensitivity have still been reported in those taking just 200mcg/day.[101] Most available chromium supplements in health-food stores provide 200mcg, but in relation to diabetes or pre-diabetes, a daily intake of 400–600mcg may be more appropriate.

I generally recommend taking 400mcg of chromium with breakfast and 200mcg with lunch for the first three months, if you have diabetes. If this doesn't considerably stabilise your blood sugar level, then you can increase up to 1,000mcg a day. But, once your blood sugar level is consistently below 6 this might be more than you need. Certainly, if you are experiencing blood sugar lows, it is probably time to experiment with taking either 400mcg or 200mcg of chromium a day to see if this is enough to keep your blood sugar level on an even keel. See Part 3, Chapter 4 for full details about taking chromium.

Stabilising blood sugar with cinnamon and chromium

In Chapter 2 of this part, I explained the diabetes-alleviating properties of cinnamon. Together with chromium, cinnamon (cassia, or Chinese cinnamon, which is the most common type sold) helps to normalise blood sugar and reduce insulin resistance. The active ingredient in cinnamon, MCHP, mimics the action of the hormone insulin, which removes excess sugar from the bloodstream. Having a teaspoon of cinnamon a day and/or supplementing a cinnamon extract high in MCHP, together with chromium, makes a lot of sense. One such extract is called Cinnulin. Supplementing 150mg of Cinnulin is equivalent to 3g of cinnamon. Cinnulin is a good choice, because it is very low in coumarin, a potentially harmful compound found in some species of cinnamon, if ingested in very large quantities. Cinnulin is guaranteed to contain less than 0.7 per cent coumarin, as well as having a high concentration of MCHP, the active ingredient. This means that if you supplemented 300mg of Cinnulin the intake of coumarin would be well below the tolerable daily intake and not remotely pose any potential health risk, while giving all the potential benefits of cinnamon. Supplementing cinnamon and chromium, together with a low-GL diet makes a lot of sense for those struggling with weight, sugar cravings or diabetes.

How much cinnamon and cinnamon extract should you take?

We need more human trials looking at the effects of cinnamon on type-2 diabetes management, but based on the available evidence I recommended on page 100 that people with type-2 diabetes include 3g of cinnamon daily (one teaspoon). I also recommend that you add 150mg of a cinnamon extract, high in MCHP – however, do bear in mind that your need for medication may decrease, so it is important to monitor your blood sugar levels and inform your primary care practitioner accordingly. See Part 3, Chapter 4 for full details about taking the supplements recommended here.

Natural support for weight control from chromium, HCA and 5-HTP

Although chromium and cinnamon are my favourites for stabilising blood sugar levels, if your goal is to lose weight my three favourite natural remedies are chromium, an extract of tamarind called HCA and the amino acid derivative 5-HTP. Unlike stimulant drugs and herbs, which work against the body's natural design, these work with it, helping to reduce hunger and carbohydrate cravings, and are therefore an additional extra, speeding up the process of weight loss, if that is your goal.

I conducted a survey on people who had followed my low-GL diet, divided into those who had taken no supplements, those who took the basics that I recommend for everybody (multivitamin–mineral, vitamin C and essential fats), and those taking the basics and at least two out of the following: chromium, HCA and 5-HTP – the 'all supplement' group. The illustration overleaf shows the average weekly weight loss for each group. Those on the diet alone lost an average of 550g (1¼lb) a week, whereas those taking these additional supplements lost an average of 900g (2lb) a week.[102]

HCA – tamarind's secret ingredient

The nutrient HCA is extracted from the dried rind of the tamarind fruit (*Garcinia cambogia*), which you may know from Indian and other Eastern cuisines. HCA works by slowing down the enzyme that converts sugar into fat. The carbohydrate in a meal is first used to provide fuel and short-term energy stores as glycogen. Any excess is then

The effects of supplements on weight loss

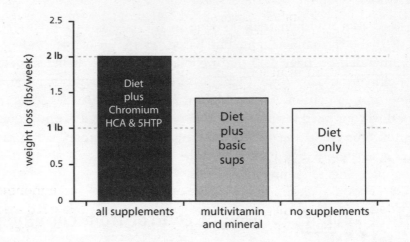

converted to fat by the enzyme ATP-citrate lyase. HCA dampens down the activity of this enzyme. It also reduces the synthesis of fat and cholesterol.

Evidence of HCA's fatburning properties has been accumulating since 1965. It has been extensively tested and found to have no toxicity or safety concerns. In terms of more recent trials, one conducted by the University of Maastricht in the Netherlands confirms that HCA acts as a powerful appetite suppressant, reducing weight with no harmful effects. In a double-blind, placebo-controlled, randomised, cross-over trial, 12 overweight men and 12 overweight women were given a tomato-juice drink three times a day for two weeks. They then had a two-week break. Following this, the group was divided up, unbeknown to them. Some participants drank tomato juice with placebo, others drank tomato juice containing 300mg of HCA, three times a day for the next two weeks.

Only those taking the HCA-loaded drink ate less – a total of 15–30 per cent fewer calories; however, they didn't report that they had tried to eat less, tried to restrict their diet or experienced any loss of enjoyment regarding their food. They just happened to eat less. They also lost more weight, averaging 450g (1lb) extra weight loss a week.[103]

A more recent trial put 60 volunteers on a 2,000 kcal diet, plus a 30-minute walking exercise programme five days a week and gave them either a placebo or 2,800mg of HCA in three equally divided doses 30 to 60 minutes before meals. At the end of eight weeks, body weight had dropped by 5.4 per cent in those taking HCA compared to placebo and their body mass index (BMI) decreased by 5.2 per cent. Food intake, total cholesterol, LDL (the bad guy), triglycerides and serum leptin levels (the hormone that triggers eating) were significantly reduced, while HDL cholesterol (the good guy), serotonin levels and excretion of urinary fat metabolites (a biomarker of fat oxidation) significantly increased. No significant adverse effects were reported.[104]

How much HCA should you take?

I recommend taking HCA, especially during the first three months of following my low-GL diet if you need to lose weight. You need at least 750mg a day for an effect. (The study above used three times this amount.) Most supplements provide 250mg per capsule, so take one capsule three times a day, ideally immediately before, or up to 30 minutes before, a main meal.

5-HTP helps you to 'think thin'

Have you ever thought about why you get hungry? You might think the obvious answer is because you haven't eaten. But that isn't always true, is it? And don't you often find yourself craving something sweet even though you just ate more than enough food?

The three most powerful controllers of your appetite are your blood sugar level, the levels of a hormone called leptin (explained on page 88) and your brain's level of serotonin, the 'happy' neurotransmitter. Serotonin is made from an amino acid, or building block of protein, called tryptophan and specifically from a form of this amino acid called 5-hydroxytryptophan, or 5-HTP for short.

Many people have low levels of this vital brain chemical and are prone to feeling low as a result, but that isn't all. Serotonin also controls appetite. The more you have, the less you eat, and the less you have, the more you eat, which is why most people eat more when they are depressed and low in serotonin. Stress, particularly in women, leads to low serotonin.

If you are low in serotonin, one of the quickest ways to restore normal levels, and normal mood, is to supplement your diet with 5-HTP. It's found in meat, fish and beans, although in rather small amounts.

Two studies show clearly that 5-HTP does work. In the first study, 20 obese volunteers took either 5-HTP (900mg) or a placebo for 12 weeks. During the first six weeks, volunteers could eat what they liked. During the second six weeks the volunteers were recommended a low-calorie diet. In both phases those taking 5-HTP consistently ate less, felt more satisfied and consequently lost weight.[105] What was particularly interesting was that they ate less carbohydrate.

The second study gave 25 overweight people with type-2 diabetes either 5-HTP or placebo for two weeks, with no dietary restriction; they could eat what they liked. In the words of the researchers, 'Patients receiving 5-HTP significantly decreased their daily energy intake, by reducing carbohydrate and fat intake, and reduced their body weight.'[106]

Furthermore, 5-HTP is often given with appetite suppressants by medical obesity specialists.[107]

CAUTION Don't take 5-HTP if you are on an antidepressant. Most of those drugs block the reuptake of serotonin, whereas 5-HTP provides the brain with the raw material to make enough in the first place. The combination increases the risk of side effects from the drug. Check with your doctor.

How much 5-HTP should you take?

I recommend a dose of 50–200mg of 5-HTP, starting with 100mg a day. See Part 3, Chapter 4 for full details about taking HCA and 5-HTP.

Summary

- I recommend chromium supplements as a core part of any plan to balance your blood glucose and reduce your need for diabetes drugs.
- Combining chromium with cinnamon should help to balance your blood glucose levels.
- For those who also want to lose weight, HCA and 5-HTP can be taken in addition to chromium.
- See Part 3, Chapter 4 on supplements for an in-depth explanation of the supplements I recommend and their doses.

7

Learn the Hard Truth about Soft Drinks, Alcohol and Coffee

What should you be drinking to minimise your risk of diabetes and help to keep your blood sugar level even? Obviously, water is a good choice, but how do different sweet drinks, including fruit juices and sugar-free drinks, affect your blood sugar control? And what about alcohol, tea, coffee, decaffeinated and caffeinated drinks?

The hard facts about soft drinks

The single biggest source of increased sugar consumption is soft drinks. Between the 1980s and 1990s there was a 41 per cent increase in the consumption of soft drinks and a 35 per cent increase in fruit drinks. In the 1990s the principal sugar in most soft drinks changed from glucose and sucrose, which was considered unhealthy, to fructose or fruit sugar, perceived to be better for you. Nowadays, as you may remember from Part 1, Chapters 1 and 3, almost all fructose in drinks is derived from high-fructose corn syrup. Although the name implies something different, high-fructose corn syrup is actually 55 per cent fructose and 45 per cent glucose. If you look at page 77 you will see that sugar (sucrose) is one fructose molecule (50 per cent) and one glucose molecule (50 per cent). So, in reality, sugar and high-fructose corn syrup are essentially the same thing as far as your body is concerned.

If you look at most cola drinks you'll find two other ingredients: caffeine, a diuretic that makes you pee more, and sodium, which makes you thirsty. Why are these added? Because they make you drink more. The more you drink the more money the soft-drink giants make. Most people in the Western world today are consuming an average of 28.5kg (63lb) of sugar per year, most of it hidden in drinks and foods sweetened with high-fructose corn syrup. A major reason for this is that this ingredient is cheap – much cheaper than sugar from sugar cane.

On the face of it, fructose sounds like a better kind of sugar to use – because it has a lower GL. Many juices, such as apple juice and orange juice, are also naturally sweet from the presence of fructose, the principal sugar in most fruits. Surely, these are not too bad for you? The difference is that in nature any offering of fructose – for example, in fresh fruit – comes 'packaged' with a lot of fibre, hence mitigating any damaging effects of too much fructose. The fibre slow-releases the sugar and makes it harder for you to consume too much. In addition, our ancestors were burning off the fructose they ate as part of the whole fruit through exercise.

Both fruit juice and soft drinks raise diabetes risk

More and more evidence is linking the regular consumption of sweetened soft drinks, and even 'natural' fruit juices, with an increased diabetes risk; for example, a large study of 59,000 African–American women, who are particularly prone to diabetes, found that drinking two or more sugar-sweetened soft drinks increases diabetes risk by 25 per cent, whereas drinking two or more fruit juice drinks increases risk by 31 per cent.[108] So, neither drinks are good news. Actually, the same increase was not observed in those drinking grapefruit juice, which has a low GL, or orange juice. Even so, you need to be careful not to overdo the orange juice, because a standard glass equals the juice of three oranges. If you then fill it up again, you could easily consume six oranges' worth of fructose and glucose. Would you *eat* that many? Few people would eat more than one orange, because the fibre helps to fill you up.

What happens to fructose in the body?

Before we even get into what the body does with fructose, it's clear that drinking any sugared juice or fruit juice exposes you to a massive and sudden increase in sugar, both glucose and fructose. In the case of glucose, 80 per cent goes to cells to burn off, provided you are physically active, leaving 20 per cent that goes to the liver. If you are not physically active and excess glucose is ingested, some of this goes into storage as glycogen; the rest turns into fat. Glucose increases insulin, increasing storage of this fat, in addition to increasing the storage of fat from food. Since fructose isn't burned for energy in the same way that glucose is – because cells can't run off fructose – the body has to do something with it, and it turns it into fat in the liver, provided again that you are not physically active. Fructose, however, does not increase insulin levels and does not promote fat storage in fat tissue from dietary fat, in the same way that glucose does.

However, every time you have a glass of fruit juice or a fructose-sweetened soft drink your liver has to work really hard. As we saw earlier in this part in Chapter 5, there is a limit to the liver's capacity to handle fructose. When stretched to the limit, the fat that your liver converted from fructose and other sugars spills out into the liver itself. This means that fat is dumped into the liver. At its extreme this creates a condition known as non-alcoholic fatty liver disease (NAFLD). This also stops insulin working in the liver. If you keep drinking these high-fructose drinks, the body has to produce more insulin. A high-GL diet or high sugar consumption is actually the second most common cause of liver failure and it inevitably leads to raised insulin levels and, in due course, insulin resistance. The consumption of soft drinks increases the prevalence of NAFLD and is also associated with a much greater risk of metabolic syndrome, weight gain and obesity.[109]

In addition, both fructose and high glucose are also turned in the liver into uric acid, which then promotes gout.[110] Uric acid also switches off something called nitrous oxide which keeps your blood pressure low. So, too much fructose is also associated with high blood pressure. But most of the fructose is turned into the bad LDL cholesterol, and is then put into storage as fat.

The bottom line is to keep any form of sugar to a minimum. Anything other than a small amount of fructose in a whole fruit is closer to a toxin than a nutrient and is best avoided completely if you have diabetes (as a general rule, don't have more than 15 grams of fructose a day). If you don't believe me, I suggest you watch the excellent YouTube seminar presented by Professor Lustig from the department of endocrinology, University of California, entitled 'Sugar, the Bitter Truth' (see Recommended Reading).

The best drinks

My recommendation is to stick to water, herb teas, teas and the occasional coffee and stay away from both sweetened soft drinks and fruit juices completely. The only exception might be a daily shot (no more) of the pure cherry juice concentrate, Cherry Active. It has a very high antioxidant content (see page 121) and the xylose in the cherries has minimal effects on your blood sugar.

Once your blood sugar is under control I have factored in a daily allowance of 5 ⓖ for drinks or desserts. If you choose to use up your allowance with a soft drink here's what 5 ⓖ equates to:

Drinks – what equals 5 ⓖ?

Tomato juice	1 pint
Carrot juice	small glass
Grapefruit juice, unsweetened	small glass
Apple juice, unsweetened	small glass diluted 50:50 with water
Orange juice, unsweetened	small glass or juice of one orange
Pineapple juice	½ small glass diluted 50:50 with water
Cranberry juice drink	½ small glass diluted 50:50 with water
Grape juice	2.5cm (1in) of liquid!

Your best pub option is a Virgin Mary, made with tomato juice, Worcester sauce, Tabasco and lemon juice.

Stay away from 'sugar-free' drinks too

Perhaps you've already switched to diet colas or other 'sugar-free' soft drinks. These drinks achieve their sweetness by the addition of aspartame as a sweetener and a caramel colourant (burnt sugar). These potentially increase insulin resistance by damaging insulin receptors and promoting inflammation.[111,112] Aspartame has also been shown to contribute to weight gain, obesity, insulin resistance and type-2 diabetes.[113]

Although aspartame has, officially, been given a clean bill of health, there are many reports of headaches, blindness and seizures with long-term, high-dose aspartame use. One study reports a raised risk of a rare kind of brain tumour called lymphoma. Clearly some people react to it badly. Although it is probably better for you than drinking drinks loaded with high-fructose corn syrup, it is not good for you. Personally, my recommendation is to avoid these drinks.

The truth about alcohol

Alcohol (ethanol) is a sugar. In many ways it behaves just like sugar. The body cannot use it for energy and hence consuming it doesn't raise your blood sugar or insulin level. But the body does have to break it down, and that job is done by the liver. As we all know, too much alcohol frequently damages the liver.

What alcohol does to the body

The liver turns alcohol into acetaldehyde, which damages the liver by generating oxidants and encouraging inflammation. The acetaldehyde then turns into acetate, which can then be 'burned' to generate some energy, but the rest is converted into LDL, thus raising your LDL cholesterol, and then into triglycerides, which are stored as fat in the body. So alcohol, like fructose, makes you fat. If the liver is producing too much fat in the body, this then accumulates in the liver as well, causing fatty liver disease as we saw above.

Too much fat in the muscles stops them from being sensitive to insulin so, in a roundabout way, alcohol does also contribute to insulin resistance even though it doesn't stimulate insulin release.

That's the bad news, and the reason why drinking a lot of alcohol leads to poor liver function and a 'beer belly'.

Too much alcohol and fructose can make you ill

The long-term effects of too much alcohol and fructose are shown below. Unlike alcohol, fructose can't be metabolised by the brain, so you don't get drunk on it, just fat. Both are treated like poisons in the body, however, and are best avoided or minimised, especially if you already have diabetes.

The long-term effects of too much alcohol and fructose

Chronic alcohol exposure	Chronic fructose exposure
Hypertension	Hypertension
Cardiovascular disease	Cardiovascular disease
High cholesterol and triglycerides	High cholesterol and triglycerides
Pancreatitis	Pancreatitis
Obesity	Obesity
Gout	Gout
Fatty liver disease	Fatty liver disease
Fetal alcohol syndrome	Fetal insulin resistance
Addiction	Habituation, if not addiction

Making changes to your alcohol drinking

If you are diabetic, it is better to avoid alcohol for the first two weeks when you begin my Anti-diabetes Diet. After that, provided your blood sugar level is stable I recommend you drink no more than two units of alcohol a week until your blood sugar balance is under control, and thereafter certainly no more than one unit a day when you have your blood sugar under control, choosing drink with the lowest GL possible. This might be a small glass of a dry red or white wine or champagne, a neat spirit or a Bloody Mary. Once past the first two weeks, you can choose if you wish to spend your 5-GL drinks or desserts portion on alcohol; however, until your blood sugar is under control, I'd still advise not having more than a couple of units of alcohol a week.

Here are the options:

⅁ and units for alcohol and your daily maximum

	⅁	Units	Daily max
Beer/lager 300ml (10fl oz/½ pint)	10	1	150ml (5fl oz/¼ pint)
Red wine 115ml (3¾fl oz)	2	1	1 glass
White wine/champagne 115ml (3¾fl oz)	1	1	1 glass
Spirits 30ml (1fl oz)	0	1	1 shot
Spirits + 125ml (4fl oz) orange juice	6	1	1 small glass
Vodka + 125ml (4fl oz) orange juice	8	1	1 small glass
(Assumes that alcohol carbs = 100 GI)			

The truth about coffee

Every day Britons drink 70 million cups of coffee – roughly two for each adult. Many get caught in the sugar–nicotine–caffeine trap, thinking this combination is good for energy. But this combination feeds increasing fatigue, anxiety and weight gain. In my own research we surveyed over 55,000 people and found that the two foods that most predict fatigue and stress are caffeinated drinks and sugary foods – both addictive substances. Many people become hooked on caffeine and sugar to 'keep going', gaining weight and losing health as a result.

If you have quit sugar, caffeine or cigarettes and feel lousy, that means you've become chemically dependent on them. Don't worry, though, you'll start feeling much better within four days.

Case Study: Kathy

Kathy, who was pre-diabetic, was drinking up to 30 cups of coffee a day to keep herself going. She also smoked 10–15 cigarettes a day. She was gaining weight and losing sleep. She wasn't fully awake when she was awake, neither was she peacefully asleep when she was asleep. Within six weeks of starting my diet and supplements Kathy had given up all caffeine, she had stopped smoking and was feeling loads better. She went to bed at 11.00 pm, instead of 2.00 am, and was waking up feeling refreshed. Three months on she had lost a staggering 19kg (3 stone/42lb) without going hungry. Her energy was greater, her skin looked much clearer and she hadn't suffered from any colds. Kathy said:

'I feel so much better. My energy levels are improved, I sleep like a baby, I don't miss coffee at all and I'm not smoking.'

Coffee and diabetes

As far as diabetes is concerned you may be pleased to know that there is now enough evidence to show that coffee actually decreases risk. In fact, there have been 18 studies involving almost half a million people that do show overall that coffee, decaffeinated coffee and tea do slightly reduce the risk of diabetes.[114] There are various theories as to why this might be the case, because taking a lot of caffeine itself isn't good for your health. Both tea and coffee are high in antioxidants, however, which is a potential benefit.

Two recent studies have shown that coffee doesn't cause the release of insulin, and may even reduce insulin resistance.[115] Interestingly, this effect is true for both coffee and decaf coffee, suggesting that it isn't the caffeine that reduces insulin resistance. In fact, decaf may even help keep insulin-producing cells healthy.

One possible explanation for coffee's protective effect is that it might help weight loss. There is some evidence for this, but it's not conclusive.[116] However, there is no question that having a coffee does tend to take the edge off hunger. This is because coffee promotes the release of the hormone glucagon, which helps raise glucose by breaking down glycogen. Coffee stimulates adrenal hormones and these, in turn, give you a burst of energy, which is your body getting you ready to hunt (adrenalin is the hormone that got our ancestors ready for 'fight or flight', although today we rarely have to do either of those). But, the trick is not to go hunting for sugar but to use your extra energy for exercising.

A coffee and a croissant is a deadly combination

Before you hit the coffee, there's something you need to know. Rather than reducing insulin resistance, if you combine coffee with a carb snack such as a croissant or a muffin, it has the opposite effect. To explore the consequence of this much-loved combination, research-ers at Canada's University of Guelph gave volunteers a carbohydrate snack, such as a croissant, muffin or toast, together with either a decaf or coffee. Those having the coffee–carb combo had triple the increase in blood sugar levels and insulin, the hormone that controls blood sugar levels, was almost halved.[117] This combination of high blood glucose levels and poor insulin function is a recipe for weight gain and increased diabetes risk, because the excess blood glucose is dumped into storage as fat. This study shows that coffee with a carbohydrate snack is a dangerous combination, even though the decaf didn't make a difference to the glycemic load of the snack.

The other problems with coffee and caffeinated drinks

There are, however, a number of downsides of drinking too much coffee or caffeinated drinks in any case. It does raise your blood pres-sure, although, once again, decaf does not.[118]

Coffee, more than tea, is also known to increase your homocysteine level – one of the best predictors of heart attack and stroke (explained on page 41). Drinking two cups of coffee a day may raise your homo-cysteine level by two points in four hours.[119] A four-point increase can double your risk of a heart attack or stroke. Decaffeinated coffee has half the effect on your homocysteine, so it is not as bad. In addition to homocysteine, other chemicals found in the body that indicate inflam-mation is occurring, such as C-reactive protein (CRP), interleukin 6 (IL-6) and tumour necrosis factor (TNF), can often indicate a risk of cardiovascular disease, arthritis, cancer and other inflammatory condi-tions. In the case of coffee, it's all bad news. A study involving 3,000 people in Greece found that those who consumed more than 200ml (7fl oz/⅓ pint) (a large cup) of coffee had a 50 per cent higher level of IL-6, a 30 per cent higher level of CRP, and a 28 per cent higher level of TNF compared to non-coffee drinkers. However, it is possible that people who drink a large amount of coffee have other bad habits that might have influenced this result.

If you want to drink coffee

The research does suggest that if you are going to drink coffee it is best to do it on its own, without either a sweetener or a carb snack, then to wait at least 30 minutes before eating. Also, it is best to not overdo it, having perhaps one or two coffees a day at most. More than this is likely to make you more stressed and agitated which, as you'll see in the next chapter, is bad for your blood sugar control. Almost all the benefits of coffee are also reported for decaf, which eliminates a fair amount of the downsides. So, a decaf a day may actually help rather than hinder your health as far as diabetes and blood sugar control is concerned. I suspect the reported benefits of coffee in relation to diabetes may be due to its relatively high antioxidant content. Having less coffee and more antioxidants from vegetables, herbs and spices makes more sense.

Drink water and eat water

There is nothing better than water. It satisfies your thirst and has no GL. So, if you are thirsty, the best thing to do is to drink a glass of water. You can also actually make the water you drink help you lose weight and stabilise your blood sugar by combining it with food.

One of the triggers for controlling appetite is stomach extension. If your meal contains plenty of fibre-rich foods and is prepared in such a way that the fibre absorbs water and is bulkier, this makes the stomach more extended. If two people eat exactly the same food, one with a glass of water and the other with the glass of water added to their food – for example, by turning the meal into soup – the latter feels more full as the stomach expands more. So, puréed soups are good news for appetite control. The water taken by the water-drinker quickly passes through the stomach. This also means that soaking your oats, or having porridge, is likely to make you feel fuller than simply pouring milk on cereal.

Whatever you do, make sure you are drinking the equivalent of six glasses of water a day (which includes herb teas and the water you add to your food). Often thirst is confused with hunger so, before you eat, have a glass of water. In Chapter 3 earlier in this part I recommend having a large glass of water, with a teaspoon of super-fibre (gluco-mannan or PGX), up to 15 minutes before you eat a meal. This will bulk up your food with more water and lower the GL of what you are eating.

Summary

It's not just the foods you eat that will affect your blood sugar level and diabetes risk, you need to consider what you are drinking too:

- Avoid drinking soft drinks, sugar-free drinks and fruit juice completely.
- Drink water, herb teas and teas throughout the day to remain hydrated.
- Eat water-rich high-fibre foods (like soups, stews and porridge).
- Have the occasional cup of regular or decaffeinated coffee (maximum 1–2 cups a day) but, of course, never with a croissant or other similar carbohydrate snack.
- Exclude alcohol especially for the first two weeks of the diet, after which you may choose to drink a maximum of one small glass a day (once you have your blood sugar under control). A glass of champagne, a small glass of wine or a single Bloody Mary have the lowest GL score.

8

Break Free from Stress and Get Enough Sleep

Stress, sugar and stimulants each have powerful effects on your blood sugar control and it's easy to get hooked into a vicious cycle. Your health is also affected by a lack of sleep. When you are tired you may look to sugary foods and caffeinated drinks for a pick-me-up. When you are stressed you may drink alcohol to calm you down. This common pattern wreaks havoc on your blood sugar balance. People with diabetes, or with metabolic syndrome, need to be especially careful of leading a stressful lifestyle or having insufficient sleep because the stress greatly exacerbates their symptoms, as I'll be explaining in this chapter.

Why stress is so bad for you

When you feel stressed your body is preparing you for 'fight or flight'. Unlike the past, when our ancestors were hunting for food or encountering wild animals, and stress helped them to react extremely quickly, 'fight' to modern people means you feel irritable, aggressive and stressed out, while 'flight' means you feel anxious and want to run away, feeling trapped in your circumstances. Do you ever feel like this?

Many people live in a state of anxiety. They arrive at work stressed out from commuting, then they have to contend with a lot of stress at work. By the time they go home they are in a state of near collapse. Unfortunately, a life of non-stop 21st-century stress takes its toll on your body's chemistry.

The chemistry of stress

In such a state of stress your body is producing two hormones: short-acting adrenalin and long-acting cortisol. Together, these hormones do everything they can to get your blood sugar level up: telling the liver to break down stores of glycogen, then turning it into glucose and pumping it into your bloodstream. This blocks the ability of insulin to take glucose back into storage. As a result, your blood sugar level goes up to get it round the body faster. You are gearing up for a fight.

If you're stressed for weeks at a time, your cortisol levels stay high and your DHEA levels – a healthy adrenal hormone – go down. This is bad news. High cortisol levels – the hallmark of the overstressed – make you even more insulin-resistant and even more prone to putting on weight. Let me explain why.

Insulin puts glucose into storage, whereas adrenalin and cortisol rapidly raise the glucose supply to muscle and brain cells for the action of 'fight or flight' – partly by blocking insulin's fat-storing effect. That sounds like good news, at least in the short term. And it is. That's why high stress and lots of stimulants, such as coffee, can keep you thin for quite a few years. (That might even be why coffee consumption is associated with a lower diabetes risk, because there is less weight gain, but the role of coffee as a stimulant is one of the reasons I'm cautious about condoning caffeine.) But when the effect of insulin is continually blocked, the body simply produces more – and the more it produces, the more insulin-resistant you become. So, over the long term, stress can actually lead to insulin resistance and weight gain.

How stressed are you?

Take a look at the symptoms below. If they sound familiar to you, then you know what I'm talking about.

- Do you have difficulty in getting up in the morning?
- Are you tired all the time?
- Do you crave certain foods?
- Do you feel anger, irritability or aggressiveness?
- Do you have mood swings?

- Are you restless?

- Do you have an energy slump during the day?

- Do you have regular feelings of weakness?

- Do you feel apathy?

- Are you depressed?

- Do you feel cold all the time?

The above symptoms suggest adrenal stress overload. Most people report experiencing a high number of these kinds of symptoms. In our 100% Health Survey, 82 per cent of respondents said that they easily became impatient, 81 per cent said they had low energy, 68 per cent said they felt they had too much to do, and 66 per cent said they became anxious or tense easily.[120]

The dangers of too much stress and cortisol

With long-term stress the adrenal hormone cortisol stays high. Meanwhile, the circulating levels of three chemicals that help you to relax decline – these are GABA, which switches off adrenalin; serotonin, which keeps you happy; and DHEA, the revitalising hormone. Your mood gets worse, your sleep gets worse, you have more and more blood sugar spikes and troughs, and produce more and more insulin as insulin resistance sets in.

Whenever your blood sugar level crashes, the body produces yet more cortisol. It thinks you are being starved and so it goes into panic mode. Your brain is literally working overtime and demanding more sugar so that your blood sugar levels stay high.[121]

If you think about it, in a real state of emergency, certainly one where you are taking physical action, the last thing you want to do is eat. Your whole body gears up to liberate its stores of energy so that you can react quickly to the emergency. When you are really pumped up, stress acts as an appetite suppressant.

Continued stress messes this up. Many people find they compulsively eat – and they eat all the wrong things, such as sugary foods. This is a recipe for disaster, because now you have cortisol trying to raise your blood sugar level, and interfering with insulin, and you have your blood sugar level rising from what you've eaten, telling your body to make more insulin. You end up with high blood glucose, high insulin and insulin resistance. This is the fast track to diabetes. Among people with diabetes, the more perceived stress the higher the cortisol levels and the more they eat sugar.[122] By the way, people under stress also gravitate towards more salt. This is another sign of adrenal overload.

What does cortisol do?

Raised levels of cortisol are strongly linked to an increased risk of heart disease, also higher cholesterol and triglyceride levels, inflammation and poorer memory, as well as a shrinking of the brain's memory-sorting centre – so says research carried out at Stanford University in California by Robert Sapolsky, professor of neuroscience.[123] This is probably why either high stress or high sugar worsens memory and concentration. After only two weeks of the raised cortisol levels of stress, the dendrite 'arms' of brain cells, which reach out to connect with other brain cells, start to shrivel up. Fortunately, such damage isn't permanent. Stop the stress and the dendrites grow back.

Prolonged stress also shuts down digestion so you get digestive problems and your immune system is less able to respond to infections – and you also gain weight.

How a low-GL diet helps you to cope with life's difficulties

The amazing thing is that if you balance your blood sugar by following my low-GL diet and take the recommended supplements, it not only affects your weight but it also has wide-reaching benefits on your health, your mood and your ability to deal with the inevitable challenges of life. When you're stressed, even molehills seem like mountains. When your energy levels are good and your mind is clear, life immediately smoothes out and calms down. People on my low-GL diet often report big improvements in mood, concentration and memory. In an eight-week trial we ran on volunteers on the Holford Diet, almost all (94 per cent) reported greater energy, two-thirds had greater concentration, memory or alertness, and half reported fewer feelings of depression and had more stable moods.[124]

The way back from stress

The only way out of the prison of stress, sugar and stimulants is:

1 To reduce or avoid all forms of concentrated sweetness, tea, coffee, alcohol and cigarettes, and start eating foods that help to keep your blood sugar level stable. By changing to the right foods, backed up with specific nutritional supplements, most people feel an amazing improvement in energy within days. It is especially important not to eat sweet foods when you feel stressed.

2 Learn how to maintain a state of balanced 'calm'. (More on this in a minute.)

3 Take exercise, which is a biochemical, physiological and psychological antidote to stress, as I'll explain in the next chapter.

Of course, it's easy to say 'reduce your stress level' but not so easy to do it – unless you know how. You might say your stresses are beyond your control – the mortgage, debts, family problems, and so on. Yet, some people seem to stay pretty calm most of the time, even when the pressure is on. How do they do this?

Often we hear advice to meditate, practise yoga, breathe deeply, and so on, but when you are tired and stressed out these things are not easy to do. Before going into practical suggestions and introducing you to techniques that work, it's worth understanding the chemistry and physiology of the different states of mind we move between.

The benefits of positivity

Doc Childre and Rollin McCraty, from the HeartMath Institute in California, have spent the last decade studying exactly what happens in the different emotional states we move between.[125] We often associate the opposite of stress as relaxation – being in a calm, quiet state. But what Childre and McCraty discovered is that countering the unhealthy effects of stress is not just about calming down but about activating a positive emotional state. They looked at the emotions that deplete us and activate the stress hormone cortisol; and then they studied the emotions that revitalise us, by stimulating DHEA, the replenishing hormone that's associated with enhanced well-being and slower rates of ageing.

If you look at the diagram below, you'll see a range of emotions plotted in four quadrants: on the right, emotions that contribute to physiological renewal, on the left those that cause depletion. Then, in the upper quadrants, those that are associated with high energy, while those in the lower are associated with lower energy. Ideally, we'd all like to spend more time experiencing the emotions on the right – happiness, enthusiasm, compassion, serenity, and so on; and less time on the left feeling frustrated, angry, fearful, depressed or bored.

Plotting your emotional state

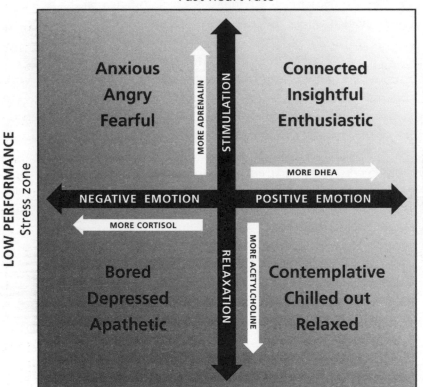

Take a few minutes to study this diagram and think about which quadrants you spend most of your time in.

Just as we take in food and transform it into energy, we transform positive emotions into buoyancy and resilience, so we become better able to cope with the difficult experiences we inevitably encounter.

Positive emotions also put us into a state of what Childre and McCraty term as 'coherence', which relates to a pattern of synchronised activity across many body systems – your heart rate, breathing, blood pressure and brainwaves.[126] In this state, cortisol levels fall and DHEA levels rise.[127] We could call it 'internal global cooling' because it actually helps to undo the 'internal global warming' that relates to metabolic syndrome, insulin resistance and, ultimately, diabetes and heart disease.

Reduce your stress by becoming 'coherent'

HeartMath teaches a simple technique that can be practised daily to help you actively reduce the stress in your life. The premise of HeartMath is different from many other approaches for relieving stress, which typically focus on calming down after the stressful event has occurred; for example, by going for a massage or having a glass of wine after a difficult day at work. With HeartMath, you learn a simple breathing technique that can help you to 'reset' your physiological reaction to stress as the event occurs. Just a couple of HeartMath breaths can help you stop the cascade that triggers the release of cortisol – and you stay coherent (that is, calm and in balance). Research has found that exercise, when practised regularly, can help you to feel better emotionally (spending more time on the right than the left of the diagram opposite), and improve your intuition, creativity and cognitive performance.[128]

Quick coherence technique

1 Heart focus Focus your attention on your heart area – the space behind your breastbone in the centre of your chest between your nipples (your heart is more in the centre than on the left).

2 Heart breathing Now imagine your breath flowing in and out of your heart area. This helps your respiration and heart rhythm to synchronise. So, focus in this area and aim to breathe evenly; for example, inhale for five or six seconds and exhale for five or six seconds (choose a timescale that feels comfortable and flows easily).

3 Heart feeling As you breathe in and out of your heart area, recall a positive emotion and try to re-experience it. This could be remembering a time spent with someone you love, walking in your favourite spot, stroking a pet, picturing a tree you admire or even just feeling appreciation that you ate today or have shoes on your feet. If your mind wanders, just bring it gently back to the positive experience.

These three steps, when practised daily for five minutes can help you to de-stress, feel calmer and more content. Once you've got the hang of the exercise, you can then use it any time you encounter a stressful event – for example, as you start to feel tense in heavy traffic, overloaded at work or sense that you are about to face a difficult emotional situation. Just a few HeartMath breaths can help you to stay calm and coherent instead of becoming stressed.

HeartMath and diabetes

Research into using HeartMath with people who have diabetes is particularly impressive. A small study[129] at the HeartMath headquarters in Boulder Creek, California involved teaching a group of 22 participants with both type-1 and type-2 diabetes the HearthMath techniques and monitoring their progress. Six months after the workshop, participants reported significant reductions in anxiety, negative emotions, fatigue and sleeplessness, along with increased feelings of vitality and improved quality of life. Changes in glycosylated haemoglobin (HbA1c) were also observed, with increased HeartMath practice associated with a reduction in HbA1c levels.

Measuring your coherence

Doing the HeartMath exercise will help you to develop greater 'coherence'. But how will you know? Childre and McCraty discovered that you could monitor your state of coherence accurately by measuring, not your heart rate (the number of beats) but the pattern of activity that exists between heart beats. This is called your heart rate variability or HRV. They developed a simple device, called an Em-Wave monitor, with an earphone that clips onto your ear lobe to pick up your HRV to track whether or not you are in this 'coherent' state in which cortisol levels rapidly decline. It is an objective measure of what works and, even the very act of knowing, through bio-feedback, helps you calm down. With each heartbeat the device flashes a colour, from red to green, and emits a tone that lets you know when you've gone into a relaxed state. By having that feedback it becomes easier to take a deep breath, or maybe have a more uplifting thought, that takes you out of the high stress/cortisol zone.

There's also an excellent book, *Transforming Stress*, which gives very effective exercises for bringing you into a coherent, de-stressed state. In the UK you can attend workshops called Transforming Stress into Resilience to really hardwire these simple stress-busting techniques (see Resources).

The importance of sleep

One of the consequences of too much stress is that you end up having sleeping problems. This is incredibly common among people with diabetes. Many people with diabetes have sleep apnoea,[130] a condition where you get an obstruction in the throat so that you stop breathing, which of course makes you wake up. Having sleep apnoea actually increases your chances of developing diabetes, and it is also linked to metabolic syndrome, insulin resistance and losing blood sugar control.[131] It creates a temporary lack of oxygen, generating oxidative stress and inflammation.[132] Lack of sleep pushes your whole system towards metabolic syndrome. One contributor is excess fat constricting the throat, so losing weight makes a big difference.

Case Study: Mary

Mary suffered from sleep apnoea and weight gain, and had many of the hallmarks of metabolic syndrome. After following my low-GL diet, she said:

'I've lost 3 stone [19kg (42lb)], I joined your low-GL Zest4Life programme eight months ago. My sleep was bad as I suffered from sleep apnoea and would wake up tired with a headache. My blood pressure was very high, my skin was flaky and I had no energy. Since I've lost the weight I sleep like a baby, my blood pressure is normal and my skin is very clear – I've loads of energy and I am very happy.'

Getting enough sleep is at least as important as eating fruit and vegetables. People who don't have enough are twice as likely to become addicted to something, twice as likely to feel anxious and four times more likely to feel depressed.[133] Anxiety caused because you can't sleep adds to the problem. Anxiety and depression increase sugar cravings, eating sweet foods to relieve these cravings upsets blood sugar balance and promotes metabolic syndrome, which we already know increases your diabetes risk.

Are you in sleep debt?

You need sleep, and good-quality sleep at that, and if you don't get enough you are in sleep debt. Sleep debt is simply the amount of sleep you require minus the amount of sleep you are getting. If you require eight hours of sleep, for example, and you're getting only five, your sleep debt is three hours.

Signs of sleep debt

The easiest way to know if you are getting enough sleep is to notice simply whether you become sleepy during the day – while driving, watching TV, or at meetings or lectures. If so, you probably have a substantial sleep debt or deprivation.

Other signs of sleep debt are frequent blinking, difficulty focusing the eyes, heavy eyelids, daytime drowsiness, impatience, irritability or being quick to anger, also having difficulty listening to what is said or understanding directions, difficulty remembering or retaining information, making frequent errors or mistakes, or if you suffer from depression or being in a bad or negative mood.

To help identify if you are suffering from excessive daytime sleepiness and poor quality of sleep complete the questionnaire below.

Questionnaire: check for excessive daytime sleepiness (the Epworth Sleepiness Scale)

Rate the chance that you would doze off or fall asleep during the following daytime situations from 0 to 3, as below:

0   means you would never doze off or fall asleep in a given situation.

1   means there is a slight chance that you would doze off or
    fall asleep.

2   means there is a moderate chance that you would doze off
    or fall asleep.

3   means there is a high chance that you would doze off or
    fall asleep.

Situation

1   Sitting and reading.

☐

2   Sitting inactive in a public place (such as a theatre, lecture
    or meeting).

☐

3   Watching TV.

☐

4   As a passenger in a car for an hour or longer without a break.

☐

5   Lying down to rest in the afternoon.

☐

6   Sitting and talking to someone.

☐

7   In a car, while stopped in traffic.

☐

Total score:

☐

Score

10 or more

You most likely suffer from excessive daytime sleepiness, a strong indication that you are sleep deprived and need to improve the quality and/or duration of your sleep. People who continue to suffer from poor sleep are more prone to depression, anxiety and drug cravings.

Causes of sleep debt and insomnia

Most researchers now agree that we need around seven to nine hours of largely uninterrupted sleep each night, ideally between 11.00 pm and 7.00 am. The use of mood-altering substances, such as alcohol and caffeine, affects your sleep, as does quitting the use of those substances, and there are other causes that contribute to sleep debt and affect your recovery. Apart from sleep apnoea, there are many disorders and conditions that deprive us of sleep, such as insomnia, restless-leg syndrome and bruxism (grinding the teeth while asleep).

The most common of some 84 different sleep disorders, insomnia is defined as:

- Difficulty falling asleep (on average taking more than 30 minutes).

- Waking up frequently during the night and having difficulty getting back to sleep.

- Waking up too early in the morning and being unable to return to sleep.

- Waking up tired or exhausted – which can persist throughout the day, making you feel irritable, anxious or depressed.

Long-term insomnia may be due to 'hyper-arousal'. Insomniacs often have a faster heart rate and higher levels of the stress hormone cortisol, which then promotes insulin resistance as we have seen. Stimulant drugs, including caffeine, can cause this state of hyper-arousal and make it difficult to go to sleep and stay asleep. In response, many people take substances that induce sleep, creating a cycle of taking stimulants to wake up and then relaxants to go to sleep. This creates more cortisol, which promotes insulin resistance.

Why sleeping pills are not the cure for sleep problems

If you can't sleep and you go to your doctor, the chances are you will be prescribed sleeping pills, also known as tranquillisers, sedatives or hypnotics. Despite having a long charge sheet of side effects,[134] hypnotic drugs still regularly feature in the top 20 most-prescribed drugs both in the UK and in the US. Not only that, but they aren't very useful, according to a report in the *British Medical Journal*[135] which concluded that there is plenty of evidence that they cause 'major harm' and that there was 'little evidence of clinically meaningful benefit'.

In fact, many of these drugs may actually suppress REM sleep (when dreaming occurs), prevent deep sleep, reduce available neurotransmitters and block the release of growth hormone, thereby aggravating low moods. You can see now why deprivation of deep sleep, plus fatigue and sleep medication often develop into a self-perpetuating cycle. A lack of restful sleep, REM and deep sleep prevents rejuvenation and the release of stress. Stress and fatigue increase the desire for sugar, alcohol, stimulants and relaxants, which lead to the inability to get restful sleep.

Just how marginally effective sleep medication is was vividly illustrated by a study by the American National Institutes of Health, which found that the newer drugs like Ambien (zolpidem) made volunteers fall asleep only 12.8 minutes faster than when they had taken a fake pill, and then to sleep for just 11 minutes longer.[136]

Despite this, sales of sleeping pills run at 4.5 billion dollars' worth in the US, because patients are very keen on them and believe they work much better than they actually do. This could be because of one of the side effects – according to the same report, the pills interfere with memory formation, so you simply forget all that tossing and turning. Sleeping pills are also very easy to become addicted to in the sense that when you try to quit them you feel lousy.

Using nutrition and supplements to promote sleep

What can you do to get a good night's sleep? If you're having sleep problems, you'll almost certainly have raised levels of the stress hormone cortisol, which, along with keeping you aroused at night, also has the effect of lowering production of the growth hormone needed for insulin to work properly. To bring cortisol down you need to introduce fish and fish oils along with vegetables into your daily diet and to follow a low-GL diet.

The main sleep hormone is melatonin (see page 160) which your body manufactures from serotonin. Although chronically raising levels of serotonin with medications can cause problems, if you provide the natural chemicals that make serotonin naturally in the body these can raise melatonin without creating excessive levels of serotonin. These raw materials include the amino acid tryptophan (found in milk, as well as chicken, turkey, seeds, nuts and cheese) and the amino acid 5-HTP, which you can take as a 100mg supplement one hour before bed.

Magnesium and B vitamins are also involved in good sleep:

Magnesium is especially calming and aids muscle relaxation. Being highly stressed or eating a lot of sugar lowers your magnesium levels.

Magnesium is found in seeds, nuts, green vegetables and seafood. You could also supplement 400mg of magnesium before bed.

B vitamins are also involved in handling stress, but, generally, they are best taken earlier in the day, as they can be energising and therefore might keep you awake.

What about taking melatonin supplements?

Produced by the pineal gland, located in the middle of the brain, melatonin regulates the sleep–wake cycle, which is why it seems the ideal sleep aid. Some sleep clinicians recommend 0.5–3mg melatonin under your tongue two hours before bed, but the results from trials have been mixed. A recent study, however, found that melatonin significantly improved the quality of sleep with alert feelings in the morning and without any side effects and no problems when it was stopped.[137]

CAUTION Melatonin's side effects include nausea, dizziness and loss of libido, and its long-term safety has not been determined. Headache and transient depression have been reported. In people who are depressed, melatonin may worsen symptoms. Melatonin is available by prescription only in the UK. In the US and South Africa you can buy it in health-food stores and pharmacies.

Using herbs

Many herbs are said to have sleep-inducing properties. Best known is valerian; others include chamomile, passionflower, lavender, hops and lemon balm. One study of 600mg of valerian, standardised, taken 30 minutes before bedtime for 28 days, found it to be as effective as oxazepam, a drug normally used to treat anxiety. Another found that the combination of valerian and lemon balm was as effective as the hypnotic Halcion, but it produced no drowsiness the next day. For more detailed advice contact the National Institute of Medical Herbalists (see Resources).

Other ways to improve your sleep

The techniques I've discussed for reducing stress also help promote a good night's sleep. Some essentially commonsense advice, rather quaintly known as 'sleep hygiene', forms part of most sleep regimes. The idea is to create regular sleep-promoting habits on the grounds that the less successful you are at getting to sleep the more you are going to worry about it:

- Keep the bedroom quiet and dark.

- Wear comfortable clothing to bed.

- Do not have a large meal before bedtime.

- Keep artificial light to a minimum in the bedroom. (Being exposed to bright light can turn off the production of melatonin, which peaks at around 1.00 am. Have a light with a low-wattage bulb in the bedroom or hallway in case you need to get up in the night.)

- Exercise regularly, but not after 7.00 pm.

- Avoid coffee from the afternoon onwards and alcohol in the evening.

Music to sleep to

New York psychiatrist Dr Galina Mindlin uses 'brain music' – rhythmic patterns of sounds derived from recordings of patients' own brainwaves – to help them overcome insomnia, anxiety and depression. The recordings sound something like classical piano music and appear to have a calming effect similar to yoga or meditation. A double-blind study by Toronto University found that 80 per cent of those getting brain music reported benefits. I have had excellent results reported by people with insomnia using Dr John Levine's CDs, *Silence of Peace* and *Orange Grove Siesta* (see Resources), played quietly as you go to sleep.

Case Study: Sue

Sue would sleep for about three hours, waking every 45 minutes or so. Here's what she says:

'The improvement happened from night one. Now, just one week later, I am sleeping for six to seven hours. I haven't heard the end of the CD yet.'

Summary

Stress If you judge that stress is playing a major part in your life and worsening health, I recommend that you:

- Follow my low-GL diet strictly.
- Avoid regular tea and coffee, probably giving all caffeine a break for one month.
- Quit smoking.
- Avoid all alcohol for two weeks and reduce your overall intake to three small glasses (no more than 2 units) a week.
- Take daily supplements (explained in Part 3, Chapter 4).
- Exercise daily (more on this in the next chapter).
- Make some positive life changes, to avoid continuously high stress levels.
- Practise the HeartMath exercise daily to become more 'coherent', perhaps monitoring your progress with an Em-Wave monitor.

Sleep There are practical steps you can take to improve your quality of sleep. Good sleep reduces cortisol levels, which in turn improves your insulin sensitivity and blood sugar control.

- Find a way to break free from living in a state of stress.
- Practise 'sleep hygiene'.
- Exercise regularly but not in the evening before sleep.
- Listen to alpha-wave-inducing music while in bed, and practise relaxation techniques.
- Eat more green leafy vegetables, nuts and seeds to ensure you're getting enough magnesium, and consider supplementing 300mg of magnesium in the evening, with or without calcium (500mg).
- Consider taking valerian, hops, passionflower, or a 'sleep formula' combining several of them, ideally including 5-HTP and magnesium. Choose a standardised extract or tincture and follow the dosage instructions.
- Take 100mg of 5-HTP, or 1–3mg of melatonin, an hour before bed.
- Eat oily fish three times a week and eat nuts and seeds daily.
- Avoid sugar and caffeine, and minimise your intake of alcohol. Don't combine alcohol with sleeping pills or anti-anxiety medication.

9

Take Regular Exercise

Being overweight is strongly associated with type-2 diabetes and many other illnesses, including heart disease and stroke. It also makes you feel uncomfortable and, in most cases, unhappy. But shifting the pounds can be extremely difficult for most people who can feel daunted by the dietary or exercise advice they have been given by health professionals. If you've been told you have to exercise to burn calories you've probably done the maths and soon realised it doesn't quite add up. Twenty minutes of jogging equals one chocolate chip cookie. How motivating is that?

There is so much more going on when you exercise than the calorie equation, however. Even if you are not significantly overweight, exercise is the final puzzle piece in the process of reversing diabetes, insulin resistance and losing weight. Let's take a look at why, and how, it works.

Why exercise?

If you haven't led a very active life, or you did once but have gradually become more sedentary, it's not surprising. Life in the West conspires against it. Cars, remote controls, food processors, home-delivered meals, 'home-entertainment centres', escalators, lifts – the list goes on. Every year, there are more gadgets and mod cons that do away with the need to expend energy. Ultimately, all roads lead straight to the sofa and, if you give in, couch-potato syndrome awaits.

Once that happens, it's all too easy to pile on the pounds. There is no doubt that part of the reason for the massive increase in the number of overweight people is that we are becoming less active.[138] Not only does less activity mean fewer calories burned but it also interferes with the body's appetite mechanisms, rate of metabolism and ability to keep blood glucose levels stable. In other words, some exercise is essential for the body's chemistry to stay 'in tune'.

According to calorie theory, exercise is a poor method of losing weight. After all, running a mile burns up only 300 calories. That's equivalent to two slices of toast or a piece of apple pie. But this argument misses six key points:

1 The effects of exercise are cumulative. OK, so running a mile a day burns up only 300 calories, but if you do that three days a week for a year, that's 22,000 calories, equivalent to a weight loss of 5kg (11lb)! Also, the number of calories you burn up depends on how fat or fit you are to start with. The fatter and less fit you are, the more benefit you'll derive from small bouts of exercise, especially exercise that increases your muscle mass, and hence the number of calories you burn.

2 Moderate exercise decreases your appetite. A degree of physical activity is necessary for appetite mechanisms to work properly. Those who do not exercise have exaggerated appetites and hence the pounds gradually creep on. Often you'll find that, after a burst of activity, you don't actually feel like eating.

3 Exercise boosts your metabolic rate. According to Professor William McArdle,[139] exercise physiologist at City University, New York, 'Most people can generate metabolic rates that are eight to 10 times above their resting value during sustained cycling, running or swimming. Complementing this increased metabolic rate is the observation that vigorous exercise will raise metabolic rate for up to 15 hours after exercise.' Your metabolic rate is also to do with how quickly the liver breaks down glycogen or fat for fuel. Exercise speeds this process up. Also, if you have eaten more carbs than you need, and the excess is dumped in the liver, exercising helps you to burn this off before you put it into storage as fat. That's why it is good to go for a stroll after a meal. It helps to stabilise your blood sugar and insulin level and stop you from making fat.

4 Exercise improves insulin sensitivity. According to Vanessa Hebditch of the British Diabetic Association, 'Being overweight reduces insulin sensitivity so the risk of developing diabetes is higher. However, there is proof that exercise increases insulin sensitivity, thereby reducing risk.' A 14-year study of nearly 6,000 men found that increased physical activity was linked to a reduction in the risk of diabetes, regardless of the level of obesity.[140] It also lowers your glycosylated haemoglobin.

When you exercise, your muscles need glucose, so exercise stimulates insulin receptors to become more sensitive, reversing insulin resistance. This means that regular exercise helps your blood sugar to become more balanced because insulin starts to work properly.

5 Exercise promotes the production of growth hormone, and also testosterone, both of which help to reduce metabolic syndrome and diabetes risk. As these hormones go up, the stress hormone cortisol, which is a major promoter of insulin resistance, goes down. (See page 112 for more on the link between testosterone deficiency and diabetes.)

6 Exercise is a great way to reduce stress. As we learnt in the last chapter, stress and weight gain go hand in hand. A great way to bring your state of mind out of stress and into coherence is to exercise.

Getting to grips with exercise as the years go by

Exercise is especially important in middle age because we are less likely to be able to maintain an even blood sugar level as we age.[141] A study of 87,000 women aged between 34 and 59 showed that those taking vigorous exercise at least once a week reduced their risk of diabetes by a third, compared with those who didn't work out.[142] Unsurprisingly, our sensitivity to insulin decreases with age, along with our control of blood sugar. But physical activity in middle and old age improves insulin sensitivity, and therefore helps to stabilise blood sugar levels and weight.[143] Athletes have vastly improved blood sugar control, enhanced insulin sensitivity and faster metabolic rates.[144]

And there's more. High-intensity exercises such as aerobics, reduces insulin levels and raises glucagon levels. This means that you improve your production of good prostaglandins (which switch off inflammation), boost your circulation (and thus the supply of oxygen and nutrients to your body's cells) and you increase your ability to burn fat. Resistance exercise, such as using weights, doesn't burn fat in the same way, but it helps you to build more muscle which, in turn, burns more fat.

To illustrate this, an Italian study, published in the *Archives of Internal Medicine*, had a group of 606 people with diabetes either join a twice-weekly aerobics group, as well as receiving advice on exercising, or be part of a control group who just received counselling. At the end of a year only those in the exercise group had lowered glycosylated haemoglobin, insulin resistance, blood pressure, cholesterol, waist circumference and BMI.[145] Another similar study, this time in Korea, reported similar benefits from a combination of diet, exercise and counselling.[146]

In short, exercise offers a huge array of benefits. If you haven't really got into it before, it opens up an undiscovered world of vitality, health and sheer enjoyment. As your energy returns on my diet you'll soon find you really do gain health and vitality through regular exercise.

The dynamic duo – diet and exercise

Combining diet and exercise is the best way to lose weight. Weight lost through restrictive dieting is often half fat and half lean tissue, such as muscle. Since muscle burns up more energy (calories) than fat, the less muscle you have, the slower your metabolism will be. Combining my low-GL diet with a good exercise programme ensures you lose fat, not lean muscle, and that you become more sensitive to insulin.

The winning combination was put to the test in a study at Case Western Reserve University, Cleveland, Ohio. The researchers put 22 pre-diabetic volunteers on an exercise training programme of one hour's exercise a day, five days a week. Half the volunteers ate a low-GL diet and the other half ate a high-GL diet of similar calories. Both groups lost an equivalent amount of weight, but only the low-GL diet group had a significant improvement in insulin sensitivity, while the high-GL diet group developed more insulin resistance.[147]

The best kind of exercises to help to burn fat efficiently arc brisk walking, jogging, cycling, swimming, aerobic dance, stepping, cross-country skiing, circuit training or any aerobic exercise that is steady, continuous and of enough intensity to get you in your heart rate zone (see page 280).

Such exercises also tone the body, reduce the risk of osteoporosis, increase muscle tissue and reduce one's body fat percentage (high ratios of body fat to lean tissue have been linked to heart disease, diabetes and some cancers). They will strengthen your heart and lungs, reduce your risk of heart disease, help control stress and improve your circulation.

Building muscle burns fat

You also need to do some exercise that helps to build more muscle. This is called 'resistance training', so named because muscle can only be built when you are resisting some force, such as lifting a weight. Having the correct balance of hormones, especially insulin (the fat-storage hormone) helps the body to use protein and, if you're exercising, to turn the protein you eat into muscle. And muscle, in its turn, burns off fat and excess sugar. Thus, your exercise regime works brilliantly with my low-GL diet, turning you into a lean and healthy fatburner.

You may need to get some advice from a fitness instructor to create your own perfect resistance-training programme – your local gym or leisure centre will probably offer an induction course at a reasonable cost. On my website (see Resources) you'll find some simple resistance exercises that you can do at home. Zest4Life groups – run by my Zest4Life team of nutritional therapists – also offer fitness training with the Zest4Fitness programme, designed by former gladiator Kate Stapleton and Olympic athlete Daley Thompson (see Resources). Rather than using gyms they get you outdoors and show you how to use your natural environment to create the perfect mix of both aerobic and resistance training.

A word of warning for the scale-watchers, though: when you start a committed exercise programme, and lose fat and gain lean muscle, you will lose inches faster than pounds. In the first month you'll look trimmer and feel fitter but may lose less weight than you wished. This is because muscle is denser and, hence, heavier than fat. In other words, 450g (1lb) of muscle takes up less space than 450g (1lb) of fat.

Remember, the enemy is not so much your weight, but having too high a body-fat percentage. So, if you have access to a body-fat monitor check this rather than just jumping on the scales to check your weight. The more lean muscle you gain, the more ability you'll have to burn fat – and that's what counts in the long run.

Aerobic and resistance exercise gets results

The combination of these two types of exercise has the best results for diabetes. A recent study published in the *Journal of the American Medical Association*, for example, compared the effects of not exercising versus aerobics exercise alone, resistance exercise alone, or a combination of the two.[148] All three lowered glycosylated haemo-globin, but only the combination of aerobic plus resistance training significantly lowered glycosylated haemoglobin compared to the non-exercising group. These volunteers also halved their need for additional medication.

How much exercise should you aim for?

Exercise shouldn't mean a fanatical struggle for some mythical level of fitness. The important thing is merely to stay within the 'training heart rate zone' for your age. Appendix 2 shows you how to work this out.

NOTE Before you start, inform your doctor that you are going to begin an exercise regime.

Summary

- Inactivity leads to increasing weight, which reduces insulin sensitivity and increases your likelihood of having diabetes.
- Regular exercise is beneficial for people with diabetes because it improves insulin sensitivity.
- In combination with a low-GL diet, exercise helps you to lose weight and keep trim.
- For maximum effect you need to do two kinds of exercise: aerobic exercise that gets you puffing and builds your stamina and a strong heart; and resistance training, which builds more muscle – and muscle burns off fat and sugar.
- What to do and how to do this is explained in Part 3, Chapter 5.

10

Treat Diabetes by Re-setting Your Genes

What we eat and the lifestyle choices that we make may have an even more complex affect on the way our bodies work than we might have imagined. If you have been told that type-2 diabetes runs in your family and that you are at a higher risk, you may feel that it is almost inevitable that you will succumb to it and that it will be difficult to treat by lifestyle and diet factors alone, although hopefully you feel more optimistic after having read the book so far. New research is showing that eating a low-GL diet and reducing the quantity of food you eat, to keep overall calories quite low, combined with taking exercise and particular nutrients, may actually help your body to switch off the genes that make you ill, thereby prolonging a healthy life.

This chapter explores these new discoveries and, although my diet stands alone, you may want to take it further and try the suggestions I make for reducing your calorie intake and 'alternate day' dieting. This research is still in its early days, but these new findings show you the significance of what you eat, how much and when you eat, for determining your immediate health, future risk of disease and healthy lifespan.

Understanding how your body works

As you have seen, the one big difference between the regular medical approach to type-2 diabetes and treating it with nutrition is that the non-drug approach involves learning a lot more about what is going wrong in your body and what you can do to change it. Few GPs have the time or the knowledge to discuss the difference between high- and low-GL carbohydrates, the links between insulin and inflammation, how stress affects blood sugar or why supplements such as chromium or cinnamon can have an effect on insulin resistance.

That's why the nutritional route gives you many more options and, because you know how they work, you are more likely to follow them. Even so, the nutritional details I've covered so far don't give the whole picture. I've talked about the hormones, insulin and cortisol, and how they affect organs like the liver and where fat and muscle cells fit into the picture, but what's missing so far is any account of what is going on at the next level down – with your genes.

This is where cutting-edge research could soon be throwing up even more precise options for handling your diabetes. So far, details have remained rather secret, but the remarkable finding is that many of the everyday things you can do to help yourself – such as changing your diet and exercising – don't just affect your organs and cells but they can also directly affect your genes, which provide the programming for how your cells are going to behave.

If drugs and all the potential profit that comes with them aren't behind new discoveries, the chances are that neither you nor your doctor will have heard much about them. Reports of new research linking a disease such as diabetes with certain genes usually end by saying that this could lead to new drug treatments. What they rarely say is that diet, exercise and certain supplements can also turn diabetes-promoting genes on and off.

A new way of looking at genes

What's involved here is a radical shift in the way we think about genes (known as epigenetics). The conventional idea is that genes are unchanging nuggets of information passed on at conception that determine your height, weight, risk of disease, and so on. So often, people believe that their diabetes runs in their family or that if you are from South Asian, African, Hispanic or Native American stock, you've got a raised risk and there's not much you can do about it.

Huge resources have been devoted to detecting such genes. A good example of this way of thinking appeared in a newspaper story in 2010 that announced: 'Doctors are closer to building a DNA profile of people who are at risk from diabetes after pinpointing another set of genes associated with the disease.'[149] This study, which discovered 12 new gene variations and involved nearly 100,000 people, was carried out at top research centres such as Oxford University and the Wellcome Trust's Sanger Institute in the UK. It identified 38 different genes linked with diabetes.

But the report admitted it would have zero impact on treatment. All 38 genes only account for an estimated 10 per cent of diabetes cases, and even if you had all of them you still wouldn't definitely develop the disease. The researchers said that the finding was: 'unlikely to have any immediate implication for screening or prevention of type-2 diabetes'.

Optimum living can change your genes for the better

The new epigenetics view of genetics sees the link between a disorder like diabetes and your genes in quite a different way. Rather than being something fixed and unchanging that you are born with, the latest research shows that genes are more like default computer settings. You get a whole array of settings at conception, but once you are up and running, all kinds of things in the environment – food, nutrients, stress and chemicals – can affect whether certain genes are turned on or off on a day-by-day basis. It looks increasingly as if many of the non-drug diabetes treatments, such as taking fish oils or following a low-GL diet, work by increasing or reducing the activity of a variety of genes and not necessarily the ones that 'cause' diabetes.

The gene for super-health

One of the clearest examples of this comes from the work of top genetic researcher Professor Cynthia Kenyon, from the University of California, who was originally trying to solve a problem that had no obvious connection with diabetes. She had become interested in a discovery made way back in the 1930s that animals fed a severely restricted calorie diet – around the equivalent of 1,200–1,500 calories a day for a human – plus a good micronutrient intake, would live about 30 per cent longer than usual and, more importantly, be very healthy too. They had clearer arteries and lower blood pressure; they were glossy, healthy specimens without a hint of diabetes or heart disease.

Professor Kenyon reasoned that the drastic drop in calories the diet entails must be changing gene activity in a way that triggers a whole range of healthy changes to the animal's metabolism. In her research, she used a type of tiny worm known as *Caenorhabditis elegans*, which is commonly used in genetic experiments because it normally only lives for about three weeks, and discovered that the key to getting all the health benefits of calorie restriction was in turning down the activity of a gene involved in controlling insulin.

'First the diet damped down the actions of a gene that is normally active in the worms all the time,' says Kenyon. 'We jokingly call it the Grim Reaper, because when it's on their lifespan is fairly short.'

Although there is no direct research on humans, Kenyon explains that a similar effect is seen in adults – turning down the Reaper turns on another gene that behaves like a kind of super-health genetic highway. 'It sends out instructs to a whole range of repair and renovation genes,' explains Kenyon.

'Your supply of natural antioxidants goes up, damping down damaging free radicals, there's a boost to compounds that make sure the skin and muscle building proteins are working properly, the immune system becomes more active to fight infection and genes that are active in cancer get turned off.' The gene's proper name is DAF 16 but it was quickly nicknamed 'Sweet Sixteen' because it turned the worms into teenagers. Subsequent research has found human versions of The Grim Reaper and Sweet Sixteen.

Low-calorie diets control insulin genes

All this research doesn't just give us some useful clues about how we might live longer, it also suggests a whole new genetically based reason why a low-GL diet is beneficial for people with diabetes. Professor Kenyon has been so impressed by the results of her own research that she now follows a pretty strict low-GL diet. 'Carbohydrates and especially refined ones like sugar make you produce lots of extra insulin so I now keep my intake really low.' She's cut right back on all starch such as potatoes, noodles, rice, bread and pasta. 'Instead I have salads, but no sweet dressing, lots of olive oil and nuts, tons of green vegetables along with cheese, chicken and eggs.'

If you eat in a way to minimise insulin levels, and reverse insulin resistance, it seems that your body can potentially turn off or turn on the actions of many genes resulting in all kinds of health benefits, such as a reduced risk of diabetes and cancer.

What convinced Professor Kenyon was seeing what happened to some of her worms that had been genetically modified to live far longer than normal when just a tiny amount of sugary glucose was added to their normal diet of bacteria. Many of their lifespan and health gains were wiped out. 'The effect was remarkable,' she says. 'The refined carbohydrate pushed up their insulin production and that blocked other genes that normally contribute to improved life span. Their own natural production of glucose dropped.'

Eating a low-GL diet is not the only way to activate the super-health highway that's linked with Sweet Sixteen. Calorie restriction, the technique for extending lifespan that first sparked Kenyon's interest, also turns it on. Unfortunately, though, it is almost impossible for humans to follow unless, like rats and mice, you are in captivity. Moreover, this type of diet is certainly not advised (restriction causes constant hunger pangs, reduced libido and a permanent feeling of cold).

The advantages of feast and famine

Another idea is that it is possible to get all of the benefits of calorie restriction with much less of the pain without having to concentrate on calorie counting. For something so revolutionary, it is remarkably simple. You can just eat less every other day. You would eat normally one day and then, to begin with, the next day you would have very little – perhaps four or five hundred calories.

The Alternate Day Diet was discovered back in 2003 by Dr Mark Mattson, a neuroscientist at the National Institute on Aging, Bethesda. Like Kenyon, he was interested in the dramatic health benefits of calorie restriction but, wondering if it could be made more palatable, he experimented with giving rats nothing one day and allowing them to eat as much as they liked the next. He found that they still got nearly all of the health benefits. After running some small trials he found that it also worked for humans, and this encouraged other scientists to run their own trials.

One of the first of these found that eating every other day could improve the wheezing and shortness of breath suffered by obese people with asthma. Not only that, but they also lost 8 per cent of their body weight in just eight weeks, their level of damaging free radicals had dropped by 90 per cent and inflammation was reduced by 70 per cent. About two weeks after coming off the diet the symptoms began to return.

The study, which involved only ten patients, was carried out by Dr James Johnson, an instructor in plastic surgery at Louisiana State

University School of Medicine[150] and author of the *Alternate Day Diet.*[151]

Lose weight and damp down inflammation

So, as well as helping asthmatics with their symptoms, the diet also produced the kind of metabolic improvements that would benefit people with diabetes. Inflammation is a central feature of diabetes, as well as other major killers such as heart disease and cancer, and one of the main sources of inflammation is obesity, especially from belly fat, also known as visceral fat, which is stored around the middle. It's known to pump out a variety of inflammatory chemicals that make your liver and cardiovascular system work less efficiently.

Another study, by Krista Varady, assistant professor of kinesiology and nutrition at University of Illinois, Chicago, has shown that eating every other day can boost levels of a protein called adiponectin, which reduces dangerous belly fat making the liver more responsive to insulin.[152] Her recently published research shows that people on an Alternate Day Diet lost weight and boosted their production of adiponectin by 30 per cent, as well as lowering the level of triglycerides in the blood, associated with increased risk of both diabetes and heart disease.

Getting the most out of eating every other day

The Alternate Day Diet doesn't just hold out the promise of being able to make improvements to the body's metabolism that are directly relevant to diabetes, it looks like being a way of getting round the biggest problem with most calorie-restriction diets (unlike the low-GL diet which isn't based on calorie counting) – that after 48–72 hours your metabolism slows down to compensate for the drop in food. The result is that when you stop the diet and eat more normally the weight goes back on even faster than before. Eating every other day seems to get round that because it allows normal eating as well.

So the severe drop in calories every other day is enough to start damping down the activity of the Grim Reaper, but the fact that you would then eat normally the second day doesn't allow your metabolism to start slowing down to compensate.

If you want to try this I would suggest you have no more than 500 calories on the fasting days for the first two weeks (however, do read the cautionary advice on page 178). Then once the metabolic benefits, like weight loss and reduced inflammation, are beginning to kick in you can up your intake on the fasting day to about 60–80 per cent of your normal diet. Of course, this is an optional idea. My low-GL diet will give you steady weight loss of around 900g (2lb) per week and re-educate you into good eating habits.

This is still a very new area of research and it is not yet clear exactly how the various mechanisms all fit together. Some researchers are experimenting with different regimes, such as eating very little every third day, but the combination of these different approaches seem to be new and effective ways of tackling diabetes. Although Kenyon has identified the Grim Reaper and Sweet Sixteen as the key genes under-lying the benefits of calorie restriction, there are almost certainly others at work.

How to switch on the 'skinny' gene

One of the best researched of these is a group of genes known as SIRTULINs, which also seems to control a cascade of health-boosting reactions, damping down or reversing many of the processes we asso-ciate with 'internal global warming': insulin resistance, metabolic syn-drome and inflammation. SIRTULINs have attracted a lot of attention because it looks as though one of them – a gene known as SIRT1 – isn't only switched on by calorie restriction; a chemical, known as res-veratrol, found in the skin of dark grapes, can also switch it on.

Like Sweet Sixteen, the benefits claimed for SIRT1 are impress-sive and could reasonably be expected to benefit people with diabetes in the same way. Activating the gene improves protection from free radical damage and boosts repair of DNA; it cuts down inflamma-tion and makes mitochondria, the tiny power plants in each of our cells, work more efficiently, burning carbohydrates rather than stor-ing them as fat. It helps protect you from diabetes, heart disease and Alzheimer's.[153]

Not only does a concentrate of resveratrol switch on the SIRTULIN gene but it also favourably affects over a hundred genes that help programme you for longevity. Dr John Pezzutto, of the University of Illinois, describes resveratrol as 'a whiff that induces a biologi-cally specific tsunami', referring to its wide range of positive effects on gene expression away from disease and towards health and youth. Resveratrol may even help you lose weight. Firstly, it inhibits fatty acid synthase, an enzyme needed to convert sugars into fat, and reduces insulin levels, which means fewer blood sugar lows and less hunger – this is why it has been dubbed 'the skinny gene'.

Resveratrol is found in green vegetables, mulberries, citrus fruits and the skins of peanuts, but it is most abundant in red grapes and good-quality red wines. A good bottle of merlot, for example, can provide 20mg, whereas cheap wines often have as little as 2mg. An alternative is to supplement it, which I do every day as part of an all-round anti-oxidant complex. I supplement 10mg and aim to eat the equivalent of 10mg. If you have diabetes or metabolic syndrome I recommend that you double this amount. Researchers at Harvard Medical School have shown that resveratrol activates the SIRT1 gene in yeast thus extending lifespan by more than 50 per cent. A trial is underway to see if a pharmaceutical version of resveratrol can lower blood sugar levels in people with diabetes.

Supplements that can boost helpful genes

This epigenetic approach to treating diabetes, which involves uncovering exactly how elements of a healthy lifestyle changes the activity of certain genes, also explains why omega-3 is such an important part of any diabetic treatment package. Recent research suggests that it may be able to do the same things as the blood glucose-lowering drug Avandia (rosiglitazone) without its potentially deadly side effects. Avandia was pulled off the market in 2010 in Europe (see Part 1, Chapter 5) after research showed it significantly increased your chances of having a heart attack.

When Avandia was launched ten years ago it was heralded as a breakthrough because it could affect the activity of a gene called PPARγ, which is involved in regulating blood sugar. Omega-3 has already been shown to affect PPARγ in a test tube, but recently a study found that it can change the way the gene behaves in mice. By boosting its level of activity it lowers their blood glucose levels.[154] Unlike Avandia, however, the fish oil also made the mice lose weight. Another serious side effect of Avandia is that it makes humans put on a lot of weight.

There are also other ways that omega-3 can help with diabetes. It reinforces one of the benefits of the Alternate Day Diet. It also lowers the level of inflammatory chemicals pumped out by belly fat, at least in obese mice, as well as improving their insulin sensitivity and lowering their blood glucose. The effect was very precise, the result of damping down the activity of a particular receptor (GPR120) found on fat cells which is known to promote inflammation.[155]

Even though this research is in its infancy it's already clear that supplements and lifestyle changes affect our genes in all sorts of beneficial ways; for example, there are hints that the effectiveness of the SIRT1 gene can be improved by increasing your niacin (vitamin B$_3$) intake, specifically if you have diabetes. A recent study involving over 400 people with diabetes, followed up for 12 years, found that the risk of dying among those who smoked went up by 50 per cent. If you had a low intake of niacin, however, that risk went up further to 230 per cent. These people had a particular variation in their SIRT1 gene which made them more vulnerable to the effects of smoking. The next step is to see if niacin reduces it.[156]

So the combination of a low-GL diet, eating less every other day, supplementing and/or eating 20mg of resveratrol plus omega-3 and niacin, is already looking like a winning formula for losing weight, reversing diabetes and living longer. And, as more research comes out, it is going to be possible to fine tune it even further.

Genes benefit from a workout too

A key element of every healthy-living programme is exercise, and it seems that it also affects our genes, although in a way that is, at first sight, rather surprising. Exercise can turn on the same genes that are affected by eating every other day. The reason this happens is probably because both expose the body to a certain amount of stress. This seems to contradict the idea that stress is harmful to people with diabetes because of its effect on the hormone cortisol, but whereas chronic stress is normally damaging, a short, sharp shock to the system seems to be beneficial.

The sudden calorie drop of a fasting day turns on the body's repair mechanisms. 'We think the genetic response to calorie restriction evolved to allow animals to survive times of famine,' says Kenyon. 'It allows them to get through the hard times so they are ready to start reproducing quickly when conditions improve.' Other examples of good stress include sudden drops in temperature and the extra strain put on the system by exercise which, while promoting adrenal hormones, are not associated with negative health consequences.

A hard workout generates dangerous free radicals and acids, as well as mildly damaging the muscle tissue. But it's good for you because, like a short fast, it stimulates the body to begin a process of repair, mopping up the free radicals and mending muscle. Exactly why long-term calorie restriction doesn't have the same effect as chronic stress isn't clear yet. Recently Dr Varady published a study showing that exercise, in the form of weight training, can boost adiponectin by the same amount as you get from the eating every other day.[157] The kind of exercise I recommend in the last chapter should have a similar effect.

How unhealthy habits can affect your children's genes

The need to target genes with nutrition and lifestyle changes may be more urgent than we could have imagined. Dramatic evidence for the possibility that a bad diet can have a harmful effect not just on our own genes but those of our children as well comes from a recent study in the journal *Nature*.

Male rats that had been made obese and diabetic with a high-fat diet were mated with normal healthy females. Even though genes are not meant to change in one generation, by six weeks the daughters of the diabetic rats had the classic signs of diabetes – insulin resistance and glucose intolerance – even though they were a normal weight. What's more the level of activity of 642 of their genes involved in producing insulin had changed.[158] This is thought to happen because genes can be switched on and off, and this switching may be passed on to our offspring. As the number of people with diabetes continues to rise, this raises at least the possibility that we will be doing something dreadful to our children. While such changes may go some way to safeguarding the health of your future children, calorie restriction or alternate-day dieting isn't appropriate for young children because they are still developing. Instead they need to have a healthy diet with plenty of protein and good-quality carbs.

An alternate-day low-GL diet

While the Alternate Day Diet recommends quite a severe calorie restriction (to 500 calories every other day for two weeks) to kick-start the process, this may not be such a great idea if you have diabetes, and could even be dangerous, giving you extreme blood sugar lows. This is therefore especially not advisable if you have type-1, insulin-dependent diabetes. If you do reduce your calories, it is vital that you are eating in a GL-balanced way so that you don't get blood sugar dips.

Part of the goal of a low-GL diet is that you don't feel hungry anyway, so you will probably be eating fewer calories in any case. But you could combine it with intermittent dieting by pushing it one day, and allowing yourself to be on the edge of hunger, and then being more lenient the next. You only need a 20 per cent drop in calories to trigger the SIRT1 effect so this could equate to 50 ⓖⓛ one day, then 40 the next, especially if you make your 40 ⓖⓛ day low in fat.

In reality, this means being really strict one day, with no drinks (other than water and teas), no desserts, and very small carbohydrate portions, and then having a little more the next day with either a larger carb portion, or a drink or dessert. This is easy to build into your Anti-diabetes Diet explained in Part 3. In order to activate the skinny genes, however, you need two weeks on the strict 40-GL diet approach, without drinks or desserts, as recommended in the Anti-diabetes Action Plan.

The Anti-diabetes Action Plan also includes resveratrol, and other anti-ageing antioxidants and foods as well as supplements of omega-3 and other nutrients that both switch off diabetes-promoting genes and reduce hunger, allowing you to eat less food without feeling hungry.

Summary

Although you can't choose the genes you inherit, you can activate particular genes through diet and lifestyle choices:

- If you have metabolic syndrome, type-1 or type-2 diabetes, follow the 40 GL Anti-diabetes Diet for two weeks, after which you can alternate between a 50 GL day and a 40 GL day. By drinking only water and tea, eating a smaller portion of carbs and avoiding dessert you can reduce your GL to 40 but avoid drops in your metabolism and blood sugar lows.
- Activate your skinny genes through exercise two to three times a week, particularly weight training or resistance training. Part 3, Chapter 5 explains how to easily include exercise into your daily activities.
- Supplementing omega-3s, niacin and resveratrol can trigger helpful genes. Read Part 3, Chapter 4 for advice on your daily supplement plan.

PART THREE

Your Action Plan for Diabetes Reversal

This part shows you exactly what you need to do to start reversing your diabetes. You will find an easy-to-use outline for your Anti-diabetes Diet, as well as supplements, exercise and lifestyle changes to rapidly stabilise your blood sugar balance, reverse insulin resistance and undo the damage caused by diabetes.

1

The Anti-diabetes Diet

Now it's time to get started on your new low-GL diet. Getting ready to start is a bit like a warm-up before you exercise, because you need a week to prepare: to restock your fridge with low-GL foods, find the best alternative foods and drinks and your nearest suppliers, and get used to eating some of the new foods.

IMPORTANT Before you start:
If you have metabolic syndrome or are wanting to avoid diabetes, you can go straight into the diet; however, if you have type-1 diabetes, or have type-2 diabetes and are currently using insulin, you need to follow the softer first-week option to help you avoid too quick a result, which could cause your blood sugar to go too low because the insulin dose you are now using is too high. This is important to avoid a hypo, especially during the night. I explain this in Part 3, Chapter 2.

After the first week, during which you will have monitored your blood sugar levels, you should be able to adjust your insulin dose with the guidance of your doctor, and can then follow my low-GL diet in full as specified in this chapter.

DON'T FORGET that it is essential to follow this diet with the support and knowledge of your doctor.

Looking at your addictions

If you're quite addicted to coffee, tea, chocolate, alcohol and/or ciga-rettes, you'll definitely get a better result by stopping these or, at least, cutting them back. Try halving your daily intake of these stimulants

– you might replace coffee and tea with naturally caffeine-free herbal teas, or eat a piece of fruit instead of your chocolate bar, for example.

Your first two weeks on 40 ⑬ a day

On your low-GL diet you will be eating carbohydrates with values that total no more than 40 ⑬ a day for the first two weeks to kick-start the diet. This means that you will not be having desserts, alcohol or even fruit juice to begin with. I'll be giving you ideas of what you can eat in this chapter. On page 69 I explained how it is important to 'graze rather than gorge' and showed you how the ⑬ are distributed during the day to spread out the carbohydrate load and avoid blood sugar dips and peaks. You will find a list of foods with their GL values in Appendix 4 and in this chapter, and you should find that it is very straightforward to work out what are the best 'value' foods to eat so that you feel full without having too many carbs.

On the third and future weeks you will have an additional 5 ⑬ quota per day for drinks or desserts – so you will be able to have a low-GL dessert, diluted fruit juice or a small glass of dry wine or spirit if you want to. If you then choose to introduce Alternate Day eating, you will need to eat 40 ⑬ one day (no drinks and desserts) and 50 ⑬ on the next.

What to eat for breakfast

First of all, never skip breakfast. It's the most important meal of your day. When you wake up your blood sugar is low because you haven't eaten, so you need to eat. But many people in the grip of a firm resolve to lose weight make the fatal mistake of trying not to eat anything for as long as possible. The following scenario may sound familiar to you: unless propped up with liquid stimulants (coffee or tea), nicotine, or instant sugar in the form of a piece of toast or a croissant, the resolve to go without food becomes weaker and weaker as the blood sugar level dips lower and lower, until the chances of making the correct food choices become smaller and smaller. Finally, you buckle under the strain and end up bingeing on high-GL foods.

Avoiding that kind of scenario is why you must eat breakfast. The only question is what to eat and how much. Nutritionists at Oxford Brookes University set out to examine this question by giving children either a low-GL breakfast or a high-GL breakfast. Then they measured who ate the most as children helped themselves to a buffet lunch. Although both breakfasts were rated as equally satisfying by the children immediately after eating, by lunchtime those who'd had the high-GL breakfast were more hungry and ate more food.[1] Exactly the same thing has been shown in adults, too.[2]

The message is clear. Eat a low-GL breakfast. It will satisfy you for longer by keeping your blood sugar level more stable, so you'll eat less later.

There are two ways to do this.

1 The simplest is to choose from any of the low-GL breakfasts listed on page 240. These are already calculated to give you no more than 10 ⒈, plus the right amount of protein and essential fats.

or

2 You can 'do it yourself'. The DIY low-GL breakfast is also very straightforward. The fundamental rules are shown in the illustration below.

The low-GL breakfast

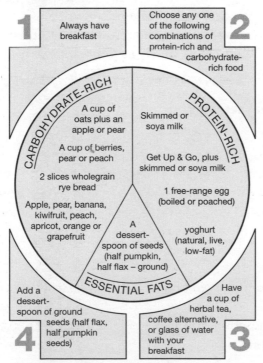

There are five fundamental breakfasts that give you the correct balance of both carbohydrate and protein. These are:

A balanced breakfast

Carbohydrates		Protein
Cereal/fruit	+	seeds/yoghurt/milk
Fruit	+	yoghurt/seeds
Fruit	+	Get Up & Go/milk
Bread/toast	+	egg
Bread/toast	+	fish (such as kippers)

We now need to look at the amount you can have of cereal, fruit, toast, and so on. Let's kick off with the cereal-based breakfast, sweetened with fruit rather than sugar.

The best cereal-based breakfasts

A good cereal-based breakfast needs to include a low-GL cereal, a low-GL fruit as a sweetener and a source of protein and essential fats. The goal, remember, is no more than 10 Ⓖ. In the chart below you'll see how much of the following six cereals you can have to total 5 Ⓖ. As you can see, the best 'value' in terms of your appetite are oat flakes, either cooked as in porridge or eaten raw, just as you would cornflakes. Basically, you could eat as much as you like, given that two servings will fill anybody up.

The Ⓖ for cereal servings

Cereal*	5 Ⓖ
Oat flakes	2 servings or cups
All-Bran	1 serving (½ bowl or 1 cup)
Unsweetened muesli	1 small serving (less than ½ bowl or ¾ cup)
Alpen	½ serving (¼ bowl or ½ cup)
Raisin Bran	½ serving (¼ bowl or ½ cup)
Weetabix	1 biscuit

*Adding a spoonful of oat bran to your cereal will lower the GL further.

In the following chart you can see how much of these six fruits you could eat to equal 5 Ⓖ.

The ⓖⓛ for fruit servings (breakfast)

Fruit	5 ⓖⓛ
Berries	1 large punnet
Pear	1
Grapefruit	1
Apple	1 small (can fit into the palm of your hand)
Peach	1 small
Banana	less than half

So your best bet out of the above foods would be to have porridge or raw oat flakes with as many berries as you could eat. Alternatively, you could have a bowl of All-Bran and a grapefruit, or a bowl of unsweetened muesli with a small grated apple. Or you can build your own breakfast using the chart in Appendix 4.

The protein element

As far as protein is concerned, there's some in milk (or in soya milk, but pick the unsweetened kind). Rice milk is high GL and best avoided. Oat milk is not bad, but not as good as soya. Yoghurt (unsweetened) is also high in protein. So, have a spoonful of yoghurt, some milk or some soya milk on your cereal if you'd like to.

Another source of protein, as well as containing countless vitamins, minerals, essential fats and fibre, is seeds. I recommend you have a tablespoon of ground seeds on your cereal as well. Ground chia seeds are the best choice because they are high in both protein and soluble fibres. Flax seeds are the next best thing but not so tasty. Pumpkin seeds are also good, and high in magnesium. Alternatively, try this mix below.

Four seed mix

1 Fill a glass jar that has a sealing lid half with chia or flax seeds (rich in omega-3) and half with sesame, sunflower and pumpkin seeds (rich in omega-6).
2 Keep the jar sealed and in the fridge to minimise damage from light, heat and oxygen. *continued*

3 Put a handful in a coffee or seed grinder, grind up and put a tablespoon onto your cereal. Store the remainder in the fridge and use over the next few days.

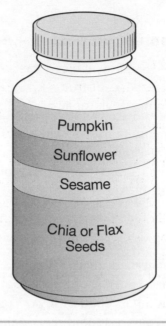

The best cereal-based breakfast is my Low-GL Muesli, made by mixing porridge oat flakes, oat bran and ground seeds, fresh berries and yoghurt. See the recipe on page 243. One serving has a GL of 8 and is completely satisfying.

The best yoghurt-based breakfasts

If you are fond of yoghurt, you could dispense with the cereal altogether and have yoghurt, fruit and seeds. Let's take a look at how this adds up. In the chart below you'll see how much yoghurt you can eat for 5 ⓖⓛ. (A small pot of yoghurt is 150g.)

The ⓖⓛ for yoghurt servings

Yoghurt	5 ⓖⓛ
Plain yoghurt	2 small pots, 330g (11½oz)
Non-fat yoghurt	2 small pots, 330g (11½oz)
Low-fat yoghurt with fruit and sugar	less than 1 small pot, 100g (3½oz)

So, provided you choose a yoghurt that doesn't have added sugar, you can eat two small pots, and sweeten it with any of the fruits you like from the fruit chart on page 187, plus a tablespoon of ground seeds. There is no need to go for the low-fat option.

Breakfasts based on Get Up & Go

Get Up & Go is a powder that you blend with a piece of fruit, choosing from any of the 5-GL servings of fruit shown on page 187, and 300ml (10fl oz/½ pint) of skimmed milk (or sugar-free soya milk if you prefer).

Get Up & Go is made from a special blend of quinoa, brown rice and soya flour, giving an excellent quality of protein. It is balanced with carbohydrate, mainly from whole apple powder, together with oat bran, rice bran and psyllium husks for added soluble fibre, plus sesame, sunflower and pumpkin seeds and some almond meal, cinnamon and natural vanilla for flavour. In addition, it has added vitamins and minerals, including 50mcg of chromium and 1,000mg of vitamin C, plus all the B vitamins.

When it's made up, it's guaranteed to fill you up until lunchtime, and yet it is only 283 calories and 5 ⒼⓁ. The best fruits to use in Get Up & Go are strawberries, raspberries, a soft pear or blackcurrants (which you can also buy canned in apple juice). You'll be looking for no more than another 5 ⒼⓁ from the fruit you blend in with it. Also add a teaspoon of cinnamon. With dairy or unsweetened soya milk this totals 8 ⒼⓁ. With oat milk it totals 10 ⒼⓁ.

Get Up & Go is available in health-food stores or by mail order (see Resources).

The best egg-based breakfasts

Although it is true that more than half the calories in an egg come from fat, the kind of fat depends on what you feed the chicken. Most eggs come from battery chickens. If you know how unhealthy they are, you won't be wanting to eat their eggs, which are high in saturated fat.

On the other hand, there are egg producers in the UK (and many more abroad) that give their chickens feed rich in fatty acids, for example flax seeds. Omega-3 free-range eggs are much better for you than ordinary eggs. I recommend you have no more than six free-range or organic eggs a week on my diet – and only these kinds of egg. Have either two small eggs, or one large egg, at one meal. Poach, boil or scramble them, but don't fry them, since the high heat damages the essential fats.

As eggs are pure protein and fat (so they have a 0 GL score), what carbohydrate can you have with them? If this is your entire breakfast you can use up your complete 10-GL quota by having any of the following bread servings.

The ⑪ for bread and bread-substitute servings for breakfast

Bread	10 ⑪
Oatcakes	4
Rye 'pumpernickel' style	2 thin slices
Sourdough rye bread	2 thin slices
Rye wholemeal bread (yeasted)	1 slice
Wheat wholemeal bread (yeasted)	1 slice
White, high-fibre bread (yeasted)	less than 1 slice (best avoided)

As you can see, your best 'value' breads are oatcakes, which are a Scottish favourite, or Scandinavian-style pumpernickel, sonnenbrot- or volkenbrot-type breads, or sourdough rye bread, made without yeast. Sourdough breads, and others like them, are real breads: substantial, fibre-rich and delicious, unlike the light, white, fluffy 'fake' breads we've been conditioned to eat, which are full of air, super-refined and nutritionally inferior. You may find the change a bit of a shock at first, but you'll discover that these breads are very satisfying.

Real breads are better for two reasons. They have far fewer additives, they use coarsely ground flours and, in the case of sourdough, they have no added yeast. All this keeps the GL score lower.

Some grains are better for you than others because of the type of carbohydrate they contain. The best are oats, followed by barley and rye, as I discussed in Part 2, Chapter 2. Whereas the GL of wheat varies depending on how long you cook it, oats are the same in any shape or form. Whole oat flakes, rolled oats or oatmeal, as used in oatcakes, all have a low glycemic effect.[3]

If you've never had an oat pancake, try the recipe on page 244.

Kippers, anyone?

Although they have gone out of fashion, kippers (smoked herring) make a fabulous low-GL breakfast that is tasty and highly nutritious.

Rich in protein and omega-3 fats, one kipper and any of the bread portions shown above will meet your needs for a healthy breakfast.

What to eat for snacks

Research shows clearly that 'grazing' (eating little and often) is healthier for you than 'gorging' (having one or two big meals in the day).[4] Grazing helps keep your blood sugar level even and this makes overeating far less likely, as you'll never experience any between-meal hunger pangs. For this reason I recommend you have a mid-morning and a mid-afternoon snack, because it helps to keep your blood sugar level stable. The ideal snack is one that provides no more than 5 🅖🅛 and also some protein, and the simplest snack food is fruit, eaten with nuts or seeds. Let's see what you'd need to eat to stay within 5 🅖🅛 for your snack.

The 🅖🅛 for fruit servings (snacks)

Fruit	5 🅖🅛
Strawberries	1 large punnet
Plums	4
Cherries	1 small punnet
Pear	1
Grapefruit	1
Orange	1
Apple	1 small (can fit into the palm of your hand)
Peach	1 small
Melon/watermelon	1 slice

Berries, plums and cherries are your best 'value' fruit snacks. Berries include raspberries, blueberries, blackberries and any others that you can get your hands on in season. You can further lower the GL score of these fruits by eating them with five almonds or a tablespoon of pumpkin seeds. Other than chestnuts, almonds are the best nut because they have the most protein compared with calories. Pumpkin seeds are also high in protein and in omega-3 fats.

Another snack option would be a bread, as listed below, with a protein-based spread. Cottage cheese, hummus and peanut butter are good examples. Hummus (see recipe on page 252) tastes great with oatcakes, on rye bread or with a raw carrot. (A large carrot is still less than 5 GL). If you like peanut butter, buy the kind with no added sugar. Or you could have sugar-free beans on toast. A slice of any of the bread servings below with either hummus or peanut butter gives you the right kind of low-GL carbohydrate with some protein to keep your blood sugar level even.

Oatcakes, and oats in general, are excellent as far as weight and blood sugar are concerned. Of all the grains, oats are the best for losing weight, and for controlling your blood sugar.[5] Watch out when buying oatcakes, though. Many contain sugar. The best are Nairn's, since not only do they have sugar-free, organic types but they also use palm fruit oil, which contains unsaturated fat, as opposed to palm oil, which is higher in saturated fat.

Alternatively, have a bowl of low-GL soup such as the Chestnut and Butterbean Soup on page 250. Also see the other low-GL snack options such as Smoked Salmon Pâté with oatcakes and crudités, and Quinoa Taboulleh.

The ⑥ for bread and bread-substitute servings for snacks

Bread	5 ⑥
Oatcakes	2 biscuits
Rye bread 'pumpernickel' style	1 thin slice
Sourdough rye bread	1 thin slice
Rye wholemeal bread (yeasted)	half a slice
Wheat wholemeal bread (yeasted)	half a slice
White, high fibre bread (yeasted)	less than half a slice (best avoided)

Here is a selection of 5-GL snacks to choose from:

- A piece of fruit, plus five almonds or a tablespoon of pumpkin seeds.

- A thin slice of rye bread or two oatcakes and ½ small tub of cottage cheese (150g/5½oz).

- A thin slice of rye bread/two oatcakes and ½ small tub of hummus (150g/5½oz).

- A thin slice of rye bread/two oatcakes and peanut butter.

- Crudités (a carrot, pepper, cucumber or celery) and hummus.

- Crudités and cottage cheese.

- A small yoghurt (150g/5½oz), no sugar, plus berries; or cottage cheese plus berries.

As you can see, you won't be bored between meals, as there's plenty of scope for mixing and matching.

What to eat for lunch and dinner

Main meals are really something to look forward to on my low-GL diet, as you'll see from the recipes and menus in Part 4. But how do you put it all together? The easiest way to get the right nutritional balance is to imagine all the different foods on a plate. I showed you this method in Part 2, and you'll find it described again below.

Half the plate will consist of very low-GL vegetables. These include peas, broccoli, carrots, runner beans, courgettes and kale, among many others. These vegetables, listed on page 197, will account for no more than 4 ⓖ, and I'm going to show you how to cook them in minutes. If you haven't been all that interested in veg up to now, you'll be amazed by how fresh and zingy they can taste when they're cooked in these ways.

The other half of your plate is divided into two, one for protein-based food such as meat, fish or tofu, and the other for more 'starchy' vegetables, which account for 6–7 ⓖ. There's a chart showing this on page 195.

So, a quarter of what's on your plate is protein-rich, a quarter is carbohydrate-rich and half is made up of very low-GL vegetables. You'll soon get the hang of it, it's dead simple.

More fish, less meat

Let's kick off with the protein serving on your plate. Remember from Part 2 that the overall amount of protein – by which I mean the protein contained in the various foods – needs to be at least 20g (¾oz) for each meal. During the first month it is fine to eat more like 30g (1oz), which is double the figure in the chart overleaf. The protein-rich food on your plate will provide 15g (½oz) of this, and the table overleaf tells you how much you need to eat of each of these to get that 15g (½oz). The one serving of carbohydrate-rich starchy vegetables and two servings of very low-GL vegetables will provide the remaining 5g (⅛oz).

In the table I've listed a lot of fish options and fewer meat options. In fact, red meat is missing entirely. White meat tends to be much lower in fat, and fish is much higher in the essential omega-3 fats so, becoming a 'fishichicketarian' is a great way to lose weight and gain health. Does this mean you can never eat red meat? Certainly not, but do stick to lean meat.

How big is a protein serving?

Food	Weight	Serving
Tofu and tempeh	160g (5¾oz)	¾ packet
Soya mince	100g (3½oz)	3 tbsp
Chicken (no skin)	50g (1¾oz)	1 very small breast
Turkey (no skin)	50g (1¾oz)	½ small breast
Quorn	120g (4¼oz)	⅓ pack
Salmon and trout	55g (2oz)	1 very small fillet
Tuna (canned in brine)	50g (1¾oz)	¼ can
Sardines (canned in brine)	75g (2¾oz)	⅔ can
Cod	65g (2¼oz)	1 very small fillet
Clams	60g (2⅛oz)	¼ can
Prawns	85g (3oz)	6 large prawns
Mackerel	85g (3oz)	1 medium fillet
Oysters	–	15
Yoghurt (natural, low fat)	285g (10oz)	½ large tub
Cottage cheese	120g (4¼oz)	½ medium tub
Hummus	200g (7oz)	1 small tub
Skimmed milk	440ml	about 15fl oz (¾ pint)
Soya milk	415ml	about 15fl oz (¾ pint)
Eggs (boiled)	–	2
Quinoa	125g (4½oz)	large serving bowl
Baked beans	310g (11oz)	¾ can
Kidney beans	175g (6oz)	⅓ can
Black-eye beans	175g (6oz)	⅓ can
Lentils	165g (5¾oz)	⅓ can

Starchy vegetables

As we saw on page 193, carbohydrate-rich starchy vegetable servings should be roughly the same size or weight as protein servings, but this does depend on how each food weighs up – for example, if you are eating chicken with rice, the serving size of rice is somewhat larger than the piece of chicken for each to be roughly the same weight because chicken is dense and heavy and rice is relatively light.

Remember, starchy vegetables will account for a maximum of 7 ⓖ of your meal (out of a total of 10 ⓖ). Let's take a look at what quantity of different starchy vegetables you can eat to keep within that limit, leaving 3 ⓖ for the very low-GL veg that occupy half the plate.

The ⓖ for starchy vegetables

Starchy vegetables	7 ⓖ
Pumpkin/squash	big serving, 185g (6¾oz)
Carrot	1 large, 160g (5¾oz)
Swede	big serving, 150g (5½oz)
Quinoa	big serving, 130g (4½oz)
Beetroot	big serving, 110g (3¾oz)
Cornmeal	serving, 115g (4oz)
Pearl barley	small serving, 95g (3¼oz)
Wholemeal pasta	½ serving, 85g (3oz) cooked weight
White pasta	⅓ serving, 65g (2¼oz) cooked weight
Brown rice	small serving, 70g (2½oz) cooked weight
White rice	⅓ serving, 45g (1½oz) cooked weight
Couscous	⅓ serving, 45g (1½oz) soaked weight
Broad beans	serving, 30g (1oz)
Corn on the cob	½ cob, 60g (2⅛oz)
Boiled potato	3 small potatoes, 75g (2¾oz)
Baked potato	½ potato, 60g (2⅛oz)
French fries	tiny portion, 45g (1½oz)
Sweet potato	½ potato, 60g (2⅛oz)

As you can see, there are some obvious winners. Wholemeal pasta – for example, spaghetti – and brown rice are much better than white pasta and white rice. (As we saw earlier, brown basmati rice has the lowest GL score of all the different types of rice.) Swede, carrot and squash are much better than potato. Boiled potato is better than baked potato, which is in turn better than French fries.

Some of these foods may be new to you. If so, try the nutty flavour of quinoa and the smooth, rich savour of the squashes. If you love pasta, switching to the wholemeal variety is painless. They cook the same, but you can eat more of the unrefined variety and stay slim.

Beans and lentils

It's telling that beans and lentils are no longer widely eaten in many of the world's fattest nations. These are the best foods for both balancing your blood sugar and giving the right mix of protein and carbohydrate. It's this rare double-whammy that keeps their GL score low. (Another reason why lentils and soya – a bean that is more usually eaten as tofu or milk – are so low is that they contain a substance that prevents the digestion of amylose, therefore slowing down its release further.) Soya also keeps your arteries healthy by lowering the 'bad' LDL cholesterol. A serving of soya a day, either as soya milk or tofu, can lower your LDL cholesterol by over 10 per cent.

With any meal containing beans and lentils you can be quite generous with the portion size because you are getting both the protein and the carbohydrate from the same food. However, when you are eating these foods as your source of protein, combine with only half the serving size of a carbohydrate-rich food, instead of an equal serving. If you were making a lentil casserole for two people, for example, you'd use a cup of uncooked lentils and half a cup of uncooked brown rice. This is, of course, because you're already getting a significant amount of carbohydrate in the lentils.

This is how much you can eat, assuming you are not eating another starchy vegetable, to stay within 7 ⒼⓁ. (Most regular cans of beans provide around 225–245g (8–8½oz) of beans.)

The ⒼⓁ for beans, chickpeas and lentils

Beans and lentils	7 ⒼⓁ
Soya beans	2 cans
Pinto/borlotti beans	¾ can
Lentils	¾ can
Baked beans	½ can
Butter beans	½ can
Split peas	½ can
Kidney beans	½ can
Chickpeas	⅓ can

NOTE A 400g (14oz) can is roughly equivalent to 75g (3oz) dried beans.

If you're not vegetarian, you may be relatively unfamiliar with beans and lentils. You may have encountered dhal, baked beans, hummus or cassoulet, but never actually thrown a packet or tin of lentils or beans into your shopping basket. These are great foods, immensely satisfying in flavour and texture, and they feature in all of the world's great cuisines – as well as kitchen classics such as beans on toast. You'll be making mouth-watering dishes with them, from hummus to Trout with Puy Lentils and Roasted Tomatoes on the Vine, Borlotti Bolognese and Chickpea Curry to name just a few.

Non-starchy vegetables

Now it's time to move on to the other half of your plate. This is made up of what I call the 'unlimited vegetables', although there are, of course, some limits, but these are vegetables for which a serving is less than 2 ⑥. A serving of peas, for instance, is a cupful.

Non-starchy vegetables

Asparagus	Kale
Aubergine	Lettuce
Beansprouts	Mangetouts
Broccoli	Mushrooms
Brussels sprouts	Onions
Cabbage	Peas
Cauliflower	Peppers
Celery	Radish
Courgette	Rocket
Cucumber	Spinach
Endive	Spring onions
Fennel	Tomato
Garlic	Watercress
Green beans and runner beans	

If you are not a fan of cabbage, say, or runner beans you will find some delicious recipes using these ingredients that I hope will change your mind – Oriental Green Beans and Broccoli, Coleslaw, and Green Bean Olive and Roasted Pepper Salad. They are brimming with vitamins, minerals and other phytonutrients so are really good for you. Aim to eat at least half your vegetables raw or lightly cooked or steamed. Cooking, burning or frying generates more AGEs (see page 8) and oxidants (see page 116).

To recap, I want you to eat two servings of non-starchy vegetables, one serving of starchy vegetables and one serving of protein-based food. Together, they'll help you feel full at the end of every meal.

Simple ways to lower the GL of a meal

- Add lemon juice (see page 85).
- Make it into a soup – it's more filling that way (see page 145).
- Soak oats or eat them as porridge.
- Chew each mouthful 20 times to further slow-release the carbohydrate.
- Sip water with your meal.
- Put your fork down between mouthfuls.
- Add a spoonful of oat bran (see page 92).
- Don't add sweet sauces.
- Wait 30 minutes before eating something sweet.
- Have dessert as a snack and include some protein.

For vegetarians

If you're a strict vegetarian, you'll need to eat more beans, lentils, soya produce (such as tofu and tempeh) and Quorn than usual to achieve the target for your protein intake. A serving size of tofu for a main meal is 160g (5¾oz), which is roughly three-quarters of a packet. Part 4 contains a tasty recipe to get you started with using tofu – the vegetarian fatburner's best friend – along with recipes using a variety of beans and lentils. Many of the recipes containing chicken or fish can be adapted by replacing them with tofu or a tofu steak.

Fats and oils

This diet is not low fat; you'll be able to eat enough to keep you satisfied. As far as fats and oils go, what's important is which fats you use, and how you use them.

Salad dressings When using seed oils for salad dressings, pick either flax seed oil or a blend of oils that gives at least one part of omega-3 fats to one part of omega-6 fats. These seed oils need to be cold-pressed and stored in a lightproof container.

A good seed oil blend is Udo's Choice, available in health-food stores (see Resources). Also good is walnut oil or a virgin pressed organic olive oil. You can lightly drizzle these oils onto vegetables instead of butter.

Cooking oils For steam-frying (see below) and sautéing, use a small amount of butter, coconut butter or olive oil. Coconut butter adds a great flavour to steam-fries.

Creams If you want to make a savoury dish creamier, try adding a teaspoon of tahini (sesame spread) or a tablespoon of coconut milk or coconut cream.

Cooking methods

All carbohydrate foods release their carbohydrate somewhat faster once cooked. The longer you cook something and the higher the temperature, the faster-releasing the food becomes. It's therefore best to eat food as close to raw as possible. Also 'wet' cooking methods, such as steaming, generate fewer AGEs than dry cooking, such as baking.[6] Crisps are especially bad news in this respect.

This doesn't mean eating endless salads. You can steam, steam-fry, boil and poach food without cooking it to death. Next best is baking, grilling, sautéing and stir-frying. Worst is frying and deep-frying.

Steaming is the best way to cook green, leafy, less starchy vegetables, since it preserves a lot of their vitamins and minimises any raising of GL. The method can be used with any food and is very successful with fish – but perhaps not ideal with starchy vegetables, which require longer cooking, or with red meat. Many different kinds of steamers are available, or you can improvise with a colander, pot and lid.

Boiling raises the GL of foods more than steaming, but less than baking. Changes can be kept to a minimum by using as little water as possible, keeping the lid on, and cooking the food as whole as possible. Also, eat all vegetables al dente – a little crisp, not soft.

Steam-frying figures large in my low-GL diet because it adds loads of taste without compromising on health. The great advantage of this style of cooking is that the lower temperature of steaming doesn't destroy nutrients to anything like the extent that frying does, and you use only a small amount of oil, if that. As with boiling and ordinary steaming, aim to keep vegetables al dente.

To steam-fry, use a shallow pan or a deep frying pan with a thick base and lid that seals well. You can steam-fry without oil by first adding two tablespoons of liquid to the pan – water, vegetable stock, soy sauce or some watered-down sauce you'll use for the dish. Once it boils, immediately add some vegetables, sauté rapidly for a minute or two, turn the heat up, add a tablespoon or two more of the liquid and clamp the lid on tightly. After a minute add the remaining ingredients. Turn the heat down after a couple of minutes and steam in this way until cooked.

Or you can add a teaspoon to a tablespoon of olive oil, butter or coconut oil to the pan, warm it, add the ingredients and sauté. After a couple of minutes, add two tablespoons of liquid as above and clamp the lid on. Steam the ingredients until done.

Poaching is like steam-frying without the sautéing. You can make delicious water-based sauces; for example, you could cook fish in vegetable broth flavoured with ginger, garlic, lemongrass, spices and wine (the alcohol boils off).

Waterless cooking requires specially designed pans in which you can 'boil' foods by steaming them in their own juice, and 'fry' foods with no oil. Both methods are excellent for preserving nutrients and flavour.

Baking is useful, especially if the food is large and has a thick skin (such as a whole or half pumpkin). Avoid coating food with oil, because the oil will oxidise with cooking, which creates free radicals (highly reactive, harmful molecules). You can roast a potato without adding oil. The higher the temperature and the longer you cook something, the higher the GL becomes.

Frying should be kept to a minimum, and deep-frying avoided altogether. When you do fry use butter, coconut oil (saturated fat) or olive oil (monounsaturated) rather than other vegetable oils (polyunsaturated oils), since these are much more prone to oxidation.

Grilling foods that contain fat is less damaging than frying, but browning or burning a food does create free radicals. Try to avoid barbecued food, or at least ensure that what you eat is not charred.

Microwaving is a problematic cooking method, although admittedly fast. As food cooks in its own water, it seems better than most cooking methods for preserving the water-soluble vitamins B and C; however, the temperatures reached in fat particles are very high, so avoid microwaving oily fish as it will destroy the essential fats it contains. And remember that microwave ovens do give off electromagnetic radiation, even 1.8m (6ft) away. It is better to use lower-voltage/heat settings for longer cooking. Cover dishes to encourage steaming, although you do need to leave some room for steam to escape.

Top tips for healthy eating

- Buy foods as fresh and unprocessed as possible and eat them soon afterwards.
- Eat more raw food. Be adventurous. Try raw beetroot and carrot tops in salad.
- Cook foods as whole as possible, slicing or blending before serving.
- Use as little water as possible for cooking, preferably steaming, poaching or steam-frying.
- Fry foods as infrequently as possible.
- Favour slow cooking methods that introduce less heat.
- Don't overcook, burn or brown food.

What to limit and what to avoid

The trick with any diet is to fill yourself up with the good stuff so there's little room left for less desirable foods. Some of the good foods, however, such as oily fish, still need to be limited because, although they contain valuable fats, too much of any fat is bad for you.

Foods to limit

The chart overleaf shows you which foods to limit and how much to limit them to. Some of these are included in the recipes in specific amounts because they contain important nutrients. Some are high in fat, whereas others are high in sugar, so do not have more than the recommended amounts.

The foods to limit

Fruit	choose fresh fruit
Coconut	can be used in small amounts to flavour dishes
Seeds	limit to two tablespoons a day maximum
Nuts	same as seeds (don't have both, and seeds are better).
Salad dressings	stick to the measures given in Part 4
Avocados	twice a week, maximum
Vegetable oil and butter	use sparingly, as in the recipes
Tahini (sesame spread)	use a small amount instead of butter
Fatty fish such as herring, mackerel, tuna, kippers	three times a week, maximum
Chicken (no skin), game	twice a week, maximum
Milk and yoghurts	stick to skimmed milk and low-fat yoghurt
Eggs	six a week, maximum

Foods to avoid

These foods are high in fat and/or fast-releasing sugar, or are devoid of nutrients, so they're best strictly avoided. Once you have attained your target weight they may be eaten on a rare occasion.

High-fat meats including beef, pork, lamb, sausages and processed meats
Lard, dripping, suet and gravy
Deep-fried foods
Cream and shop-bought ice cream
High-fat spreads and mayonnaises
All cheeses except cottage cheese, low-fat quark or fromage frais, and half-fat
Cheddar cheese such as Shape
Rich sauces made with cream, cheese or eggs
Sugar, sugar-laden sweets and foods with added sugar
Pastries, cakes and biscuits
White bread
Snack foods such as crisps
Dried fruit

Desserts

During the first two weeks it is best to avoid all desserts, as well as sweets and sweetened drinks, even fruit juice. Once your blood sugar level is more stable you have a daily 5 GL allowance for drinks or desserts. In Part 2, Chapter 7 I explained which drinks are possible within the 5 GL rule. But what about desserts?

If you are used to eating a lot of desserts, or if you are insulin-resistant, you will probably crave something sweet at the end of each meal. It is very important to break this habit because, if you don't, it will keep your blood sugar level seesawing. It takes only three days in most cases to stop the craving. So, after your initial stimulant- and sugar-free period, limit desserts to one a week, perhaps at the weekend.

You'll find wonderful recipes for low-GL desserts in Part 4, including Chocolate Ice Cream and Kiwi and Coconut Pudding. These don't exceed 5 ⓖⓛ and aren't loaded with saturated fats. You could also choose a low-GL bar such as a Fruitus Oat and Fruit bar, which is about 5 ⓖⓛ, but don't go over this limit.

Don't have desserts when you are eating out (see page 208), because almost all restaurant desserts are heavily loaded with sugar and saturated fat.

When to eat

As I've already emphasised, breakfast is the most important meal of the day and you want to make sure you eat a breakfast containing plenty of protein – for example with eggs. If you do go for a grain cereal such as oats, make sure you have ground seeds and a protein-based milk with it. This helps reduce your appetite later on in the day.

At the other end of the day, aim to finish eating dinner at least two hours before you go to sleep. It is very important to eat a low-GL dinner, with sufficient protein. Having beans, lentils or chickpeas as your 7 GL 'carb' portion really helps keep your blood sugar level stable. This will actually lower the GL of your breakfast the next day. Don't eat after dinner. That means no snacks or drinks other than water or non-sweetened herb teas. The only exception to this is for people with type-1 diabetes or those currently using insulin, in which case follow the recommendations in the next chapter.

Otherwise, aim for eleven hours without eating between dinner and breakfast. Do make sure you get enough sleep because research has found that a lack of sleep also disrupts your appetite hormones.[7] Part 2, Chapter 8 explained how to get a good night's sleep.

2

Diet and Supplements for People with Type-1 Diabetes and those Taking Insulin

If you have type-1, insulin-dependent diabetes, or have type-2 diabetes and are currently taking insulin, you need to build up to the full Anti-diabetes Diet explained in the last chapter, plus supplements, more gradually. The reason for this is to avoid hypos and to give you time to adjust your insulin dose accordingly. Once you are on the full diet and supplement programme you can hope to have much more control over your blood sugar levels, although those with type-1 diabetes will still need to inject insulin, although at a reduced dosage.

IMPORTANT Before you start:
Before you start the diet you must inform your doctor that you are going on a strict low-GL diet and keep him or her informed so that they can make the necessary changes to your medication or insulin dose. All changes must be with your doctor's approval – do not adjust your medication doses without informing him or her.

It is possible that your doctor will be sceptical about the kind of reductions you can achieve; however, it is important to seek their guidance and support as you take control of your health and blood sugar balance.

Your first week

The most critical time for you is the long haul from dinnertime to breakfast time. Therefore, for the first week I recommend you follow the Anti-diabetes Diet given in the previous chapter but rather than have one of the low-GL dinners, continue eating your usual dinner. As an exercise you could calculate roughly what the GL of your current dinner is using the charts in Appendix 4. If you wish, you can experiment with one of my low-GL dinners but you should add an appropriate number of ⑩ to be equivalent to what you are currently eating. You can do this by either increasing the carbohydrate proportion (such as having more rice, potatoes or pasta) or by adding a dessert from the recipes in this book (that's another 5 ⑩) or have a 5 GL snack before bed (either some fruit or a Fruitus bar). But the most important thing is to avoid having a hypo during the night. Make sure you have available some glucose tablets or Lucozade in case you do.

I also recommend that you don't have any of the super-fibres or supplements during the first week.

Keep a record of your glucose levels

Monitor your glucose levels at noon and at 6.00 pm. You goal is to achieve stable glucose levels (between 5–5.7mmol/l), having adjusted your insulin levels accordingly, before moving on to the next stage. If you do not achieve this during the first week, then keep going with this strategy until you do.

It will help you and your doctor to keep a record of changes. You can do this by photocopying and completing the chart in Appendix 5, which has the following headings:

Date   Time of meal
Time   Meal consumed
Blood glucose level   Supplements taken
Type and amount of insulin injected

On page 303 you'll find an example of a completed chart.

With your doctor's supervision you will be adjusting your short-acting insulin doses (such as Humalog or Novorapid) accordingly; for example, if you took 10 units at 8.00 am and your blood glucose level is 4mmol/l at noon, you would be advised to lower your insulin dose to 8 units the next day.

Short-acting insulins affect your blood sugar levels for up to four hours. But you will also be on long-acting insulin which affects your blood sugar level for up to 24 hours. Generally, you will probably be needing to lower this by 20 per cent, but again do this with your doctor's guidance.

The trickiest part comes when you go on to the full low-GL diet, by including your low-GL evening meal. Don't start this second phase before you have (a) attained stable blood glucose levels at noon and 6.00 pm; and (b) reduced long-acting insulin by at least 20 per cent.

In most cases you should achieve this within one to three weeks.

Phasing in supplements

In the second week you can start phasing in the supplements. (It is best to read Chapter 4 later in this part now so that you know what you are trying to achieve.) Here's how.

Once you have stabilised your noon and 6.00 pm glucose levels on the diet, add in the basics (page 214). Do this for at least three days before adding in chromium. Start with a chromium dose of 200mcg for one week (with or without cinnamon extract), taken with breakfast. This may require you to further adjust your insulin levels. Once you have, again, attained stability, double the chromium dose to 400mcg, taking 200mcg at breakfast and 200mcg at lunch. Again, you are likely to need to adjust your insulin levels accordingly. Then increase the chromium dose to 400mcg with breakfast and 200mcg with lunch. Adjust your insulin requirement accordingly. Once you are stable, you could go a final step and take 200mcg of chromium at dinner, but by now you must be on less long-acting insulin, so don't do this without your doctor's guidance. Also, make sure you have glucose tablets available in the night in case of a hypo.

It will probably take you the best part of a month to find the right balance on the low-GL diet, plus supplements – chromium being the key since it makes you more responsive to insulin.

Phasing in super-fibres

Once you have achieved your maximum chromium dose (600–800mcg), and are stable on the diet, you can start adding in 5g of either glucomannan or PGX 15 minutes before a meal. Start with breakfast, monitor your blood glucose at noon, and then adjust your next morning's insulin accordingly.

Then, add 5g of a super-fibre before lunch, monitor your 6.00 pm glucose and adjust the next day's insulin at noon accordingly.

Once you have done this for a week, and have stable glucose levels at noon and 6.00 pm, add 5g of super-fibre before dinner. By now you'll have a good idea of what effect this has on your insulin requirement and will need to have adjusted both your short-term and long-acting insulin doses accordingly.

It is important to keep a record of your levels as you make these changes, using the form in Appendix 5. This will help you and your doctor to adjust your insulin requirements accordingly.

The ultimate goal

Once you are on your low-GL diet, including your evening meal, with the 5 GL drink or dessert option, eating three meals and two snacks a day, your insulin requirement will have reduced considerably.

If you have type-2 diabetes and take insulin you should get to the point, within three to nine months, when you no longer need insulin. You will probably still be on metformin, which is the best of the diabetes drugs, but even this may become unnecessary.

If you have type-1 diabetes you are likely to achieve, at least, half your current requirement of insulin and, in many cases, one-third your requirement, but you will not be able to stop your requirement for insulin completely. You will also have much more control over your blood sugar levels.

3

Eating Out

You don't need to stay in every night, slaving over a hot stove (or a salad bowl) on your low-GL diet. But when it comes to eating out you will need to be choosy. I travel the world on lecture tours and I always find excellent restaurants as I go, simply by choosing Chinese, Japanese, Malaysian or Thai establishments.

The reason I do this is that these countries have the leanest, healthiest people, and much of that is down to the way they eat. Because the Chinese, for example, have emigrated to so many countries around the world, it's usually possible to find a Chinese restaurant at least, whether in the US, Canada, Australia, Continental Europe, South America – or the Far East! But this doesn't mean you can't eat French, Italian, Mexican, Indian or other foods. You just need to know what to order.

Eating well, the low-GL way

The trick, as ever, is to fill yourself up with the good stuff. That means having a starter and a main course, or just a main course, but not a dessert. It also means avoiding any breads, prawn crackers or the like. In fact, it's best to ask the waiter to take those away, thus removing the temptation. Instead, ask them to bring some olives or a dish of hot pickles. Order water and say you won't be drinking anything else.

When you are choosing items from the menu, watch out for the hidden sugar and high-GL carbohydrates in sauces, pickles and dips. All Thai restaurants, for example, do very tasty fishcakes and spring rolls. The fishcakes are better than the spring rolls because they have more protein. Both come with a sweet sauce, and you'll need to leave this on the side.

Where possible, choose food that hasn't been deep-fried. So, go for boiled noodles rather than fried, or boiled rice rather than fried rice. Share a portion between two or even three people. Remember, you want about as much weight of the carbohydrate food as the protein-rich food, such as a steamed or poached fish.

Japanese restaurants are great, especially if you like fish. All offer wonderful fish dishes, such as teriyaki salmon and sashimi. This can be very satisfying without filling you up with fast-releasing carbohydrates or saturated fat. (Sushi isn't as good because it includes a lot of sweet white rice.)

Always order some vegetable dishes, whether it's a salad or a side order of green beans or broccoli. Make sure you eat your greens and, if you haven't had enough, order some more.

By the time you get to the end of your main course you should be full. This is the time to make your exit, asking for the bill and letting your waiter know that the food was so good and so filling that you don't want coffee or dessert!

Most of all, remember who is in charge of what goes into your mouth. Think of the menu as only a small selection of what's on offer, opening up the possibility of ordering 'off menu'. If you like the sound of the fish, but not the cream sauce, ask for it without, or swap to another method of cooking. Ask what's in various dishes and have a look around at what other people are eating.

Be careful of hidden fat and sugar

Indian food uses a lot of vegetables, beans and lentils, but there's also a lot of hidden sugar and fat in some of the sauces. You have to choose very carefully indeed in an Indian restaurant, so I'd recommend going there only as an occasional treat. The same applies to cheaper Italian restaurants that specialise in pizza and pasta. These dishes are based on high-GL carbohydrates and the pasta can come with fatty cheese or cream sauces, so they're best avoided. In contrast, authentic Italian and French restaurants will have plenty of excellent main dishes, such as grilled chicken, plus good salads and vegetables, so be on the lookout for these.

Here are some typical items from Chinese, Thai, Japanese, Malaysian or Indian restaurant menus to choose, or avoid.

Choose
Sashimi (Japanese raw fish dish)
Fish/chicken teriyaki
Tom yum soup
Thai fish/chicken/prawn tikkas, curries (but avoid the creamier ones listed under 'Avoid' below)
Fish/chicken satay (peanut-based sauce)
Indian bhunas or baltis – ask for less oil
Steamed fish and other non-fried fish dishes
Tofu-based dishes
Omelettes
Noodles with vegetables, such as chop suey (share a portion)
Vegetable dishes such as chana masala or dhal (Indian) or stir-fried beansprouts, bamboo shoots, water chestnuts or mushrooms (Chinese)

Avoid
Fried fish/meat
Sweet-and-sour dishes
Creamy curries such as kormas and masalas
Rice (unless brown – share a portion)
Potato dishes
Bread such as naans and chapattis
Prawn crackers

The fallback in any restaurant is to choose something simple, without sauces with unknown ingredients. So you can't go wrong with grilled fish or chicken and vegetables or salad.

Food and the new you

Restaurants are a good proving ground for your new relationship with food. Now that you understand so much more about how food affects your blood sugar, and the way you feel, make good food your friend. Become the master of your own weight and blood sugar balance by becoming the master of your diet.

The best way to do this is to prepare your own meals. Experiment. Make mistakes. Try new foods. Get involved with creating a way of eating that really works for you and test what they do to your blood sugar.

Choose to follow this diet because it is best for your health and it can make a real difference to the medication you will have to take. Make this your diet, and simply use what's in this book as a springboard to changing your eating patterns for the future. That means finding the balance between eating out and eating in.

4

Your Daily Supplement Programme

In Part 2 I examined the evidence on a number of nutrients and their proven effects in helping to reverse diabetes and blood sugar imbalance. The science shows without a shadow of a doubt that taking optimal doses of nutritional supplements works, so whether you have type-1 or type-2 diabetes, or if you are trying to avoid diabetes, I recommend that you follow one of the supplement programmes in this chapter, alongside your low-GL diet.

The optimal level of a nutrient necessary to help bring your system back into balance is almost always far greater than the amount you need to maintain health. This is clear from the research, and it is also a fundamental principle of nutritional medicine. Nutrients, in large amounts, do correct underlying disease processes. There is also another reason why supplementation is so essential. Most people with diabetes pee a lot because of worsening kidney function. The more you pee the more nutrients you lose in your urine. So, for this reason alone, it's important to be continually replacing those lost nutrients.

Your helpful nutrients

The following are the nutrients that the research has shown have the effect of lowering blood glucose levels, glycosylated haemoglobin and/or improving insulin resistance:

Vitamins
Vitamin D (15–50mcg)

Vitamin C (1–2g)
Vitamin E (100–300mg)
B complex (B_1, B_2, B_3, B_6, B_{12}, folic acid) (depending on your homocysteine level)

Minerals
Chromium (200–1,000mcg)
Zinc (10–20mg)
Magnesium (150–300mg)

Others
The super-fibres, glucomannan and PGX
Omega-3 (EPA and DHA)
CoQ_{10} (10–100mg)
Alpha lipoic acid (10–600mg)
Glutathione and N-acetyl cysteine (50–500mg)
Resveratrol and anthocyanidins (10–40mg)
5-HTP (100–300mg)
HCA (750–2,250mg)
Glutamine (5–10g)

Herbs
Milk thistle (600mg)
Gymnema sylvestre (400mg)
Cinnamon (3–6g) or Cinnulin (500–1,000mg)

If you are new to nutritional supplements, this probably looks like a very long list and it might conjure up images of handfuls of pills and big bills. In truth, most of the above you can get from fewer than six combination formulas.

The figures in brackets are the minimal to maximal intakes required to have an effect. Bear in mind that levels used in research are often quite high to weight the study towards producing an effect. Only when lots of studies with different doses have been carried out does it become possible to tease out the optimal amounts. Also, when synergistic nutrients are given together you may not need such high levels to get the maximum effect. The level you need also depends on how out of control your blood sugar balance is and how much damage or inflammation you currently have.

Bearing this in mind, I've created four different supplement pro-grammes depending on where you are along the curve. As your health and vital statistics improve, your need to supplement will become less. All these recommendations are 'ideal' for those who wish to have the most rapid recovery. You can also recover with diet alone, but it will take much longer and you may not make as complete a recovery. In terms of cost, you are looking at something between the cost of a daily paper and a fancy cup of coffee.

Working with a nutritional therapist

If you have diabetes and have some concerns about interactions between the drugs you are taking and nutritional supplements, I recommend you work with a nutritional therapist who is trained in the nutritional medicine approach to diabetes and can work alongside your doctor. In Resources I show you how to find a nutritional therapist near you.

The basics

There are three basic supplements, the foundation of any good supple-ment programme, that are recommended for *everybody* with or without diabetes. These are:

- An 'optimum nutrition' multivitamin–mineral
- An essential omega-3 and 6 supplement
- Extra vitamin C, plus other immune-boosting nutrients

I take these every day to maintain good health and recommend you do the same. But how do you know which formulations to choose?

The best multis

Any decent multivitamin and mineral will tell you to take two a day, preferably one at breakfast and one at lunchtime. Firstly, because you cannot get enough of all the nutrients in one pill; and secondly, because the water-soluble vitamins B and C are in and out of your body in four to six hours, so you get twice the benefit by taking them twice a day.

Many multivitamin–minerals skimp on the minerals. A hallmark of good ones is that they provide at least 150mg of magnesium, 10mg of zinc plus 25mcg of selenium and chromium. A good multivitamin will also have at least 15mcg of vitamin D and around 100mg of vitamin E. In the supplement programmes that follow, this is called a 'high-strength multivitamin–mineral', not to be confused with the very basic, and ineffective, RDA-level multis.

The best essential-fat supplements

The most potent forms of omega-3 are called EPA, DPA and DHA. These are found in oily fish. The most potent omega-6 is called GLA. This is found in borage and evening primrose oil. Since we need more, and are more deficient in, omega-3, you want at least ten times more omega-3 than 6. (Add up the total EPA, DPA and DHA in a supplement and divide by the total GLA. This figure should be over 10.) In all you are looking for at least 600mg of combined EPA, DPA and DHA a day for general health maintenance. It is not worth supplementing the vegetarian form of omega-3, alpha linolenic acid such as linseed oil capsules. This you can get from eating seeds, together with fibre. It is much less potent than omega-3s derived from fish oil. In the supplement programmes that follow, this is called an 'essential omega-3 fish oil'.

The best vitamin C supplements

The form of vitamin C itself doesn't make as much difference as people make out. You will see ascorbic acid, ascorbate and 'ester' C – they all work. But there are other nutrients and herbs that support health and immunity. These include zinc, black elderberry extracts and anthocyanidins (for example, in bilberry, which are rich sources of anthocyanidins). (Vitamin C products that contain significant amounts of anthocyanidins will have a purple hue.) A vitamin C supplement that also contains these synergistic ingredients will therefore give you more bang for your buck. Ideally, you want something like 2,000mg of vitamin C in total a day, but you can eat 200mg if you eat six or more servings of the right fruits and vegetables a day. So that leaves 1,800mg – or 900mg taken twice a day. That's a good level for general health maintenance. In the supplement programmes below, this is called a 'vitamin C 1g complex'.

You can also get these basics in a daily pack or strip, which makes life a lot easier. I refer to these three supplements as 'the basics'.

Strip of vitamins

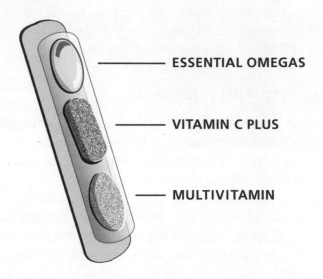

ESSENTIAL OMEGAS

VITAMIN C PLUS

MULTIVITAMIN

Other important combination formulas

Quite a few of the nutrients listed on pages 212–13 are antioxidant nutrients. There are a number of good antioxidant complex formulas that include many of these in one supplement (see Resources).

Look for formulas that provide:

- Glutathione or N-acetyl cysteine (NAC), alpha lipoic acid, vitamin E, vitamin C (not so essential as it's included in the basics above), CoQ_{10}, resveratrol, anthocyanidins, carotenoids and vitamin A. (I take one of these every day for maintaining good health. I will refer to this in the supplement programmes as an 'antioxidant complex'.)

- Chromium is sometimes supplied with either cinnamon, *Garcinia cambogia* (which is high in HCA) or 5-HTP. These last two principally help weight management, although 5-HTP has a very beneficial effect on your mood too, so if that is an issue you might want chromium combined with 5-HTP. I shall call any of these a 'chromium 200mcg plus'. The critical issue is the amount of chromium you take, ranging from the minimal effective dose of 200mcg up to the maximal effect dose of 1,000mcg. (The upper safety level is 10,000mcg a day.) You should not need the high dose for more than a month. Most chromium supplements provide 200mcg per capsule.

Your personal supplement programme

Each programme below is based on a glucose and glycosylated haemoglobin score. Use your scores to choose the right programme for you, but note: these are what you would score if not on medication. If you *are* on medication, and have to keep your blood sugar levels in check, or if you have type-1 diabetes and are dependent on insulin, go for the 'maximum recovery' programme using the gradual ascent as explained in Chapter 2 earlier in this part, and monitor your blood sugar levels carefully, as your need for your medication is likely to reduce rapidly.

If you have type-2 diabetes, but are not taking insulin, start with the 'maximum recovery' programme and work towards the 'maintenance' programme.

If you are trying to reduce your diabetes risk, follow the 'maintenance' programme.

REMEMBER Keep your doctor informed so that he or she can advise you on reducing your drug doses. This is especially important if you are on insulin. Remember also that too many supplements plus medication can over-lower your blood sugar leading to a hypo, so you need to adjust your supplement programme as explained later in this chapter.

IMPORTANT Remember, if you are dependent on insulin, I recommend a more gradual ascent to the 'maximum recovery' programme as explained on page 206. This will give you at least a week to stabilise your insulin needs on your new low-GL diet, before adding the 'maintenance' supplements, then working up to the 'maximum recovery' level so you can learn how to adjust your insulin requirement accordingly.

Choose the best programme for you

Supplements	When to take them
MAINTENANCE (glucose below 5.5; glycosylated haemoglobin below 5.5)	
The basics	twice a day, with meals
Antioxidant complex	once a day, with breakfast or lunch

Chromium 200mcg plus	once a day, with breakfast or lunch
Cinnamon	½ teaspoon or 250mg of extract in chromium pill
Glucomannan or PGX	5g/heaped teaspoon once daily up to 20 minutes before, or just before, dinner with a large glass of water

NEARLY THERE (glucose is between 5.6 and 6.5; glycosylated haemoglobin is between 5.6 and 6)

The basics	twice a day, with meals
Antioxidant complex	twice a day, with breakfast or lunch
Chromium 200mcg plus	twice a day, with breakfast or lunch
Cinnamon	a teaspoon or 500mg of extract in chromium pill
Glucomannan or PGX	5g/heaped teaspoon twice a day up to 20 minutes before, or just before, main meals with a large glass of water

IN RECOVERY (glucose is between 6.6 and 7.5; glycosylated haemoglobin is between 6.1 and 7.5)

The basics	twice a day, with meals
Antioxidant complex	twice a day, with breakfast or lunch
Chromium 200mcg plus	three times a day, with breakfast, lunch and dinner
Cinnamon	a teaspoon or 500mg of extract in chromium pill
Glucomannan or PGX	5g/heaped teaspoon three times a day, up to 20 minutes before, or just before, main meals with a large glass of water

MAXIMUM RECOVERY (glucose above 7.5; glycosylated haemoglobin above 7.5)

The basics	twice a day, with meals
Antioxidant complex	twice a day, with breakfast or lunch
Chromium 200mcg plus	four times a day, two with breakfast, one with lunch and dinner
Cinnamon	a teaspoon or 500mg of extract in chromium pill
Glucomannan or PGX	5g/heaped teaspoon three times a day up to 20 minutes before, or just before, main meals with a large glass of water

Optional extras

You can also add, especially in the 'maximum recovery' category, the following single supplements:

- Alpha lipoic acid (600mg) if you have any signs of neuropathy (explained on page 123).

- CoQ_{10} (90mg) if you are on statins (cholesterol-lowering drugs).

- Milk thistle (600mg) if you have any signs of decreased liver function.

- *Gymnema sylvestre* (400mg) – if your glycosylated haemoglobin is above 7.

- Glutamine powder 5–10g/1–2 heaped teaspoons – if you crave sugar, but this is not advisable if you have advanced liver or kidney disease. Extra amino acids, although helpful, are extra work for these organs of elimination. Otherwise, you could add to your daily fibre drinks.

- Homocysteine-lowering B vitamins (containing at least B_{12} 500mcg, folic acid 500mcg and B_6 20mg) – good to take if your homocysteine level is high, above 9. Certainly don't take more than this if you have advanced kidney disease, colorectal cancer polyps or cancer. This also protects you from the side effects of metformin.

- 5-HTP 100mg – good to take if you are overweight or suffer from low moods and sugar cravings. Don't take if you are on antidepressant medication.

- HCA (*Garcinia cambogia*) 2,000mg – good to take if you are overweight and often hungry. Often comes with chromium.

- High dose niacin (B_3) 1,000mg – good to take if you have high cholesterol and low HDL. Forms that make you blush can destabilise blood sugar, so experiment cautiously.

CAUTION If you are on any other medication, it is advisable to let your doctor know what supplements you are taking in case there is anything that would interfere with it.

In the Resources section I list formulas that contain or combine these nutrients at appropriate doses.

Adjusting your supplement programme

It is important to keep monitoring your daily glucose levels, on rising, as you start to introduce supplements. You can use this to learn what works best for you, both in terms of the diet and the supplements (more on this in Part 3, Chapter 6).

As your glucose levels stabilise you should move from the maximum recovery level towards the maintenance level. Bear in mind that glycosylated haemoglobin is an average of the last three months, so its rate of decrease may lag a bit behind the actual improvement happening in your body. I would suggest you test it every two months until you are in the healthy zone, with a score below 5.5 per cent.

None of these supplements are harmful, but if you are taking medication as well it is possible that too many supplements, plus medication, can over-lower your blood sugar, leading to a hypo. Therefore, it is best to lower the medication first until you need none, then the supplements, especially chromium. Most former diabetics benefit from 200mcg a day on a regular basis as part of their maintenance programme.

Metformin is the least harmful drug, especially if you didn't suffer from any gastrointestinal side effects, and some doctors would recommend staying on this drug, albeit at the lowest dose of 500mg once a day. If so, make sure you monitor your homocysteine level once a year and, at least, take a high-strength multivitamin–mineral containing at least 20mg of vitamin B_6, 10mcg of B_{12} and 200mcg of folic acid.

5

Building Daily Exercise into Your Life

To avoid developing diabetes, or to help reverse it, you need to build exercise into your weekly routine, as I explained in Part 2, Chapter 9. The combination of the optimal diet and optimal exercise is a winning formula. According to a comprehensive review by the American Diabetes Association you need to do two types of exercise – aerobic and resistance:[8]

Aerobic exercise

'To improve glycemic control, assist with weight maintenance, and reduce risk of CVD [cardiovascular disease], we recommend at least 150 minutes per week of moderate-intensity aerobic physical activity [meaning, in your training heart-rate zone, see overleaf].

The physical activity should be distributed over at least 3 days per week and with no more than 2 consecutive days without physical activity.'

Even better is doing slightly shorter sessions, maybe high-intensity exercises three times a week, but you'll need to follow the guidance of a fitness instructor if you have diabetes.

Resistance exercise

'In the absence of contraindications, people with type 2 diabetes should be encouraged to perform resistance exercise three times a week, including all major muscle groups, progressing to three sets of 8–10 repetitions at a weight that cannot be lifted more than 8–10 times.'

These two kinds of exercise, aerobic and resistance, have two different effects. You can think of them as the difference between a long-distance runner and a sprinter. The long-distance runner is lean, while the sprinter has more muscle. The ideal is a bit of both, because you want to burn fat, and when you build muscle you naturally raise your level of growth hormone, which helps to improve insulin sensitivity as well as giving you more muscle to burn more fat.

NOTE Before starting your exercise regime don't forget to check with your doctor, and remember to start off gently and build up as you get fitter. If you join an exercise class of any kind the trainer will advise you how to begin. The advantage of an exercise class is that, contrary to what you might believe, most people are not super-fit but just ordinary people of all fitness levels working hard to improve their fitness, and the classes are often very friendly.

The type of exercise is as important as the duration

If you are doing the right kind of exercise (that is, a mixture of aerobic and resistance), all you need to do is 20–30 minutes a day. And this will be enough both for losing weight and helping to reverse diabetes. If you want to confine your exercising to five days a week, you can do 30 minutes a day with two days off. If you are doing less strenuous exercise you may need to increase your daily time of exercising to 30–45 minutes a day, but it is important to build up the intensity. My advice is to make an appointment in your diary to exercise, just like you would to attend a meeting or see a friend. Then, don't break it.

Aerobic exercise

Depending on your current level of fitness, aerobic exercise can be anything from brisk walking to playing golf, going for a swim or a bike ride or joining an exercise class, but the key is that you get your heart rate into your 'training heart-rate zone'. Turn to Appendix 2 to work this out.

An overweight, out-of-condition person may reach their training heart-rate zone by walking just a few hundred yards. A fitter, leaner person may have to walk briskly for at least five minutes to push their pulse up to their training zone. This is why you need to monitor your pulse while exercising to make sure you do not over- or under-exercise, and to achieve the best benefits for burning fat. As you get fitter and leaner, you'll find that you will have to push harder – perhaps by walking faster or adding more hill walking to your programme – to reach your training zone.

Resistance exercise

Resistance exercise is akin to building muscle, but you don't need to be lifting a whole ton of weight to do this! To understand why this type of exercise is important it's good to know that there are three different kinds of muscle fibres and, ideally, you want more of all three. These are:

1 Slow (red muscle, which contains more oxygen)

2 Fast (white muscle)

3 Super-fast (white muscle)

Your aerobic exercise is working mainly the slow muscle. When you work the fast or, even better, the super-fast muscle – for example in a sprint – this is beyond your oxygen capacity and is called 'anaerobic' exercise – at the end you'll be puffing and panting.

The interesting thing is that if you do the right kind of high-intensity exercise – using and developing super-fast muscle – you don't need to do it for long. It can literally be a 30-second burst of intense exercise, five to eight times. That's it. Do this three times a week and you'll get a great result. It makes your heart muscle work hard, so you'll be really panting at the end of your 30 seconds, and this can increase your growth hormone level by up to five times, which then both re-sensitises you to insulin, and builds muscle.

One of the original proponents of this type of exercising is Phil Campbell, author of *Ready Set Go!* (see Recommended Reading) which is a great book to read if you want to go into this in more detail. He's a trainer of top athletes and sportsmen, but don't be put off by that – the principles are really simple. You can see for yourself by watching the YouTube video, made by Dr Joseph Mercola, who describes a version of these principles as the Peak 8 system (see Resources). This is based on eight sprints, in this case done on an exercise bike, but you can do it with any kind of exercise – sprinting, swimming or cycling, for example. The basic guidelines are as follows:

1 You warm up for three minutes.

2 Now exercise as hard and fast as you can for 30 seconds. You should feel like you couldn't possibly go on for another few seconds.

3 Recover for 90 seconds.

4 Then do it again.

5 Repeat this cycle a total of eight times.

That's the goal, but Rome wasn't built in a day, and it is really important to build up to this if you are currently not in good shape. That might mean doing the sequence only two or three times first time, then adding a repetition as you become more able. At the first level, for example, you might be walking for three minutes, then have a 30-second burst of walking or jogging as fast as you can, then you stop. You want to get your heart rate up into the top end of your training heart-rate zone.

You know you've reached it when it's hard to breathe and talk due to the temporary oxygen debt – you start to sweat, you feel hot and you get some muscle ache. But simply doing this three times a week will make a big difference to your health, building muscle, burning fat and helping restore blood sugar control. This whole sequence takes 20 minutes.

Your weekly routine

Choose the kind of training that appeals to you, making sure the aerobic exercise will raise your heart rate into the training zone. Don't try to do too much to start with. If you are very unfit or overweight it is good to get some professional guidance and support at the beginning. Now plan your week ahead. A typical weekly routine might look like this, but you will need to build up to it if you are very unfit:

Monday – resistance training (20 minutes)
Tuesday – aerobic exercise (30-plus minutes)
Wednesday – resistance training (20 minutes)

Thursday – aerobic exercise (30-plus minutes)
Friday – resistance training (20 minutes)
Saturday – aerobic exercise (30 minutes)
Sunday – day off

If you are working with a fitness instructor, make sure he or she includes both aerobic and resistance training. You are aiming to exercise for at least 150 minutes a week, or 20–30 minutes every day, or 30 minutes five times a week.

When to exercise

The best time to exercise is two hours after eating. No self-respecting animal would eat before exercising. From an evolutionary perspective the purpose of exercise is to get food to eat. If you exercise first thing in the morning, make sure you have breakfast straight after. When you eat after exercising your muscles and liver are geared up to deal with the carbohydrates in your food so you don't get such big spikes in your blood sugar.

Having said that, going for a stroll after a main meal – for example after Sunday lunch – then having your dessert after the walk, also helps to stabilise blood sugar levels.

Don't exercise late at night. Also, if possible, exercise in natural day-light because you'll make vitamin D, which strengthens bones.

Warm up before aerobic exercise by starting off slowly, and before resistance exercises warm up by walking or stretching.

Increase your base-line activity

One great way to increase your general level of exercise is simply to get more active generally. Use the stairs instead of the lift. Walk or cycle instead of driving everywhere. Run around with your kids, or take up a sport. There are many ways in a day to develop fitness, and soon this way of living becomes a habit.

Get fit by taking the alternative way

The fat way	The fit way
Take a lift	Use the stairs
Use a trolley when shopping	Use a hand basket
Drive to work	Walk or cycle some of the way
Drive to the shops	Walk to the shops
Spend the night watching TV	Take up an active hobby
Get other people to bring you one too!	Get up and do it yourself
Use powered tools for gardening or DIY work	Use manual tools when it's just as quick
Go upstairs as little as possible at home	Run upstairs as often as possible
Use automatic car washes	Wash the car yourself
Stick children in front of TV	Actively play with them
Have business meetings inside	Go for a walk where possible

6

Charting Your Progress

You are unique and the best way for you to learn what works for you in terms of diet, supplements, exercise and lifestyle strategies is to monitor what happens to your blood sugar levels as you make changes.

Food is complex, and the GL of a meal is going to be different if, for example, you add more protein or take super-fibres or chromium before a meal. Only by monitoring what happens can you adjust accordingly. If, for example, you find that chromium and super-fibres make a big difference and you are at a function where it is very hard to stick to the 10 GL rule, you can learn that having a fibre drink and supplementing chromium can effectively lower the GL of the meal you are about to eat.

Also, you won't need high doses of chromium for ever if you follow this regime. So, how do you know when 600mcg of chromium is too much? The answer is when your drug-free blood glucose levels are dipping too low. You can then experiment with cutting back to 400mcg (one with breakfast, one with lunch). If your blood sugar level is still on the low side, then cut back to 200mcg as a maintenance dose. Most people are able to cut back to this maintenance dose within six months. But the only way for you to find out is to chart your progress.

In Appendix 6, page 304, you will find a chart, which you are free to photocopy, to help you keep track of your results.

On page 305, you will also see an example of how to use the chart. In the space for diet notes you can use abbreviations; for example, 'GUG' might mean Get Up & Go, or 'porridge' might mean your morning porridge, plus seeds and berries. If you try out a new recipe or combination, it's good to write this down to see what effect it has on your blood sugar level. You won't want to fill out everything you eat every day, but it is useful to do so for the first couple of weeks and whenever you start to make significant changes, perhaps adding or changing your supplements or medication.

The space for notes is there for you to write down something you have learnt or noticed.

Keeping these records of your glucose levels will also help you to monitor your progress. From these notes you can plot your glucose graph over a month, noting significant changes. This kind of information is most useful for your doctor or other health-care provider that you are working with. It also helps you see what works for you.

7

Keeping Yourself Free from Diabetes

Some people, enthused and inspired by the realisation that they can reverse diabetes, get stuck in, following the diet and supplements to the letter, exercising regularly and, sure enough, getting great results. Some stick at it for a month or two and then slip back to old habits. Others find it hard to get going despite knowing the vast stakes involved if you don't do anything. There are two reasons for this. The first is that change isn't easy. We are creatures of habit. The second is that there are very often underlying issues behind our eating habits. These usually revolve around your self-image, your self-esteem and emotional and psychological issues in life and relationships.

Sometimes, as you start to lose weight these issues and feelings come to the surface. As you start to take control of your diet and health it gives you the power to start to take control of your life. If there was a way to package it in a book I'd like to offer you psychological support as you start the process of reclaiming your life. An alternative is to see a psychotherapist to help explore the barriers that stop you really taking care of yourself. This is well worth doing if you are stuck – you know you need to change but just can't do it.

Join a Zest4Life group

Another excellent way forward is to join one of my Zest4Life groups, based on my GL principles. These are run throughout the UK and Ireland, as well as in South Africa and Dubai, and are fast spreading into other countries. To find a group near you go to www.zest4life.eu (also see Resources). A Zest4Life group is run by a fully qualified and registered nutritional therapist who has been trained by my team in coaching, motivational techniques and how to uncover, and help you work through, the barriers and obstacles that stop you achieving your goals. Each group runs for ten weeks and you attend once a week for two hours. They run groups in the evenings and in the daytime, so whether you are a mum with kids at school or are at work during the day you'll find a group that works for you.

Most people who join a Zest4Life group want, among other things, to lose weight. Some have diabetes, some have cardiovascular disease, some have low energy and mood. Whichever way, the process is very successful. In a recent audit of 295 people in a Zest4Life group, over a period of six weeks, these were the results:

- over 95 per cent lost weight
- 47 per cent lost more than 3.2kg (7lb)
- 9 per cent lost over 6.3kg (1 stone/14lb)
- 95 per cent reported greater energy levels
- 83 per cent reported greater concentration, memory and alertness
- 79 per cent reported improved sleep quality
- 73 per cent experienced reduced stress levels
- 73 per cent reported improved skin and hair health

Here's what a few of the diabetic participants had to say after only six weeks:

> *'Due to the fact that I have been able to control my blood sugar levels on this programme, I have been able to halve my diabetes medication – my goal would be to dispense with them all. This is the best diet regime I have experienced and the only one where I have felt I am changing my eating habits for ever.'*
>
> *'Very happy, and insulin levels have gone back to normal, so no need for medication!'*

If you prefer to work one to one, my website www.patrickholford. com contains a directory of nutritional therapists trained in delivering results with the low-GL diet.

Results from the Zest4Life Diabetes Trial

We recently completed a 12-week project to assess the impact of the Zest4Life low-GL diet on a group of 21 patients at a GP surgery in Berkshire. All the participants had been identified as being at high risk of developing diabetes and/or heart disease, and exhibited one or more of the following risk factors:

- impaired fasting glucose
- elevated glycosylated haemoglobin (HbA1c)
- waist-to-hip ratio greater than 1 for men or 0.85 for women
- elevated blood pressure
- elevated LDL, and HDL and triglycerides outside target range

Patients were encouraged to follow the low-GL eating plan and were supported in making lifestyle changes, including exercise and developing new habits. Nutritional supplements were not used as we wanted to test the effects of the diet plus lifestyle changes alone. The clinical markers for chronic disease listed above were measured at the beginning of the programme and again at the end of 12 weeks, and weight and body composition were tracked during the 12 weeks.

The results speak for themselves. Everyone taking part lost weight and nine of the 21 participants lost over a stone (7kg). For the majority of participants, there was a clinically significant reduction in most of the markers.

Health markers	Before	After 12 weeks	% reduction
Average weight	202lb	187lb	7.42%
	92kg	85kg	
Average HbA1c	6.9	5.9	14.5%
Average fasting glucose	6.3	5.6	11.1%
Average total cholesterol	5.27	4.59	12.9%
Cholesterol/HDL ratio	4.12	3.69	8.7%

The average reduction in HbA1c results at the end of 12 weeks was approximately 14.5 per cent; the most significant individual reduction observed was 29 per cent, going from 7.8 to 5.5. Most of the fasting glucose results had improved, as had cholesterol and blood pressure. Henry is a great example – at the start he weighed 19 stone 2lb, his HbA1c was 6.8 and his blood pressure was 131/84. By the end of 12 weeks Henry had lost 31lb (14kg) and weighed 16 stone 13lb, his HbA1c was down to 5.8 and his blood pressure was 116/66. His cholesterol ratio had also reduced from 4.2 to 3.7. He said, 'My levels of energy were noticeably higher even after only a few weeks and the health improvements in both my body and mind have given me the incentive to maintain these changes for life.'

Such comments were representative of the whole group. Everyone felt they had gained significant benefit from the programme in a range of ways, including improved energy levels, elevated mood or a lifting of depression, better sleep, less stress and anxiety, and even improved confidence and self-esteem. The GPs and practice nurses supporting the programme have been impressed with the results and plans are underway to determine how to take this forward.

The Zest4Life team of nutritional therapists was lead by Ann Garry, who commented, 'In week one of the programme the patient group appeared defeated, resigned and exhausted but over the weeks we have witnessed a dramatic transformation. They became lively, energetic, engaged and positive and I'm confident that they are now equipped with the knowledge to continue their journey to optimum health.'

The 3/6/36 rule

You may know that it takes roughly three weeks to break a habit, six weeks to make a habit, and 36 weeks to hardwire a habit. That is why it is most important to commit to your Anti-diabetes Action Plan for at least six weeks. If you can hardwire these changes to your diet and lifestyle over 36 weeks (about nine months), there's very little chance you'll slip back into bad habits. This should be your long-term goal.

Personalising your GL

Even though, in the early phases, I've recommended you eat 40–45 ⓖ a day in total, the truth is that your ideal daily GL is whatever keeps your blood sugar level in check. Also, it will vary according to your height and the amount of exercise you do. The chart below shows you your ideal daily GL to lose weight and stabilise your blood sugar, according to your height and frequency of exercise.

Your ideal daily GL intake to lose weight according to your height and activity level

		Average exercise per day (mins)						
		0	**15**	**30**	**45**	**60**	**90**	**120**
	5 ft (1.52m)	35	35	40	45	45	50	55
	5 ft 3 (1.60m)	40	40	40	45	50	55	60
	5 ft 6 (1.67m)	40	40	40	45	50	55	60
Height	5 ft 9 (1.75m)	40	40	45	50	55	60	65
	6 ft (1.83m)	45	45	50	55	60	65	70
	6 ft 3 (1.91m)	50	50	55	60	65	70	75
	6 ft 6 (1.98m)	55	55	60	65	70	75	80

Once you achieve your ideal weight and get your blood sugar balance under control, you can move on to a maintenance level of ⓖⓛ. For most people this is 60 ⓖⓛ rather than 45. This might mean a 10-GL serving of carbohydrates with each main meal and 10-GL snacks rather than 5-GL snacks. That gives you an additional 15 ⓖⓛ each day. By monitoring your glucose levels and your weight you'll be able to find the best diet for you. You should be neither hungry nor eating more than you need. If you do find yourself slipping, go back on the diet strictly for two weeks.

Another great way to keep yourself informed and motivated is to join my on-line 100% Health Club. That way we will stay in touch and, if you have any questions you can ask them in our diabetes forum. See the details on page 325, at the end of this book.

Your feedback is most welcome

In my experience the combination of the right nutrients, together with diet and exercise, is what really works. These recommendations are constantly being adjusted as new studies become available and I receive feedback. You can leave your feedback, read and share comments, and ask questions at www.patrickholford.com/diabetes

Now I leave you with Part 4, giving you a wide choice of recipes for breakfast, main meals, starters and snacks. I hope you will find them tempting as you start to enjoy balancing your blood sugar level and feeling well again.

Wishing you the very best of health and happiness.

Patrick Holford

PART FOUR

Recipes for Reversing Diabetes

The two comments I hear again and again from people on my low-GL diet are, firstly, that the recipes are delicious and, secondly, after a few months they say, 'It's not a diet, it's just become how I eat.' This is really important for you to know, because the only long-term solution has to be something you enjoy and something that becomes second nature. In this part you will find tempting recipes for breakfast, lunch, snacks, starters, main meals, side vegetables and desserts, as well as menu suggestions.

1

The Sample Menus

The reason people find my diet so easy to incorporate as part of their lives, I believe, is that the low-GL principles really are in sync with how we are designed as human beings. Your body will love this food and you will love the effects of eating this way – the clear-headedness, the emotional stability, the big increase in energy, and the effortless weight loss, if you have weight to lose.

I am deeply indebted to my wonderful 'kitchen wizard', Fiona McDonald Joyce, who trained with me at the Institute for Optimum Nutrition, and knows how to design delicious menus applying the principles in this book. Over the past decade we have built up a library of delicious recipes – many are so simple to make that you can prepare a meal in under two minutes. Others you could serve at any dinner party and get star ratings even if the guests had no idea the meal was low-GL and super-healthy.

We now have three books full of low-GL recipes: *The Low-GL Diet Bible*, *The Low-GL Diet Cookbook* and *Food GLorious Food*. Between them there are over 300 delicious recipes to choose from for every occasion, from a quick snack or lunch to a three-course dinner. In *Food GLorious Food* we collected low-GL recipes from around the world – including Indian, Thai, Middle Eastern, African and Mediterranean. Not all of these recipes are as low as those in the *Low-GL Diet Cookbook*, so they may not be your first choice in the first month on this diet, but once your blood sugar level has stabilised and you move into the maintenance phase, they will be perfect.

The recipes in this book are here to get you started and to show you how, in real terms, to apply the low-GL principles. I've created three days of menus so that you can also see how to put the recipes together to make a day of low-GL eating, scoring 40 ⒼⓁ. These recipes include the extra 5 ⒼⓁ reserved for drinks or desserts; however, in the first two weeks you need to leave these out (unless you have type-1 diabetes or are currently injecting insulin), as described in Part 3, Chapters 1 and 2.

Make your own recipes

You can also make your own low-GL recipes and menus. All you need is to refer to the list showing the ⒼⓁ of foods in Appendix 4, or you can access the Low-GL Counter on my website www.holforddiet.com. This allows you to enter the ingredients of a recipe, see what the total GL adds up to, and then you can adjust the proportion of the ingredients to achieve 10 ⒼⓁ for a main meal and 5 ⒼⓁ for a snack.

Sample Menus

Day 1
Breakfast	Scots oats with apple compote and seeds
Mid-morning snack	Pear with pumpkin seeds
Lunch	Artichoke and Red Pepper Tortilla with a green leaf salad
Mid-afternoon snack	Smoked Salmon Pâté with toasted rye bread
Dinner	Chickpea Curry with brown basmati rice
Drink or dessert★	Chocolate Ice Cream

★(not in the first two weeks)

Day 2
Breakfast	Get Up & Go
Mid-morning snack	Sardines on rye toast
Lunch	Green Bean, Olive and Roasted Pepper Salad with feta cheese and a green leaf salad
Mid-afternoon snack	An apple and 5 almonds
Dinner	Sesame Chicken and Soba Noodle Steam-fry
Drink or dessert★	Kiwi and Coconut Pudding

★(not in the first two weeks)

Day 3

Breakfast	Scrambled, boiled or poached eggs and oatcakes
Mid-morning snack	Fruit and Yoghurt Shake
Lunch	Quinoa Taboulleh and steamed green beans
Mid-afternoon snack	A pear and 5 walnuts
Dinner	Pesto-crusted Salmon with Roast Squash and Sweet Potatoes with Shallots and steamed broccoli
Drink or dessert*	Plum Amaretti Slices

*(not in the first two weeks)

2

Breakfasts

Never skip breakfast. It's an essential start to the day.

Apple and Cinnamon Compote

Apples are full of fibre and vitamins and are one of the lowest GL fruits. This compote is delicious with muesli or porridge oats. Serves 2

1 Bramley (cooking) apple, unpeeled, cored and diced
¼ tsp ground ginger or ½ tsp cinnamon
1 tsp xylitol
2 tsp lemon juice

Put all of the ingredients in a pan, cover and gently stew until the apples soften and start to disintegrate (this takes about 10 minutes), stirring from time to time so that they do not stick to the pan base.

ⓖ per serving: 5
Serving suggestion: serve with Low-carb muesli (see page 243) or porridge, or as a pudding with a scoop of ice cream or crème fraîche.
Variations: use other low-GL fruits such as apricots, plums, berries or pears instead of the apple.
Allergy suitability: gluten, wheat, dairy, yeast free.

Boiled, Poached or Scrambled Egg and Toast

This simple breakfast makes a wholesome start to the day. Eggs are good for you – they don't raise cholesterol! Choose organic, free-range eggs, preferably omega-3 eggs. Serves 1

    1 or 2 free-range eggs
    ground black pepper
    knob of butter
    1 thin slice wholegrain rye toast or 4 oatcakes

1 Cook the egg to your taste – boil for 3–4 minutes for a soft egg *or* crack the egg into a pan of simmering water and poach for 3–4 minutes. Alternatively, beat the egg with a dash of skimmed or soya milk and cook slowly in a small pan with a small knob of butter, stirring constantly. Sprinkle liberally with black pepper before serving.
2 Serve with one very lightly buttered thin slice of wholegrain rye toast or oatcakes.

ⓖ per serving: 8; 6 with 3 oatcakes
Serving suggestion: add a small slice of smoked salmon. Add some chopped parsley or chives to the scrambled egg.

Fruit Yoghurt or Yoghurt Shake

Low-fat, live, natural yoghurt is a first-class food containing friendly bacteria that have a spring-cleaning effect on your digestive system, as well as being a good source of protein. In yoghurt the sugar (lactose) is converted into lactic acid which lowers the GL of the meal. Serves 1

> 280g (10oz) very low-fat live yoghurt
> 1 tsp xylitol
> 1 serving of fruit (apple, pear, berries, kiwi)
> 2 tsp ground flax and pumpkin seeds

Combine all the ingredients or, if you prefer, make a shake by processing the mix in a blender.

ⓖ per serving: 7

Allergy suitability: gluten, wheat, yeast free.

Get Up & Go

Healthy Get Up & Go is a powdered breakfast drink, which is blended with skimmed milk or soya milk and berries. Nutritionally speaking, it is the ultimate breakfast: each serving gives you more fibre than a bowl of porridge, more protein than an egg, more iron than a cooked breakfast and more vitamins and minerals than a whole packet of cornflakes. In fact, every serving of Get Up & Go gives you at least 100 per cent of every vitamin and mineral and a lot more of some key nutrients. For example, you get 1,000mg of vitamin C – the equivalent of more than 20 oranges.

Get Up & Go contains no sucrose, no additives, no animal products, no yeast, wheat or milk, and it tastes delicious. Each serving, with 300ml (10fl oz/½ pint) skimmed milk or soya milk and some fruit, provides 3 ⓖ and fewer than 300 calories and, when mixed up, only 8 ⓖ, making it ideal as part of your Anti-diabetes Diet. If you use oat milk, a serving equals 10 ⓖ. It is nutritionally superior to any other breakfast choice and is totally suitable for adults and children alike. It is fine to have this for breakfast every day, if you choose.

Make it up with berries such as strawberries, raspberries or blueberries, or a soft pear. If you use banana use no more than a third of a decent-sized banana. Get Up & Go is widely available in health-food stores (see Resources). Serves 1

300ml (10fl oz/½ pint) skimmed milk or low-fat soya milk
2 heaped tbsp berries or a soft pear
2 tsp ground chia seeds (optional)
1 serving Get Up & Go powder

Blend the milk, fruit, seeds and Get Up & Go powder.

Ⓖ per serving: 8
Allergy suitability: dairy, wheat, yeast free (contains soya, nuts, sesame seeds, gluten).

Low-GL Muesli

A chewy, satisfying recipe that is lower in carbs than standard muesli, my low-GL version features more nuts and seeds than grains and has no dried fruit (which is very high in sugar). It is also wheat- and sugar-free, unlike most of the shop-bought ones available, but you can use a little xylitol to sweeten it, if you like. Serves 2

115g (4oz) whole oat flakes
50g (2oz) ground or flaked almonds
2 tbsp pumpkin seeds
2 tbsp macadamia nuts, roughly chopped
2 tbsp sunflower seeds
1 tsp xylitol (optional)

Stir all the ingredients together until well mixed.

Ⓖ per serving: 4
Serving suggestion: serve with 1 tbsp blueberries per person, or fruit compote (see page 240) and live natural yoghurt or soya yoghurt, or skimmed milk, soya milk or nut milk.
Variations: vary the nuts (such as pecan nuts or hazelnuts instead of the macadamia nuts).
Allergy suitability: wheat, dairy, yeast free.

Oat Pancakes

Once you've eaten an oat pancake they'll become your favourite. Made by putting oat flakes in a grinder, this simple combination of oat flour and egg, with cinnamon, is a delicious and simple low-GL breakfast, served with berries and yoghurt. Makes two large pancakes, or four small ones. Serves 2

> 75g (3oz) oat flakes (a full mug's worth), ground in a grinder
> 1 large egg
> 125ml (4fl oz) milk or soya milk, diluted with a little water
> 1 tsp cinnamon
> knob of butter or 1 tsp olive oil

1 Combine all the ingredients and whisk (or mix in a blender).
2 Heat a little butter or olive oil in a frying pan on a medium heat, then drop in a large dollop of the mixture. Allow to cook on the underside for a few minutes before turning over.
3 Repeat until all the mixture is cooked.

ⓖ per serving: 5
Serving suggestion: lightly butter with a sugar-free berry jam or agave syrup or a hint of honey. Serve with a cup of berries, such as blueberries or strawberries, and 1 tbsp yoghurt. Total: 9 ⓖ
Allergy suitability: dairy, wheat and yeast free.

Plum Yoghurt Crunch

This recipe is based on the fruit and yoghurt cups with a granola topping that you can get in sandwich shops and coffee bars, but it is lower in saturated fat and sugar. Plums are one of the lowest GL fruits, but they still have a lovely natural sweetness, while the live yoghurt contains probiotic bacteria for digestive health. Serves 2

> 2 plums, stoned and chopped
> 200g (7oz) live natural yoghurt
> ½ tbsp hazelnuts
> ½ tbsp macadamia nuts
> 1 tbsp ground chia seeds (or flax seeds)
> ½ tbsp pumpkin seeds

1 tbsp flaked almonds
½ tsp xylitol

1 Put the chopped plums in two short glasses and spoon the yoghurt on top.
2 Grind the hazelnuts, macadamia nuts, chia and pumpkin seeds, and stir in the flaked almonds and xylitol.
3 Sprinkle on top of the yoghurt and serve.

Ⓖ per serving: 4
Variations: vary the nuts and seeds on top. Use 1 pear, 2 apricots or a portion of fruit compote (see page 240) instead of the plums.
Allergy suitability: gluten, wheat, yeast free.

Scots Rough Porridge with Cinnamon and Apple

On a cold winter's day nothing can be more warming than porridge. Oats contain beta-glucans which stabilise your blood sugar. If you add oat bran you get an even better blood-sugar stabilising effect. Serves 1

300ml (10fl oz/½ pint) water
300ml (10fl oz/½ pint) skimmed or soya milk
55g (2oz) porridge oats
1 heaped tsp oat bran
½ tsp cinnamon
2 tsp ground chia, flax and pumpkin seeds
½ apple, grated
½ tsp honey or 1 tsp xylitol

1 Put the water and half the milk in a pan and sprinkle in the oats, oat bran and cinnamon.
2 Bring to the boil and simmer for 3–5 minutes, stirring all the time.
3 Serve with milk, seeds, grated apple and a little honey or xylitol.

Ⓖ per serving: 6
Variations: vary the fruits. Add a handful of berries or one sliced pear instead of the apple.
Allergy suitability: gluten, wheat, yeast free.

Smoked Trout Omelette

The combination of egg and oily fish makes a perfect low-GL meal, with plenty of omega-3s and protein to fill you up. Serves 1

> 2 medium eggs
> a pinch of Solo or sea salt
> 1 slice smoked trout, chopped
> 1 tbsp coconut oil or olive oil
> ground black pepper

1 Beat the eggs with the salt and pepper and add the smoked trout pieces.
2 Melt the oil in an omelette pan or medium frying pan then pour in the beaten egg mixture. Quickly stir the omelette to allow the raw egg to come into contact with the pan base and start to set.
3 Let the omelette cook through until it is set at the edges and starting to set on top (this will take a couple of minutes) then carefully insert a heatproof spatula underneath and push it around the pan to detach the omelette. Flip it over (this is easiest done by inverting it onto a plate then sliding it back into the pan) to allow the other side to set (this will only take 30 seconds or so). Remove from the heat and serve.

ⓖⓛ per serving: 0
Serving suggestion: either serve it by itself or fold it up and place it in a toasted pitta bread pocket or on toasted rye bread and serve with grilled tomatoes.
Variations: melt 1 tbsp crème fraîche with some chopped chives or parsley and spoon it into the middle of the omelette once it is on the plate.
Other omelette ideas include: smoked salmon and chive omelette, Parmesan with pumpkin seeds omelette, roasted pepper and artichoke omelette, pea and ham omelette, courgette and cherry tomato omelette, onion and mushroom omelette, mushroom and crème fraîche omelette (sauté mushrooms, add crème fraîche and allow to melt, stir in chopped herbs).
Allergy suitability: gluten, wheat, dairy, yeast free.

Smoked Kippers with Pumpernickel Bread

The kipper here provides omega-3 essential fats and good-quality protein. With pumpernickel bread or oatcakes this will fill you up for hours to come. Serves 2

75g (3oz) smoked kipper
1 slice pumpernickel bread, lightly buttered

1 Warm the kippers according to the pack instructions.
2 Serve on lightly buttered toasted pumpernickel bread.

ⓖ per serving: 5
Serving suggestion: try with oatcakes – they become soft with the juices from the kipper.

3

Snacks, Starters and Light Lunches

Remember that it's good for you to eat little and often, so snacks and a light lunch are important ways to keep your blood sugar level even.

Artichoke and Red Pepper Tortilla

Although potatoes have a fairly high GL, the protein from the eggs balance out the overall GL score. This version uses antipasti vegetables but you could experiment with anything you have in the fridge.
Serves 2

120g (4¼oz) baby new potatoes (about 6), scrubbed, cut into small cubes
1 tbsp coconut oil or olive oil
2 garlic cloves, crushed
2 roasted red peppers, about 150g (5½oz), cubed
2 tbsp marinated artichoke hearts, drained and mashed or chopped into
   chunks
4 medium eggs
½ tsp dried oregano
Solo or sea salt and ground black pepper

1 Put the potatoes in a small pan and just cover with cold water. Bring to the boil and simmer, covered, for 10 minutes, or until the potatoes are soft. Drain and set to one side.
2 Heat the oil in a medium frying pan (or use a small pan if you are making this for one person) and fry the garlic for 30 seconds. Add the potatoes and sauté for 5 minutes or so.
3 Stir the peppers and artichokes into the pan and reduce the heat.
4 Beat the eggs with the pepper, a little salt and the oregano. Pour evenly over the vegetable mixture in the pan and stir to expose the egg on top to the heat on the base of the pan. Leave the tortilla cooking over a low to medium heat for 6 minutes or until the eggs are set (the edges and base should be set, with the top still a little soft, as it carries on cooking after you remove it from the heat).
5 Remove the pan from the heat and loosen the edges and base with a palette knife. Turn the tortilla out onto a plate. Serve hot or cold.

ⒼⓁ per serving: 9
Serving suggestion: all this needs is a simple tomato and red onion salad and perhaps some lettuce.
Variations: omit the artichokes if you like, and use double the amount of peppers, or add some pitted black olives or sunblush tomatoes.
Allergy suitability: gluten, wheat, dairy free.

Chestnut and Butterbean Soup

A tasty soup that is an all-time favourite at our cookery demonstrations. Chestnuts have the lowest fat content of all nuts and a pleasantly sweet flavour that goes well with the smooth texture from the butterbeans. This is very filling and cooks quickly with minimal effort on your part. Serves 2

> 200g (7oz) cooked and peeled chestnuts (available vacuum-packed in
>   boxes, cans or jars)
> 400g (14oz) can butterbeans, drained and rinsed
> 1 medium white onion, chopped
> 1 large carrot, chopped
> 3 tsp Marigold reduced-salt vegetable bouillon powder dissolved in 600ml
>   (1 pint) water
> ground black pepper

1 Put all the ingredients (except for a handful of the chestnuts) in a pan, cover with a lid and bring to the boil, then simmer gently for 15–20 minutes.
2 Purée the soup until smooth, then season with pepper.
3 Sprinkle the reserved chestnuts on top to serve.

ⓖⓛ per serving: 6
Allergy suitability: gluten, wheat, dairy, yeast free.

Green Bean, Olive and Roasted Pepper Salad

A Spanish-style salad that goes well stuffed in a pitta bread pocket. Or, optionally, add some black-eyed beans (5 ⓖⓛ per ½ cup). Serves 2

> 2 medium eggs
> 200g (7oz) French beans, topped and tailed
> 1 tsp red wine vinegar
> 1 tbsp olive oil
> 1 small red onion, finely chopped
> 2 roasted red peppers, finely chopped
> a handful black olives, stoned and halved
> Solo or sea salt and ground black pepper

1 Hard-boil the eggs for 8 minutes, then cool rapidly under cold water until they are cold. Shell and slice.
2 Steam the beans until al dente, then refresh under cold running water to keep the deep green colour. Dry well on kitchen paper and put in a bowl.
3 Whisk the vinegar into the oil and season, then toss over the beans.
4 Put the beans in a serving dish, stir through the onion, red pepper and olives, then gently scatter the egg over the top.

ⓖⓛ per serving: 3
Variations: use runner beans or sugar snap peas instead of French beans.
Allergy suitability: gluten, wheat, dairy, yeast free.

Hot Smoked Trout with Pumpkin Seed Pesto and Watercress Open Sandwich

This recipe is bursting with essential fats and is absolutely delicious.
Serves 2

> 2 slices of thin pumpernickel-style rye bread (check the packet to make
>   sure it is wheat-free, as some brands sneak wheat in)
> 1 tbsp pumpkin seed pesto (see overleaf)
> 1 hot smoked trout fillet, flaked
> 1 handful of watercress, roughly chopped
> ground black pepper

1 Toast the rye bread and spread with the pesto.
2 Put the flaked fish on top and scatter with watercress.
3 Season with black pepper and serve.

ⓖⓛ per serving: 6
Variations: use hot smoked salmon instead of trout, or normal (cold) smoked salmon or trout rather than hot smoked fish.
Allergy suitability: Wheat, dairy free.

Pumpkin Seed Pesto

This can be stirred through soup or pasta, spread onto rye bread or added to bean or lentil salads. It tastes amazing and, unlike standard pesto, it does not contain any Parmesan. Plus the pumpkin seed butter and Udo's Choice or olive oil provide a rich source of essential fats. Serves 2

25g (1oz) pumpkin seeds
40g (1½oz) pumpkin seed butter
15g (½oz) flat-leaf parsley leaves
15g (½oz) basil leaves
1 garlic clove, crushed
1 tsp lemon juice
½ tbsp Udo's Choice oil blend or cold-pressed extra virgin olive oil

1 Grind the pumpkin seeds until roughly chopped.
2 Put the pumpkin seed butter into a small blender or food processor with the pumpkin seeds, herbs, garlic and lemon juice. Blitz until the mixture is well combined.
3 Add the olive oil and mix until the pesto is an even consistency.

Ⓖ per serving: 1
Allergy suitability: gluten, wheat, dairy, yeast free.

Hummus

Chickpeas have a unique taste, which combines well with tahini, a paste of ground sesame seeds. You may prefer to buy ready-made hummus, which is widely available in supermarkets. Serves 2

400g (14oz) can chickpeas, drained and rinsed
2 garlic cloves, crushed
2 tbsp olive oil
juice of ½ lemon
2 tsp tahini
Solo or sea salt
pinch of cayenne pepper, plus extra to garnish

1 Put all the ingredients into a food processor or blender and blend until smooth and creamy, adding a little water if necessary. Check the flavour and adjust according to preference.
2 Garnish with a little cayenne pepper.

gl per serving: 5
Serving suggestion: serve with oatcakes, rye bread or crudités.
Allergy suitability: gluten, wheat, dairy, yeast free.

Quinoa Taboulleh

Using quinoa instead of bulgur wheat provides first-class protein for this Middle Eastern dish. You could double up the quantities and keep some in the fridge to take to work. Serves 2

140g (5oz) quinoa
vegetable bouillon (2 parts liquid to 1 part quinoa)
¼ cucumber, sliced lengthways into quarters, then finely sliced horizontally (making tiny triangles)
2 good handfuls cherry tomatoes, chopped to the same size as the cucumber
4 spring onions, finely sliced
good handful fresh mint, finely chopped
good handful fresh flat-leaf parsley, finely chopped
1–2 tbsp olive oil
1 tbsp lemon juice
2 tsp balsamic vinegar, or to taste
Solo or sea salt and ground black pepper

1 Bring the quinoa to the boil in a pan with the bouillon, then cover, reduce the heat and simmer for 10–15 minutes or until the liquid is absorbed and the grains are fluffy. Put the quinoa in a bowl and leave to cool.
2 When at room temperature, mix in the chopped vegetables and herbs, then add the oil, lemon juice and vinegar. Season.
3 Put in the fridge for at least an hour to allow the flavours to develop.

ⓖⓛ per serving: 8
Variations: replace the cucumber, cherry tomatoes and spring onions with chickpeas tossed in cumin, garlic and the zest and juice of ½ lemon, roasted at 200°C/400°F/Gas 6 for 30 minutes.
Allergy suitability: gluten, dairy, yeast free.

Sardines on Toast

This may take you back to your childhood. Sardines are endowed with lashings of omega-3 fats, and make a fast, delicious meal served this way. Just add a big green salad. Serves 2

    2 slices of rye bread
    2 tbsp olive oil
    2 tomatoes, sliced
    175g (6oz) sardines in brine, drained
    ground black pepper

1 Toast the bread and drizzle with the olive oil.
2 Put the tomato slices and sardines on the toast and season with black pepper.

ⓖⓛ per serving: 8
Allergy suitability: dairy free.

Smoked Salmon Pâté

This could be a great dinner party starter. The cannellini beans provide long-term energy and are a healthier alternative to the cream in most fish pâtés. Serves 2

    200g (7oz) smoked salmon trimmings
    200g (7oz) canned cannellini beans, rinsed and drained
    juice of ½ lemon
    a drizzle of water or olive oil (to loosen if the mixture is too thick)
    1 tbsp chopped fresh parsley
    1 tbsp chopped fresh dill
    Solo or sea salt and ground black pepper

Blend all the ingredients in a food processor or blender until the mixture is really smooth, adding a little oil or water to loosen the mixture if you like, then chill and serve.

Ⓖ per serving: 5
Allergy suitability: gluten, wheat, dairy, yeast free.

Spicy Pumpkin and Tofu Soup*

A wonderfully warming soup that is a completely balanced meal, with hidden protein power from the tofu. Serves 4

1 tbsp olive oil
1 large onion, finely chopped
2 garlic cloves, crushed
2 large butternut squash, diced
1½ tsp cumin
1 tsp dried coriander
¼ tsp chilli powder
½ tsp freshly grated nutmeg
1 tsp fresh thyme, chopped
3 vegetable stock cubes dissolved in 1 litre (1¾ pints) hot water
1 packet of Cauldron Organic Tofu, drained
Solo or sea salt and ground black pepper to taste
parsley and chives, freshly chopped, to garnish

1 Heat the olive oil in a large pan. Add the chopped onion and garlic, and gently cook over a low heat until the onion has softened.
2 Add the diced squash, cumin, coriander, chilli, nutmeg, thyme and stock. Bring to the boil, turn down the heat and simmer for 15 minutes.
3 Blend the tofu in a food processor and set aside.
4 Once the soup has simmered for 15 minutes, allow to cool slightly, then liquidise and return to the pan.
5 Whisk in the tofu using a balloon whisk, a tablespoon at a time, and gently reheat. Season to taste, then add the fresh herbs and serve.
* Courtesy of Cauldron Foods.

Ⓖ per serving: 6
Allergy suitability: gluten, dairy, yeast free.

Walnut and Three-bean Salad

No foods are better than beans for satisfying your appetite and giving stamina. It helps if they're served in a delicious, crunchy salad such as this one. Serves 2

400g (14oz) canned mixed beans (such as haricots, chickpeas and flageolet beans), rinsed and drained
a handful of walnuts, roughly chopped
½ apple, cubed
2 tsp chopped fresh flat-leaf parsley or chives
1 tbsp olive oil
1 tbsp walnut oil or olive oil
juice of ½ lemon
1 celery stick, finely chopped
Solo or sea salt and ground black pepper

Combine all the ingredients and serve with mixed salad leaves (such as baby spinach, rocket and watercress).

Ⓖ per serving: 3
Allergy suitability: gluten, wheat, dairy, yeast free.

4

Main Meals

I think you'll find that my main meal recipes are far from dull. They are low in ⓖ but full of flavour and variety.

Borlotti Bolognese

This, a mouth-watering vegan alternative to the classic Spag Bol, is packed with fibre and lycopene (an antioxidant found richly in cooked tomatoes). It can be prepared in batches and frozen for convenience. Serves 2

> 2 tsp coconut oil or olive oil
> 2 garlic cloves, crushed
> 1 onion, chopped
> 115g (4oz) button mushrooms, sliced
> 1½ tsp Marigold reduced-salt vegetable bouillon powder
> 1 tsp herbes de Provence
> 1½ tbsp tomato purée
> 200g (7oz) canned tomatoes
> 400g (14oz) can of borlotti beans, drained and rinsed
> Solo or sea salt
> ground black pepper

1 Heat the coconut or olive oil and cook the garlic and onion gently for 2 minutes then add the mushrooms and cook until fairly soft (about 5 minutes).
2 Add the vegetable bouillon powder, dried herbs, tomato purée, canned tomatoes and beans, season and simmer for about 10 minutes to allow the vegetables to soften and the sauce to thicken.

ⓖ per serving: 7
Serving suggestion: serve with steamed Tenderstem or broccoli and wholemeal spaghetti.
Variations: use kidney beans or pinto beans instead of borlotti beans.
Allergy suitability: gluten, wheat, dairy, yeast free.

Cashew and Sesame Quinoa

This is unbelievably tasty and contains ample protein from the quinoa. The raw vegetables also substantially increase the vitamin and antioxidant levels. Serves 2

140g (5oz) quinoa
400ml (14fl oz) water
1 tsp Marigold reduced-salt vegetable bouillon powder
3–4 tbsp fresh or frozen petits pois
2 tbsp cashew nuts
2 tsp sesame oil
1 tbsp tamari or soy sauce
2 tsp lemon juice
1 large carrot, julienned (finely sliced lengthways)
6 spring onions, finely sliced
ground black pepper

1 Add the quinoa, water and vegetable bouillon powder to a pan and bring to the boil. Cover and simmer for about 13 minutes, or until all the water has been absorbed and the quinoa grains are soft and fluffy.
2 Add the peas and stir through then remove from the heat (they will cook or soften slightly in the residual warmth).
3 Combine with all other ingredients, tossing thoroughly to mix all the flavours.

ⓖⓛ per serving: 6
Variations: omit the cashew nuts if you have an allergy to them – the quinoa provides complete protein on its own.
Allergy suitability: gluten, wheat, dairy free (use tamari instead of soy if you cannot eat wheat).

Chickpea Curry

You could throw this curry together in about 5 minutes flat. It is full of valuable nutrients, from the antioxidants in the garlic, onion and curry powder to the calcium and magnesium in the almonds and the phytoestrogens in the chickpeas. Serves 2

    1 tsp coconut oil or olive oil
    2 garlic cloves, crushed
    1 onion, diced
    2 tsp curry powder
    300ml (10fl oz) water
    2 tsp Marigold reduced-salt vegetable bouillon powder
    2 tbsp tomato purée
    400g (14oz) can chickpeas, rinsed and drained
    2 tbsp ground almonds

1 Heat the oil in a large frying pan or wok and fry the garlic and onion for 2 minutes.
2 Add the curry powder and cook until the onion softens.
3 Pour in the water and add the bouillon powder, tomato purée, chickpeas and ground almonds. Simmer and stir for a minute or so to let the mixture thicken.

ⓖⓛ per serving: 7
Serving suggestion: serve with quinoa or with brown basmati rice if you have reached the 'Maintenance' phase.
Variations: omit the almonds if you like, or if you have a nut allergy.
Allergy suitability: gluten, wheat, dairy, yeast free.

Cod roasted with Lemon and Garlic

A delicious, no-fuss fish dish that is perfect for a light summer supper, served with new potatoes. Serves 2

½ tbsp olive oil
½ tbsp chopped fresh parsley
2 garlic cloves, crushed
2 cod fillets (or other white fish)
1 lemon, sliced thinly
Solo or sea salt and ground black pepper

1 Mix together the oil, parsley, garlic and seasoning and rub over fish. Set it aside to marinate for 10 minutes. Preheat the oven to 180°C/350°F/ Gas 4.
2 Put the fish on a baking tray and arrange the lemon slices on top. Cook in the oven for 8–10 minutes (or according to the instructions for the fish) until just cooked and the flesh flakes easily.
3 Serve with a Green Bean, Olive and Roasted Pepper Salad (3 ⓖⓛ – see page 250).

ⓖⓛ per serving: 0
Serving suggestion: Serve with buttered, boiled new potatoes – two small ones, cut into four halves, per serving (6 ⓖⓛ in total).
Allergy suitability: gluten, wheat, dairy, yeast free.

Nick's Beefburgers

Created by Fiona's husband, this burger is seriously delicious served with salad in a toasted pitta bread (5 ⓖⓛ per half-slice). Serves 2

1 tbsp tamari or soy sauce
1 tsp Worcestershire sauce
1 tbsp finely chopped fresh coriander
¼ red onion, finely chopped
½ a beaten egg
½ tsp Solo or sea salt
½ tsp ground black pepper
225g (8oz) extra-lean minced beef

1 Mix all the flavouring ingredients together, then add to the mince.
2 Knead the mixture thoroughly, then divide into four and flatten into burger shapes.
3 Put on a plate and cover, then put in the fridge to firm for 10 minutes or until required.
4 Grill under a medium heat for about 7 minutes per side or to taste.

GL per serving: 1
Serving suggestion: try with Oriental Green Beans and Broccoli (see page 269)
Allergy suitability: gluten, dairy, yeast free.

Pesto-crusted Salmon

The strong flavours of the pesto work well with salmon, which is high in omega-3. This is a very quick supper that is perfect if you are having friends round and you don't want the cooking to interrupt the conversation. Serves 2

2 salmon fillets
2 portions of pesto (choose from the recipe opposite or use a classic ready-made pesto of basil and pine nuts)

1 Preheat the oven to 180°C/350°F/Gas 4 and grease a baking tray.
2 Put the salmon on the baking tray and spread the pesto on top.
3 Bake for 18 minutes or until the flesh flakes easily when pressed.

GL per serving: 2
Serving suggestion: serve with Roast Squash and Sweet Potatoes with Shallots 10 GL (see page 269).
Allergy suitability: gluten, wheat, dairy, yeast free (I hate to state the obvious but please choose a dairy-free pesto if you're avoiding dairy products).

Sun-dried Tomato and Black Olive Pesto

The full-flavoured sun-dried tomatoes and olives make up for the lack of cheese in this pesto. Serves 2

50g (2oz) sun-dried tomato paste (available in jars or tubes from supermarkets)
50g (2oz) pitted black olives
50g (2oz) pine nuts
15g (½oz) flat-leaf parsley leaves
25g (1oz) basil leaves
2 garlic cloves, crushed
1 tsp lemon juice
1 tbsp olive oil
ground black pepper

Put all the ingredients in a small food processor or mini chopper and blend until fairly smooth.

Ⓖ per serving: 2
Allergy suitability: gluten, wheat, dairy free.

Poached Haddock with Cannellini Bean Mash

This is a sort of deconstructed fish pie, with a low-GL, using high-fibre beans instead of potato mash. Serves 2

2 medium undyed smoked haddock fillets
300ml (10fl oz) skimmed milk, soya milk or nut milk (or enough to cover the fish in the pan to poach)
300ml (10fl oz) water
2 portions Cannellini Bean Mash (see overleaf)

1 Poach the haddock by putting the fillets into a deep frying pan and covering them with the milk and water. Bring to the boil then simmer gently for 7–8 minutes until cooked (the flesh should flake easily when pressed).
2 Warm through the bean mash and serve with the fish.

Ⓖ per serving: 8
Serving suggestion: serve with some steamed broccoli.
Allergy suitability: gluten, wheat, dairy, yeast free.

Cannellini Bean Mash

Serve this mash with fish or meat. It is delicious warm but could also be served cold. Serves 2

    400g (14oz) can cannellini beans, rinsed and drained
    1 tbsp skimmed milk, soya milk or nut milk
    1 tsp Marigold reduced-salt vegetable bouillon powder
    1 tbsp olive oil
    ground black pepper

1 Purée the beans roughly using a blender.
2 Put in a pan with the rest of the ingredients and heat through, mashing until fairly smooth.

ⓖⓛ per serving: 5
Variations: use butterbeans instead of cannellini beans.
Allergy suitability: gluten, wheat, dairy, yeast free.

Smoked Mackerel Kedgeree with Barley

Kedgeree is traditionally made with haddock and rice but this variation is both exceedingly tasty and high in omega-3s, antioxidants and soluble fibres. It keeps for a few days in the fridge so make enough to last for a couple of days. Serves 6

    3 cups pearl barley
    700ml (1¼ pints) boiling water
    3 tsp tamari
    3 tsp tahini
    350g (12oz) peas
    1 tsp turmeric
    1 tsp cumin
    ½ tsp medium curry powder or cayenne
    ½ tsp coriander
    1 tbsp coconut oil or olive oil
    2 garlic cloves, crushed
    3 red onions, chopped

3 smoked mackerel in peppercorns, about 250g (9oz) total weight, skinned
and flaked into pieces (any bones removed)
a handful of olives
3 eggs, hard-boiled and chopped

1 Put the barley and boiling water into a pan, bring to the boil, then
simmer for 40 minutes until soft and chewy. Drain and add the tamari
and tahini.
2 Meanwhile, boil the peas.
3 Dry-fry the spices for a minute in a large frying pan.
4 Add the oil and garlic, and fry for 30 seconds then add the onions and
sweat until they soften. Add the fish pieces and stir in to absorb the flavour. Add in a handful of olives, the peas and the chopped egg. Stir in
the barley and serve.

Ⓖ per serving: 8
Serving suggestion: delicious with 1 tsp of brinjal pickle and
mayonnaise.
Variations: this is also delicious with rice and you can vary the veg-
etables that you add.
Allergy suitability: wheat, dairy free.

Sesame Chicken and Soba Noodle Steam-fry

Soba noodles are made from buckwheat, a gluten-free grain. They
cook quickly in 4–6 minutes and make an interesting change to wheat
or egg noodles. Serves 2

2 tsp coconut oil or olive oil
2 garlic cloves, crushed
2 tsp chopped fresh root ginger
2 chicken breasts, trimmed of skin and fat and sliced into strips
4 handfuls chopped mixed vegetables (such as peppers, carrots, baby corn,
mangetouts, broccoli)
2 tsp Marigold reduced-salt vegetable bouillon powder
2 tbsp water
100g (3½oz) soba (buckwheat) noodles
2 tsp sesame oil

1 Melt the oil in a wok and stir-fry the garlic, ginger and chicken over a medium heat for 2 minutes or until the meat is coloured on both sides.
2 Add the vegetables, bouillon powder and water to the wok and put the lid on for 5–7 minutes to let the vegetables soften and the meat finish cooking.
3 Meanwhile, cook the noodles: put in a pan of boiling water, cover and boil for 4–6 minutes, drain and rinse under cold water (take care not to overcook).
4 Tip the noodles into the wok and add the sesame oil, then stir it all together and serve.

ⓖ per serving: 10
Allergy suitability: gluten, wheat, dairy, yeast free (make sure you choose 100 per cent buckwheat soba noodles if you are gluten intolerant – some of them also contain wheat).

Trout with Puy Lentils and Roasted Tomatoes on the Vine

A simple but sophisticated dish that is perfectly balanced. Smart enough to serve at a supper party. Serves 2

85g (3oz) dried Puy lentils, washed
1 tsp Marigold reduced-salt vegetable bouillon powder
1 tsp mixed dried herbs (such as Herbes de Provence)
2 trout fillets, fully prepared
cherry tomatoes on the vine (½ bunch, or 5–6 tomatoes per person)
2 slices of lemon
a handful of fresh flat-leaf parsley
ground black pepper

1 Cover the lentils with cold water and bring to the boil, then simmer for 20 minutes or until the water is more or less absorbed, adding the bouillon powder and mixed herbs when the lentils are soft to the bite. (Don't worry if the lentils seem hard – Puy lentils retain their shape and have a satisfyingly chewy texture even when cooked.) Preheat the oven to 190°C/375°F/Gas 5.
2 Put the fish in a non-stick roasting tin and lay the tomatoes around them, then bake for 12–15 minutes or according to the instructions for the fish.

3 Lay the fish on a dollop of lentils, with a slice of lemon and chopped parsley on top of each fillet and the tomatoes on the side. Sprinkle with black pepper.

ⓖ per serving: 11
Allergy suitability: gluten, dairy, yeast free.

Chicken with Cherry Tomatoes

This is an easy yet impressive dish. The tomatoes cook down to release their juice, which combines with crème fraîche to make a creamy sauce.
Serves 2

2 tbsp olive oil
2 chicken breasts, trimmed of fat and skin
225g (8oz) cherry tomatoes
1½ tbsp low fat crème fraîche
1 tbsp basil leaves, chopped or roughly torn
Freshly ground black pepper

1 Preheat the oven to 180°C/350°F/Gas 4.
2 Pour the oil into a shallow ovenproof dish and add the chicken breasts, coating in the oil.
3 Place the whole cherry tomatoes around the chicken in the dish and cook for around 30-35 minutes or until the chicken is cooked, basting occasionally.
4 When the chicken is cooked, place the dish on the hob and add the crème fraîche. Heat gently until it starts to bubble, then simmer for a moment until the sauce thickens.
5 Stir in the basil and season with black pepper.

ⓖ per serving: 4
Serving suggestion: serve with 3 small boiled baby new potatoes or half a baked potato and a green salad (total ⓖ 11).
Allergy suitability: gluten, wheat free.

5

Side Vegetables

You can have these with a main meal or as your light lunch, snack or starter.

Coleslaw

Cabbage is packed with vitamins and minerals. So are carrots, which are high in vitamin A, and onions, high in sulphur-rich amino acids. This coleslaw is nothing like the limp supermarket variety – it really packs in the power and crunch. Serves 2

    200g (7oz) red or white cabbage, finely shredded
    85g (3oz) carrots, grated
    ½ small onion, finely chopped
    1 tbsp low-fat mayonnaise
    1 tbsp fat-free live yoghurt

Mix all the ingredients well in a large bowl.

Ⓖ per serving: 3
Allergy suitability: gluten, wheat, yeast free.

Oriental Green Beans and Broccoli

Tender green beans and broccoli go well with this dressing. This recipe works brilliantly with tofu steam-fries. Serves 2

250g (9oz) young green beans, cut in half crossways
175g (6oz) broccoli, broken into florets
1 garlic clove, crushed
1 tbsp tamari
1 tsp sesame oil
1 tsp sesame seeds, dry-roasted in a pan until golden (shaking occasionally)

1 Steam the beans and broccoli gently for about 3 minutes, or until tender.
2 Put the remaining ingredients in a bowl and stir together, then toss over the beans and broccoli, and serve warm.

Ⓖ per serving: 2
Allergy suitability: gluten, wheat, dairy, yeast free.

Roast Squash and Sweet Potatoes with Shallots

Orange fruits and vegetables, like squashes and sweet potatoes, are a good source of beta-carotene, which your body converts to vitamin A. They are also absolutely delicious and cook down to a wonderfully squidgy consistency that melts in the mouth. Serves 2

½ small butternut squash, about 325g (11½oz) pre-prepared weight, cut into bite-sized chunks
1 sweet potato, cut into bite-sized chunks
8 shallots
1 tbsp olive oil
ground black pepper

1 Preheat the oven to 200°C/400°F/Gas 6.
2 Put the squash, sweet potatoes and shallots in a roasting tin and drizzle with oil, shaking them around to coat evenly.
3 Put in the oven and cook for about an hour, shaking the tray again half-way through.

4 When the squash and sweet potatoes are fairly soft when pierced with a knife remove from the oven and season with black pepper.

GL per serving: 8
Serving suggestion: serve with Pesto-crusted Salmon (see page 262).
Allergy suitability: gluten, wheat, dairy, yeast free.

Steamed Savoy Cabbage with Crème Fraîche

Savoy cabbage makes an interesting change from white cabbage, and has a superior nutritive content. Serves 2

½ a savoy cabbage (approximately 200g/7oz), outer leaves removed and
   the rest rinsed, dried and thinly sliced
3 tbsp crème fraîche
½ tbsp fresh flat-leaf parsley, finely chopped
Pinch of low-sodium salt or sea salt
Freshly ground black pepper

1 Steam the cabbage for 6 minutes then remove from the heat and place in a pan.
2 Stir the crème fraîche and parsley into the cabbage, allowing the crème fraîche to melt, or loosen in the heat from the cabbage, and season with salt and pepper.

GL per serving: 2
Serving suggestion: serve with chicken or fish – it's particularly good with smoked fish.
Allergy suitability: gluten, wheat free.

6

Desserts

After the first two weeks of your low-GL diet you can have a drink or dessert (unless you have type-1 diabetes or are currently injecting insulin, in which case you can have a dessert when you first start the diet – see Part 3, Chapter 2, page 205). Most desserts are very high in ⑩ but here you will find some that will fit into your GL allowance and still taste wonderful too.

Recipe	Page	⑩
Apple and Almond Cake	271	5
Carrot and Walnut Cake	273	5
Chocolate Ice Cream	274	6
Plum Amaretti Slices	275	5
Kiwi and Coconut Pudding	276	6

Apple and Almond Cake

We all want to be able to have our cake and eat it, and this delicious recipe is proof that you can do just that. This cake has all the taste and texture of the traditional Dorset Apple Cake, on which it is based, but is free from gluten, sugar and dairy, and it's full of fibre and minerals. Delicious as a snack with a lemon tea. Serves 4

55g (2oz) coconut oil or butter (at room temperature)
55g (2oz) xylitol
55g (2oz) organic soya flour
½ tsp baking powder
55g (2oz) ground almonds
55g (2oz) flaked almonds, plus 1 tbsp for sprinkling on top
150g (5½oz) Bramley apples (cored weight), unpeeled and diced
2 medium eggs

1 Preheat the oven to 180°C/350°F/Gas 4. Grease and line a 10cm (4in) mini cake tin.
2 Cream the coconut oil or butter and xylitol together until soft and smooth.
3 Stir in the flour and baking powder and the ground almonds until the mixture resembles breadcrumbs.
4 Mix in the flaked almonds and apples, then stir in the eggs (but don't beat the mixture).
5 Spoon into the prepared tin and sprinkle flaked almonds on top. Bake for 25 minutes or until the top is golden and set. Remove from the oven and cover the top with a sheet of foil then return to the oven for a further 20 minutes or until the cake is cooked; insert a skewer into the middle – if it comes out fairly clean then the cake is cooked, if it is still runny then it needs a bit longer.

Tips: you can buy mini cake tins from kitchen shops. They make cakes that are perfect for anyone on a diet who doesn't want the temptation of leftover cake hanging around.

If you want to make a full-sized cake, multiply the quantities by 4 and use a standard 23cm (9in) cake tin.

GL per serving: 5
Variations: replace the apple with pears. You could also use quinoa flour (another high-protein flour from health-food stores) instead of soya flour, although the flavour is not as good.
Allergy suitability: gluten, wheat, dairy, yeast free (use coconut oil rather than butter if you cannot eat dairy).

Carrot and Walnut Cake

A fabulous tea-time treat that you can enjoy without feeling guilty. The walnuts, carrots and eggs in this cake lower the GL score and provide plenty of nutrients. This is really delicious with a cup of peppermint tea as an afternoon snack. Serves 4

55g (2oz) coconut oil or butter (at room temperature)
55g (2oz) xylitol
55g (2oz) organic soya flour
½ tsp baking powder
55g (2oz) ground walnuts
55g (2oz) chopped walnuts, plus 2 tbsp chopped walnuts for decoration
   (optional)
1 medium carrot, about 85g (3oz), finely grated
2 medium eggs

For the cream cheese frosting (optional):
55g (2oz) low-fat cream cheese
¼ tsp vanilla extract
1 tsp xylitol

1 Preheat the oven to 180°C/350°F/Gas 4. Grease and line a 10cm (4in) mini cake tin (see Tips opposite).
2 Cream the coconut oil or butter and xylitol together until soft and smooth.
3 Stir in the flour and baking powder, then the ground walnuts until the mixture resembles breadcrumbs.
4 Mix in the chopped walnuts, carrot and eggs (do not beat the eggs).
5 Spoon into the prepared cake tin and sprinkle the chopped walnuts on top, if you like. Bake for 35 minutes or until the top is risen and golden. Remove from the oven and cover the top with foil, then bake for a further 20 minutes or until the cake is cooked; insert a skewer into the middle – if it comes out fairly clean, the cake is cooked, if it is still runny it needs a bit longer. Allow to cool.
6 For the frosting (if using), mix together the cream cheese, vanilla and xylitol and spread over the top of the cake.

ⓖⓛ per serving: 5

Variations: You could also use quinoa flour (another high-protein flour from health-food stores) instead of soya flour, although the flavour is not as good.

Allergy suitability: gluten, wheat, dairy, yeast free (use coconut oil rather than butter if you cannot eat dairy products and opt for the chopped nuts topping rather than the cream cheese frosting).

Chocolate Ice Cream

This luscious ice cream shines if made with the highest-quality cocoa powder.

  75g (2¾oz) xylitol
  225ml (8fl oz) milk
  1 egg
  40g (1½oz) dark chocolate cocoa powder
  450ml (16fl oz) double cream, lightly whipped
  1 tsp vanilla extract

1 Mix the xylitol, milk and egg together in a bowl, then pour into a small pan and cook over a medium low heat, stirring constantly, until the mixture thickens – this takes about 10 minutes. Take care not to let it boil.
2 Remove from the heat and add the cocoa powder, stirring until the cocoa dissolves and is mixed in well.
3 Leave to cool for 15 minutes at room temperature before adding the cream and vanilla extract. Chill then freeze for 2 hours, whisk with an electric beater or fork to break up the ice crystals then freeze for another 2½ hours. Remove from the freezer 5 minutes before serving.

ⓖⓛ per serving: 6

Allergy suitability: gluten, wheat, yeast free.

Plum Amaretti Slices

This soft macaroon-style tray-bake is seriously scrummy served as a pudding or just with afternoon tea. What's more, it is free from wheat, gluten, sugar and dairy products, yet high in essential fats and low-GL – for guilt-free nibbling. You could also substitute cherries or apricots instead of plums, or omit them entirely. Makes enough to fit one standard baking tray (23 × 31cm; 9 × 12½in). Serves 12

310g (11oz) ground almonds
200g (7oz) xylitol
115g (4oz) cornflour
2 tsp almond extract (not artificial almond flavour)
4 eggs
1 can of plums, cherries or apricot halves in unsweetened fruit juice, drained (or 400g/14oz fresh apricots, plums or cherries in season)
3 good handfuls of flaked almonds

1 Preheat the oven to 180°C/350°F/Gas 4 and line a 23 × 31cm (9 × 12½in) baking tray.
2 Combine the ground almonds, xylitol, cornflour, almond extract and eggs, and mix thoroughly until smooth. Spoon into the baking tray and smooth out.
3 Lightly press the plums evenly into the base then sprinkle the flaked almonds on top.
4 Bake for 20–25 minutes or until the top is light golden (check after 20 minutes). Cut into 12 slices.

ⓖⓛ per serving: 5
Allergy suitability: gluten, wheat, sugar, dairy, yeast free.

Kiwi and Coconut Pudding

The easiest pudding ever, yet special enough for entertaining. This can be made in advance and kept in the fridge until needed. Serves 2

    2 ripe kiwi fruits, peeled and cut into thin slices
    4 tbsp Rachel's Organic Coconut Greek-style Live Yoghurt

1 Divide the kiwi slices between two bowls or ramekins (glass dishes look best, because you can see the different layers of the finished pudding).
2 Spoon the yoghurt on top of the fruit.

ⓖⓛ per serving: 6
Allergy suitability: gluten, wheat, yeast free.

Appendix 1

Body Mass Index (BMI)

Even better than knowing your ideal weight for your height is to calculate your body mass index, or BMI, a measure of fat based on your height and your weight. Your BMI is a reliable indicator of total body fat. The score is valid for both men and women, but it does have some limits:

- It may overestimate body fat in athletes and others who have a muscular build.

- It may underestimate body fat in older people and those who have lost muscle mass.

Your BMI can be used to work out whether you are overweight or obese. Here are the scores:

Underweight = 18.5 or less
Normal weight = 18.5–24.9
Overweight = 25–29.9
Obese = 30 or more

Body Mass Index table – Imperial version

Body weight (pounds)

Height (inches) / BMI	Normal							Overweight				Obese										Extreme obesity														
BMI	19	20	21	22	23	24	25	26	27	28	29	30	31	32	33	34	35	36	37	38	39	40	41	42	43	44	45	46	47	48	49	50	51	52	53	54
58	91	96	100	105	110	115	119	124	129	134	138	143	148	153	158	162	167	172	177	181	186	191	196	201	205	210	215	220	224	229	234	239	244	248	253	258
59	94	99	104	109	114	119	124	128	133	138	143	148	153	158	163	168	173	178	183	188	193	198	203	208	212	217	222	227	232	237	242	247	252	257	262	267
60	97	102	107	112	118	123	128	133	138	143	148	153	158	163	168	174	179	184	189	194	199	204	209	215	220	225	230	235	240	245	250	255	261	266	271	276
61	100	106	111	116	122	127	132	137	143	148	153	158	164	169	174	180	185	190	195	201	206	211	217	222	227	232	238	243	248	254	259	264	269	275	280	285
62	104	109	115	120	126	131	136	142	147	153	158	164	169	175	180	186	191	196	202	207	213	218	224	229	235	240	246	251	256	262	267	273	278	284	289	295
63	107	113	118	124	130	135	141	146	152	158	163	169	175	180	186	191	197	203	208	214	220	225	231	237	242	248	254	259	265	270	278	282	287	293	299	304
64	110	116	122	128	134	140	145	151	157	163	169	174	180	186	192	197	204	209	215	221	227	232	238	244	250	256	262	267	273	279	285	291	296	302	308	314
65	114	120	126	132	138	144	150	156	162	168	174	180	186	192	198	204	210	216	222	228	234	240	246	252	258	264	270	276	282	288	294	300	306	312	318	324
66	118	124	130	136	142	148	155	161	167	173	179	186	192	198	204	210	216	223	229	235	241	247	253	260	266	272	278	284	291	297	303	309	315	322	328	334
67	121	127	134	140	146	153	159	166	172	178	185	191	198	204	211	217	223	230	236	242	249	255	261	268	274	280	287	293	299	306	312	319	325	331	338	344
68	125	131	138	144	151	158	164	171	177	184	190	197	203	210	216	223	230	236	243	249	256	262	269	276	282	289	295	302	308	315	322	328	335	341	348	354
69	128	135	142	149	155	162	169	176	182	189	196	203	209	216	223	230	236	243	250	257	263	270	277	284	291	297	304	311	318	324	331	338	345	351	358	365
70	132	139	146	153	160	167	174	181	188	195	202	209	216	222	229	236	243	250	257	264	271	278	285	292	299	306	313	320	327	334	341	348	355	362	369	376
71	136	143	150	157	165	172	179	186	193	200	208	215	222	229	236	243	250	257	265	272	279	286	293	301	308	315	322	329	338	343	351	358	365	372	379	386
72	140	147	154	162	169	177	184	191	199	206	213	221	228	235	242	250	258	265	272	279	287	294	302	309	316	324	331	338	346	353	361	368	375	383	390	397
73	144	151	159	166	174	182	189	197	204	212	219	227	235	242	250	257	265	272	280	288	295	302	310	318	325	333	340	348	355	363	371	378	386	393	401	408
74	148	155	163	171	179	186	194	202	210	218	225	233	241	249	256	264	272	280	287	295	303	311	319	326	334	342	350	358	365	373	381	389	396	404	412	420
75	152	160	168	176	184	192	200	208	216	224	232	240	248	256	264	272	279	287	295	303	311	319	327	335	343	351	359	367	375	383	391	399	407	415	423	431
76	156	164	172	180	189	197	205	213	221	230	238	246	254	263	271	279	287	295	304	312	320	328	336	344	353	361	369	377	385	394	402	410	418	426	435	443

Source: Adapted from Clinical Guidelines on the Identification, Evaluation, and Treatment of Overweight and Obesity in Adults: The Evidence Report.

Body Mass Index table – metric version

Body weight (kgs)

BMI Height (cms)	Normal						Overweight					Obese										Extreme obesity															
	19	20	21	22	23	24	25	26	27	28	29	30	31	32	33	34	35	36	37	38	39	40	41	42	43	44	45	46	47	48	49	50	51	52	53	54
147	41	43	45	48	50	52	54	56	58	61	63	65	67	69	72	74	76	78	80	82	84	87	89	91	93	95	98	100	102	104	106	108	111	112	115	117
150	43	45	47	49	52	54	56	58	60	63	65	67	69	72	74	76	78	81	83	85	88	90	92	94	96	98	101	103	105	108	110	112	114	117	119	121
152	44	46	49	51	54	56	58	60	63	65	67	69	72	74	76	79	81	83	86	88	90	93	95	98	100	102	104	107	109	111	113	116	118	121	123	125
155	45	48	50	53	55	58	60	62	65	67	69	72	74	77	79	82	84	86	88	91	93	96	98	101	103	105	108	110	112	115	117	120	122	125	127	129
158	47	49	52	54	57	59	62	64	67	69	72	74	77	79	82	84	86	89	92	94	97	99	101	104	107	109	112	114	116	119	121	124	126	129	131	134
160	49	51	54	56	59	61	64	66	69	72	74	77	79	82	84	87	89	92	94	97	100	102	105	108	110	112	115	117	120	122	126	128	130	133	136	138
163	50	53	55	58	60	63	65	68	71	74	77	79	82	84	87	90	93	95	98	101	103	106	108	111	113	116	119	121	124	127	129	132	134	137	140	142
165	52	54	57	60	63	65	68	71	73	76	79	82	84	87	90	93	95	98	101	103	106	109	112	114	117	119	122	125	128	131	133	136	139	142	144	147
168	54	56	59	62	64	67	70	73	76	78	81	84	87	90	93	95	98	101	104	107	110	112	115	118	120	123	126	129	132	135	137	140	143	146	149	152
170	55	58	61	64	66	69	72	75	78	81	84	87	90	93	96	98	101	104	107	110	113	116	118	122	124	127	130	133	137	139	142	145	147	150	153	156
173	57	59	63	65	68	72	74	78	80	83	86	89	92	95	98	101	104	107	110	113	116	119	122	125	128	131	134	137	140	143	146	149	153	155	158	161
176	58	60	64	66	70	73	77	80	83	86	89	92	95	98	101	104	107	110	113	117	119	122	126	129	132	135	139	141	144	147	150	153	156	160	162	166
178	60	63	66	69	72	76	79	82	85	88	92	95	98	101	104	107	110	113	117	120	123	126	129	132	136	139	142	145	148	152	155	158	161	164	167	170
180	62	65	68	71	75	78	81	84	88	91	94	98	100	103	107	110	113	117	120	123	127	130	133	137	140	143	147	150	153	156	159	162	166	169	172	175
183	64	67	70	73	77	80	83	87	90	93	96	100	103	107	110	113	117	120	123	127	130	134	137	140	143	147	150	154	157	160	164	167	171	175	178	182
185	65	68	72	75	79	82	86	89	93	96	99	103	106	109	113	116	120	123	127	130	134	137	141	144	148	151	154	158	161	165	168	171	175	178	182	185
188	67	70	74	78	81	84	88	92	95	99	102	106	109	113	116	120	123	127	130	134	137	141	145	148	152	155	159	162	166	169	173	176	179	183	187	190
191	69	73	76	80	83	87	91	94	98	102	105	109	112	116	119	123	126	130	134	137	141	145	148	152	156	159	163	166	170	173	177	181	185	188	192	196
193	71	74	78	82	86	89	93	97	100	104	108	112	115	119	123	127	130	134	138	142	145	149	152	156	160	163	167	171	175	179	182	186	190	193	197	201

Appendix 2

Working Out Your Training Heart-rate Zone

The best way to know that you are exercising at an intensity that will burn fat and boost your metabolism is to measure your pulse while exercising. If it is within your training heart-rate zone for 15 minutes or more, then your exercise is having a fatburning effect.

To find your training heart-rate zone, you need to subtract your age from 220, then calculate 65 per cent of this amount for the lower end of your training zone and 80 per cent for the upper limit:

220 – [age] × .65 = lower limit
220 – [age] × .80 = upper limit

For example, for a 30-year-old:
220 – 30 = 190 × .65 = lower limit = 124 beats per minute
220 – 30 = 190 × .80 = upper limit = 152 beats per minute

To find your pulse rate, you will need a watch with a second hand. There are two main points at which the pulse can be felt easily: the neck (the carotid pulse) on either side of the Adam's apple; or the wrist (the radial pulse). To find your pulse, apply light pressure with your fingers. Normally, for medical examinations your pulse is taken for 60 seconds. But to find your pulse while exercising, stopping for this long would lower your pulse and give you a false reading. So, take your pulse for only 10 seconds and multiply the result by 6 to give you the number of beats in one minute without giving your heart rate a chance to slow down. This will be your exercising pulse rate.

When you first embark on your aerobic exercise sessions, you will need to stop briefly every 10–15 minutes to monitor your pulse. After a while you will become familiar with how the correct pulse feels for you. See the chart below to find your exercise heart rate for your age.

Training heart-rate zone chart (while exercising)

Age	65–80 per cent of maximum heart rate (beats in 1 minute)	(beats in 10 sec.)
20	130–160	22–27
22	129–158	22–26
24	127–157	21–26
26	126–155	21–26
28	125–154	21–26
30	124–152	21–25
32	122–150	20–25
34	121–149	20–25
36	120–147	20–25
38	118–146	20–24
40	117–144	20–24
45	114–140	19–23
50	111–136	19–23
55	107–132	18–22
60	104–128	17–21
65	101–124	17–21
70	98–120	16–20

The centre column shows how many beats you should have in one minute; beginners should aim for the lower figure on the left-hand side (that is, 65 per cent of their maximum heart rate for their age), then slowly increase to 80 per cent. Do not exceed this higher level. The column on the far right gives you how many beats you should have in a 10-second pulse count. Again, beginners should stay at the lower end of their exercise range.

Appendix 3

How to Work Out the Glycemic Load of Foods

Glycemic index

The glycemic index is about the quality of the carbohydrate within a food, not the quantity. In other words, the glycemic index (GI) of a food remains the same whether you eat 10g (¼oz) or 100g (3½oz). It is a comparison of how one type of carbohydrate (for example, that in bread) compares to another type of carbohydrate (for example, in sugar). It's worked out by feeding volunteers however much of the food in question they would need to eat to consume 50g (1¾oz) of 'available' carbohydrate. (Some carbohydrate, such as fibre, is not available to the body for its energy needs.) If, for example, half a food's carbohydrate is 'available', the volunteers would be fed 100g (3½oz) of the food to obtain 50g (1¾oz) of the available carbohydrate. The extent to which this raises blood sugar levels (see the diagrams on page 73), compared to the extent to which 50g (1¾oz) of glucose does, determines its GI score. Glucose, by definition, scores 100 on the GI index. So, if a food creates half the increase in blood sugar compared to glucose, its GI score will be 50. This means that you could eat twice as much carbohydrate in the form found in this food to match the effect of glucose on your blood sugar level.

Glycemic load

The glycemic load of a food (GL) is basically the GI of a food multiplied by the serving size. So, the GL actually tells you what that specific serving, for example a biscuit or slice of bread, will do to your blood sugar. The GL of a food is worked out as follows: GI score divided by 100, multiplied by the available carbohydrate (carbohydrates minus fibre) in grams. So, in our example above this would be:

50 (GI score) ÷ 100 × 50 (50g/1¾oz of carbohydrate in 100g/3½oz serving) = 25

So a 100g (3½oz) serving of our example food has a GL of 25.

Take watermelon as another example. Its glycemic index (GI) is pretty high, about 72. According to the calculations by the people at the University of Sydney's Human Nutrition Unit, in a serving of 120g (4¼oz) it has 6g (⅛oz) of available carbohydrate per serving, so its glycemic load is pretty low, 72 ÷ 100 × 6 = 4.32 (rounded to 4). So, as long as you know the glycemic index of a food, the size of the serving you wish to use, and the amount of available carbohydrate in the food, you can calculate the GL yourself; however, I have calculated the GL for a comprehensive range of foods, which can be found in the chart in the following appendix.

Appendix 4

The GL Index of Hundreds of Foods

The most accurate way to gauge whether or not you should eat a food is its glycemic load, which is a calculation based on both the quantity of carbohydrate in a food and the quality of that carbohydrate.

A GL of 10 or less is good, and is shown in **bold**
A GL of 11–14 is OK, shown in normal text
A GL of 15 or more is bad, shown in *italics*

Even this is only a guide, however, because the amount you eat of a food will obviously alter its effect on your blood sugar, and hence your weight. So, while generally I say you can liberally eat the bold foods with low ⒼⓁ, limit the normal-text foods and avoid the italic foods, what is most important is to limit the *total glycemic load* of your diet. If you want to lose weight and feel great, eat no more than 40 ⒼⓁ a day. This means roughly 10 for breakfast, 10 for lunch, 10 for dinner and 5 each for your two snacks, mid-morning and mid-afternoon. You can also drink 5 ⒼⓁ, or have a 5-GL dessert, after the first two weeks or from the start of the diet if you are on insulin, so your total daily intake from food and drink is 45.

If you choose the good, low-GL foods you'll be able to eat more food. If you choose the bad high-GL foods you'll have to eat much less. In the chart on page 286 mainly select from the bold foods, then use the right-hand column to work out how much to eat for 5, which is the serving for a snack, or 10, which is a serving for a main meal. If you are not sure what a 'serving' means look at the amounts of grams given for 5 and check the grams on the packet of the food in question. Foods containing no carbohydrate, composed entirely of protein or fat (meat, fish, eggs, cheese, mayonnaise) have, in effect, a GL of 0, and are not included in this chart. Please note that the glycemic index for some foods has not been published. In these instances we have estimated the GL based on the GI for very similar foods. These foods are marked 'E'. As the ⓖⓛ of more foods are calculated, this table will be updated on www.theholforddiet.com. You can also input a selection of foods into this database and it will calculate the GL of a particular recipe for you.

THE GLYCEMIC LOAD OF COMMON FOODS

Bakery products

Item	Serving size (in g)	GLs per serving	10 GLs	5 GLs	5 GLs
Muffin – apple, made without sugar	**60**	**9**	**1 muffin**	**½ muffin**	**33g**
Muffin – apple muffin, made with sugar	60	13	1 small muffin	½ small muffin	23g
Crumpet	50	13	1 crumpet	½ crumpet	19g
Muffin – apple, oat, sultana, made from packet mix	50	14	1 small muffin	½ small muffin	18g
Muffin – bran	57	15	½ muffin	¼ muffin	18g
Muffin – blueberry	57	17	½ muffin	¼ muffin	17g
Muffin – banana, oat and honey	50	17	½ muffin	¼ muffin	15g
Muffin – carrot	57	20	½ muffin	¼ muffin	14g
Banana cake, made without sugar	80	16	1 small slice	⅓ slice	25g
Croissant	57	17	½ croissant	¼ croissant	17g
Doughnut	47	17	½ doughnut	¼ doughnut	14g
Sponge cake, plain	63	17	½ slice	¼ slice	19g

Breads

Item	Serving size (in g)	GLs per serving	10 GLs	5 GLs	5 GLs
Rye kernel (pumpernickel) bread	30	6	2 slices	1 slice	25g
Sourdough rye	30	6	2 slices	1 slice	25g
Volkenbrot, wholemeal rye bread	30	7	2 slices	1 slice	21g
Rice bread, high-amylose	30	7	2 small slices	1 small slice	21g
Rice bread, low-amylose	30	8	2 thin slices	1 thin slice	19g
Wholemeal rye bread	30	8	2 thin slices	1 thin slice	19g
Wheat tortilla (Mexican)	50	8	1½ tortillas	Less than 1 tortilla	31g
Chapatti, white wheat flour, thin, with green gram	50	8	1½ chapattis	1 chapatti	31g
White, high-fibre	30	9	1 thick slice	1 thin slice	17g
Wholemeal (wholewheat) wheat flour bread	30	9	1 thick slice	1 thin slice	17g
Gluten-free fibre-enriched	30	9	1 thick slice	½ thick slice	17g
Gluten-free multigrain bread	30	10	1 slice	½ slice	15g
Light rye	30	10	1 slice	½ slice	15g
White wheat flour bread	30	10	1 slice	½ slice	15g
Pitta bread, white	30	10	1 pitta	½ slice	15g
Wheat flour flatbread	30	10	1 slice	½ slice	15g
Gluten-free white bread	30	11	1 slice	½ slice	14g

Item	Serving size (in g)	GLs per serving	10 GLs	5 GLs	5 GLs
Corn tortilla	50	12	1 tortilla	½ tortilla	21g
Middle Eastern flatbread	*30*	*15*	*⅔ slice*	*⅓ slice*	*10g*
Baguette, white, plain	*30*	*15*	*1/20 baton*	*1/40 baton*	*10g*
Bagel, white, frozen	*70*	*25*	*½ bagel*	*¼ bagel*	*14g*

Breakfast cereals

Item	Serving size (in g)	GLs per serving	10 GLs	5 GLs	5 GLs
Low-GL Muesli (see page 243) (E)	**30**	**1**	As much as you like	As much as you like	100g
Porridge made from rolled oats	**30**	**2**	As much as you like	1 very large bowl	75g
Get Up & Go with strawberries and ½ pint milk (E)	30	5	½ pint drink	½ pint drink	5fl oz/ 150ml
All-Bran™	**30**	**6**	2 small servings	1 small serving	25g
Muesli, gluten-free	**30**	**7**	2 small servings	1 small serving	21g
Muesli (Alpen)	**30**	**10**	1 serving	½ serving	15g
Muesli, Natural	**30**	**10**	1 serving	½ serving	15g
Raisin Bran™ (Kellogg's)	30	12	1 small serving	⅓ serving	13g
Weetabix™	30	13	2 biscuits	1 biscuit	12g
Bran Flakes™	30	13	1 small serving	⅓ serving	12g

Item	Serving size (in g)	GLs per serving	10 GLs	5 GLs	5 GLs
Sultana Bran™ (Kellogg's)	30	14	1 small serving	½ serving	11g
Special K™ (Kellogg's)	30	14	1 small serving	½ serving	11g
Shredded Wheat	30	15	1 biscuit	½ serving	10g
Cheerios™	30	15	1 very small serving	⅓ serving	10g
Frosties™, sugar-coated cornflakes (Kellogg's)	30	15	1 very small serving	⅓ serving	10g
Grapenuts™	30	15	1 very small serving	⅓ serving	10g
Golden Wheats™ (Kellogg's)	30	16	1 very small serving	⅓ serving	9g
Puffed Wheat	30	16	1 very small serving	⅓ serving	9g
Honey Smacks™ (Kellogg's)	30	16	1 very small serving	⅓ serving	9g
Cornflakes, Crunchy Nut™ (Kellogg's)	30	17	1 very small serving	⅓ serving	9g
Coco Pops™ (cocoa-flavoured puffed rice)	30	20	½ serving	¼ serving	8g
Rice Krispies™ (Kellogg's)	30	21	½ serving	¼ serving	7g
Cornflakes™ (Kellogg's)	30	21	½ serving	¼ serving	7g

Cereal grains

Item	Serving size (in g)	GLs per serving	10 GLs	5 GLs	5 GLs
Semolina	150	6	1 very large serving	small serving	125g
Taco shells, cornmeal-based, baked (Old El Paso)	20	8	2 shells	1 shell	13g
Quinoa	150	8	1½ cups	⅔ cup	94g
Cornmeal	150	9	1 very large serving	1 small serving	83g

Item	Serving size (in g)	GLs per serving	10 GLs	5 GLs	5 GLs
Kamut (E)	150	9	1 very large serving	1 small serving	83g
Pearl Barley	150	11	1 serving	½ serving	68g
Cracked wheat (bulgur/bourghul)	150	12	1 serving	½ serving	63g
Brown basmati rice	150	13	1 small serving	½ serving	58g
Buckwheat	150	16	1 small serving	⅓ serving	47g
Rice, brown	150	18	1 small serving	⅓ serving	42g
Rice, long grain, white, precooked microwaved 2 min. (Express Rice, Uncle Ben's)	150	19	½ serving	¼ serving	39g
Basmati, white, boiled	150	22	½ serving	¼ serving	34g
Couscous	150	23	½ serving	¼ serving	33g
Rice, white	150	23	½ serving	¼ serving	33g
Long grain, boiled	150	23	½ serving	¼ serving	33g
Millet, porridge	150	25	½ serving	¼ serving	30g

Crispbreads and crackers

Item	Serving size (in g)	GLs per serving	10 GLs	5 GLs	5 GLs
Oatcakes	25	8	4 oatcakes	2 oatcakes	16g
Digestives	25	10	1 biscuit	½ biscuit	13g
Cream cracker	25	11	2 biscuits	1 biscuit	11g
Rye crispbread	25	11	2 biscuits	1 biscuit	11g

Item	Serving size (in g)	GLs per serving	10 GLs	5 GLs	5 GLs
Water cracker	25	17	2 biscuits	1 biscuit	7g
Puffed rice cakes	25	17	2 biscuits	1 biscuit	7g

Dairy products and alternatives

Item	Serving size (in g)	GLs per serving	10 GLs	5 GLs	5 GLs
Plain yoghurt (no sugar)	200	3	3 small pots	1½ small pots	333g
Non-fat yoghurt (plain, no sugar)	200	3	3 small pots	1½ small pots	333g
Milk, full-fat	250ml	3	833ml	416ml	416ml
Milk, skim (Canada)	250ml	4	625ml	312ml	312ml
Soya yoghurt (Provamel)	200	7	2 small pots	1 small pot	150g
Soya milk (no sugar)	250ml	7	2 small cups	1 small cup	178ml
Custard, homemade from milk	100ml	7	1 small cup	½ cup	71ml
Ice cream, regular	50ml	8	2 scoops	1 scoop	31ml
Soya milk (sweetened with apple juice concentrate)	250ml	8	2 small cups	1 small cup	156ml
Soya milk, reduced-fat (1.5%), 120mg calcium	250ml	8	2 small cups	1 small cup	156ml
Soya milk (sweetened with sugar)	250ml	9	1½ small cups	⅔ small cup	138ml
Low-fat yoghurt, fruit, sugar, (Ski™)	200	10	1½ small pots	⅔ of small pot	100g
Rice milk, E	250ml	14	1 small cup	½ cup	90ml
Milk, condensed, sweetened (Nestlé)	50ml	17	1 tsp	½ tsp	14ml

Fruit and fruit products

Item	Serving size (in g)	GLs per serving	10 GLs	5 GLs	5 GLs
Blackberries E	120	1	2 large punnets	1 large punnet	600g
Blueberries E	120	1	2 large punnets	1 large punnet	600g
Raspberries E	120	1	2 large punnets	1 large punnet	600g
Strawberries, fresh, raw	120	1	2 large punnets	1 large punnet	600g
Cherries, raw	120	3	2 punnets	1 punnet	200g
Grapefruit, raw	120	3	1 large	1 small	200g
Pear, raw	120	4	2 large pears	1 large pear	150g
Melon/cantaloupe, raw	120	4	1 small melon	½ small melon	150g
Watermelon, raw	120	4	2 big slices	1 big slice	150g
Peaches raw (or canned in natural juice)	120	5	2 peaches	1 peach	120g
Apricots, raw	120	5	8 apricots	4 apricots	120g
Oranges, raw	120	5	2 large	1 large	120g
Plum, raw	120	5	8 plums	4 plums	120g
Apples, raw	120	6	2 small	1 small	100g
Kiwi fruit, raw	120	6	2 kiwis	1 kiwi	100g
Pineapple raw	120	7	2 thin slices	1 thin slice	85g
Grapes, raw	120	8	20 grapes	10 grapes	75g

Item	Serving size (in g)	GLs per serving	10 GLs	5 GLs	5 GLs
Mango, raw	120	8	½ mango	1 slice	75g
Apricots, dried	60	9	6 apricots	3 apricots	33g
Fruit Cocktail, canned (Delmonte)	120	9	Small can	Half a small can	66g
Pawpaw/papaya, raw	120	10	Half a small papaya	1 slice	60g
Prunes, pitted	60	10	6 prunes	3 prunes	30g
Apple, dried	60	10	6 rings	3 rings	30g
Banana, raw	120	12	1 banana	½ banana	50g
Apricots, canned in light syrup	120	12	Less than 1 small can	⅓ small can	50g
Lychees, canned in syrup and drained	120	16	½ 200g can	¼ 200g can	37g
Figs, dried, tenderised, Dessert Maid brand	60	16	2 figs	1 fig	19g
Sultanas	60	25	20	10	12g
Raisins	60	28	20	10	11g
Dates, dried	60	42	2 dates	1 date	7g

Jams and spreads

Item	Serving size (in g)	GLs per serving	10 GLs	5 GLs	5 GLs
Pumpkin seed butter E	16	1	3 large pots	1½ large pots	765g
Peanut butter (no sugar) E	16	1	3 large pots	1½ large pots	765g
Blueberry spread (no sugar) E	30	4	4 tbsp	2 tbsp	21g
Apricot fruit spread, reduced sugar	30	7	8 tsp	4 tsp	21g

Item	Serving size (in g)	GLs per serving	10 GLs	5 GLs	5 GLs
Orange marmalade	30	9	8 tsp	4 tsp	17g
Strawberry jam	30	10	2 tbsp	2 heaped tsp	15g

Legumes and nuts

Item	Serving size (in g)	GLs per serving	10 GLs	5 GLs	5 GLs
Hummus (chickpea dip)	30	1	4 large tubs	4 small tubs	765g
Soya beans	150	1	6 cups	3 cups	750g
Peas, dried, boiled	150	2	3 cups	1½ cups	375g
Pinto beans, boiled in salted water	150	4	2 cups	1 cup	187g
Borlotti beans, boiled, canned	150	4	1½ cans	⅔ can	187g
Lentils	150	5	2 cups	1 cup	150g
Butter beans	150	6	1½ cups	⅔ cup	125g
Split peas, yellow, boiled 20 min.	150	6	1½ cups	⅔ cup	125g
Baked beans, canned	150	7	½ can	¼ can	107g
Kidney beans, canned	150	7	¾ can	⅓ can	107g
Chickpeas (Bengal gram), boiled	150	8	1½ cups	⅔ cup	94g
Chickpeas, canned in brine	150	9	¾ can	⅓ can	83g
Chestnuts, cooked E	150	8	1½ cups	⅔ cup	94g
Flageolet beans, canned in brine E	150	8	¾ can	⅓ can	83g
Haricot/navy beans, canned	150	12	½ can	¼ can	62g
Black-eyed beans, boiled	150	13	1 cup	½ cup	58g

Pasta and noodles*

Item	Serving size (in g)	GLs per serving	10 GLs	5 GLs	5 GLs
Ravioli, durum wheat flour, meat filled, boiled	90	7.5	½ packet	1 small serving	60g
Vermicelli, white, boiled	90	8	1 large serving	½ large serving	56g
Spaghetti, wholemeal, boiled	90	8	1 large serving	½ large serving	56g
Pasta, wholemeal, boiled	90	8	1 large serving	½ a serving	56g
Fettuccine, egg, boiled	90	9	1 serving	½ a serving	50g
Spirali, durum wheat, white, boiled to *al dente* texture	90	9	1 serving	½ serving	47g
Spaghetti, white, boiled	90	9	1 serving	½ serving	47g
Instant noodles	90	9	1 serving	½ serving	47g
Spaghetti durum wheat, boiled 10–15 min,	90	10	1 serving	½ serving	43g
Gluten-free pasta, maize starch, boiled 8 min.	90	11	1 small serving	½ small serving	41g
Macaroni, plain	90	11	1 very small serving	½ very small serving	39g
Rice noodles, dried, boiled	90	11	1 very small serving	½ very small serving	39g
Udon noodles, plain (buckwheat/wheat)	90	15	⅔ serving	⅓ serving	30g
Corn pasta, gluten-free	90	16	1 small serving	½ small serving	28g
Gnocchi	90	16	1 very small serving	½ small serving	27g
Rice pasta, brown, boiled 16 min.	90	17	1 very small serving	½ small serving	26g

Snack foods (savoury)

Item	Serving size (in g)	GLs per serving	10 GLs	5 GLs	5 GLs
Olives, in brine E	50	1	4 cups	2 cups	270g
Peanuts	50	1	1 large pack	1 medium or 2 small packs	250g
Cashew nuts, salted	50	3	1½ small packs	Less than 1 small pack	83g
Popcorn, salted, no sugar	20	8	1 small pack	½ small pack	12g
Potato crisps, plain, salted	50	11	1½ small packs	⅔ small pack	23g
Pretzels, oven-baked, traditional wheat flavour	30	16	8 pretzels	4 pretzels	9g
Corn chips, plain, salted	50	17	13 chips	7 chips	15g

Snack foods (sweet)

Item	Serving size (in g)	GLs per serving	10 GLs	5 GLs	5 GLs
Fruitus apple cereal bar E	35	5	2 bars	1 bar	35g
Rebar fruit and veg bar E	50	8	1 bar	½ bar	25g
Muesli bar containing dried fruit	30	13	Less than 1 bar	Less than ½ bar	12g
Chocolate, milk, plain (Mars/Cadburys/Nestlé)	50	14	Less than ½ bar	Less than ¼ bar	18g
Apricot fruit bar (dried apricot filling in wholemeal pastry)	50	17	1 bar	½ bar	15g

Item	Serving size (in g)	GLs per serving	10 GLs	5 GLs	5 GLs
Twix ® Cookie Bar, caramel (M&M/Mars, USA)	60	17	1 stick	½ stick	18g
Snickers Bar ®	60	19	⅔ bar	⅓ bar	16g
Polos – peppermint sweets	30	21	8 polos	4 polos	7g
Jellybeans, assorted colours	30	22	4 jellybeans	2 jellybeans	7g
Pop Tarts™, double choc	50	24	21g	10g	10g
Mars Bar ®	60	26	½ bar	¼ bar	13g

SOUPS

Item	Serving size (in g)	GLs per serving	10 GLs	5 GLs	5 GLs
Tomato soup	250	6	1 can	½ can	208g
Minestrone	250	7	1 can	½ can	179g
Lentil, canned	250	9	⅔ can	⅓ can	139g
Split pea, canned	250	16	½ can	¼ can	78g
Black bean, canned	250	17	½ can	¼ can	74g
Green pea, canned	250	17	½ can	¼ can	74g

Sugars

Item	Serving size (in g)	GLs per serving	10 GLs	5 GLs	5 GLs
Xylitol	20	2	6 tbsp	3 tbsp	50g
Blue agave cactus nectar (liquid sweetener in drinks)	20	2	100ml	50ml	50g

Item	Serving size (in g)	GLs per serving	10 GLs	5 GLs	5 GLs
Fructose	20	4	3 tbsp	5 tsp	25g
Sucrose	*20*	*14*	*3 tsp*	*1½ tsp*	*7g*
Honey	*20*	*16*	*2 tsp*	*1 tsp*	*6g*
Glucose	*20*	*20*	*2 tsp*	*1 tsp*	*5g*
Maltose (malt)	*20*	*22*	*2 tsp*	*1 tsp*	*5g*

Vegetables

Item	Serving size (in g)	GLs per serving	10 GLs	5 GLs	5 GLs
Tomato E	70	2	5 medium	2½ medium	175g
Broccoli E	100	2	5 handfuls	2½ handfuls	250g
Kale E	75	1	10 handfuls	5 handfuls	375g
Avocado E	190	1	10	5	950g
Onion E	180	2	5 medium	2½ medium	450g
Asparagus E	125	2	5 handfuls	2½ handfuls	315g
Green beans E	75	1	10 handfuls	5 handfuls	375g
Carrots	80	3	2 carrots	1 carrot	133g
Green peas	80	3	5 tbsp	2–3 tbsp	133g
Pumpkin	80	3	3 servings	1½ serving	133g
Beetroot	80	5	4 beets	2 beets	80g
Swede	150	7	½ swede	1 serving	107g

Item	Serving size (in g)	GLs per serving	10 GLs	5 GLs	5 GLs
Banana/plantain, green	**120**	**8**	1 small	½ small	**75g**
Broad beans	**80**	**9**	89g	1 tbsp	**44g**
Sweetcorn	**80**	**9**	1 serving	½ serving	**44g**
Parsnips	80	12	1 small	½ small	33g
Yam	150	13	1 small serving	½ small serving	58g
Boiled potato	150	14	107g	1 small	53g
Microwaved potato	150	14	107g	1 small	53g
Mashed potato	*150*	*15*	*2 tbsp*	*1 tbsp*	*50g*
New potato, unpeeled and boiled 20 min.	*150*	*16*	*4 very small*	*2 very small*	*47g*
Instant mashed potato	*150*	*17*	*88g*	*2 tsp*	*44g*
Sweet potato	*150*	*17*	*1 small*	*½ small*	*44g*
Baked potato, white, baked in skin	*150*	*18*	*83g*	*⅔ medium*	*42g*
French fries	*150*	*22*	*68g*	*4–5*	*34g*
Baked potato, baked without fat	*150*	*26*	*½ a medium*	*¼ a medium*	*29g*

TABLE OF GLYCEMIC LOAD (GL) OF COMMON DRINKS

DRINKS

Item	Serving size in ml	GL per serving	10 GLs	5 GLs	5 GLs
Tomato juice, canned, no added sugar	250	4	625ml	½ pint	315ml
Yakult ®, fermented milk drink with Lactobacillus casei	65	6	108ml	⅔ × 65ml bottle	30ml
Smoothie drink, soya, banana	250	7	357ml	⅔ × 250ml carton	175ml
Smoothie drink, soya, chocolate hazelnut	250	8	313ml	⅗ × 250ml carton	150ml
Carrot juice, freshly made	250	10	250ml	⅕ pint or ⅓ cup	125ml
Grapefruit juice, unsweetened	250	11	227ml	⅕ pint or ⅓ cup	115ml
Apple juice, pure, unsweetened	250	12	208ml	⅙ pint or ⅓ cup	105ml
Orange juice	250	13	192ml	⅙ pint or ⅓ cup	95ml
Cordial, orange, reconstituted	250	13	192ml	⅙ pint or ⅓ cup	95ml
Smoothie, raspberry	250	14	179ml	⅖ 250ml carton or ⅓ cup	90ml
Pineapple juice, unsweetened	250	16	156ml	¼ pint or ½ cup	80ml
Cranberry juice drink, Ocean Spray®	250	16	156ml	¼ pint or ½ cup	80ml
Coca Cola ®, soft drink/soda	250	16	156ml	⅕ × 330ml can	80ml
Fanta ®, orange soft drink	250	23	109ml	⅙ pint or ⅓ cup	50ml
Lucozade ®, original	250	40	63	⅛ pint or ¼ cup	30ml

Most of the GL values of foods listed here are derived from research published in 2002 by K. Foster-Powell, S.H. Holt and J. C. Brand-Miller in 'International table of glycemic index and glycemic load values: 2002', *American Journal of Clinical Nutrition* Vol. 76(1) (2002), pp. 5–56 or from the University of Sydney online database at http://www.glycemicindex.com/ (database pages created by A/Prof. Gareth Denyer and Scott Dickinson using data collected by Professor Jennie Brand-Miller & SUGIRS). Last modified: 13 December 2005.

Notes

Serving sizes:

* All pasta serving sizes are for cooked food. For the equivalent of dry weight, halve the amount – so, if you're cooking spaghetti and the serving size is 120g, that means you put 60g in the pan.

Appendix 5 Glucose Monitoring Charts

Template for recording changes during first week

Date	Time	Blood glucose level	Type and amount of insulin injected	Time of meal	Meal consumed/Supplements taken

Example day during first week

Date	Time	Blood glucose level	Type and amount of insulin injected	Time of meal	Meal consumed/ Supplements taken
17/4/11	7.55 am	4.4	3.5 units Humalog	8.00 am	Cheese and mushroom omelette Redbush tea no milk
	10.00 am	4.9			
	12.55 pm		4 units Humalog	1.00 pm	Prawn cocktail, tuna pate, Greek salad mineral water coffee with cream
	3.00 pm	4.6			
	6.25 pm		6.5 units Humalog	6.30 pm	Roast chicken in cream sauce, cabbage, linseed bread with cheese
	10.00 pm	5.0		10.05 pm	200ml red wine
	10.30 pm		5 units Levimir (before bed)		

Appendix 6 Results Monitoring Chart

	Morning				Noon						Evening					
	8am	9	10	11	12	1pm	2	3	4	5	6	7	8	9	10	11
Diet notes:																
Supplements (inc. fibre):																
Medication/dose:																
Exercise:																
Glucose score:																
Approx GL score:	Breakfast:					Lunch:			Dinner:			Snacks:			Total:	
Notes:																

Example results monitoring chart

	Morning					Noon						Evening				
	8am	9	10	11	12	1pm	2	3	4	5	6	7	8	9	10	11
Diet notes:	Scrambled egg on toast			oat cakes and humus		Walnut + 3-bean salad			Apple and almonds			Pesto-crusted salmon + mashed potatoes				
Supplements (inc. fibre):		1 strip Optimum Nutrition pack / 2 chromium / 1 tsp glucomannan fibre				1 strip Optimum nutrition pack / 2 chromium / 1 tsp glucomannan fibre						1 tsp glucomannan fibre				
Medication/dose:	Metformin 500mg															
Exercise:	30 min brisk walk															
Glucose score:	5.5					6										
Approx GL score:	Breakfast: 9				Lunch: 3				Dinner: 16				Snacks: 4			Total: 32
Notes:	Energy very good throughout the day. No sugar cravings at all!															

References

Introduction

1 See http://www.diabetes.org.uk/About_us/News_Landing_Page/One-million-people-in-UK-unaware-they-have-Type-2-diabetes/

2 Diabetes Prevalence by Age Group, http://www.data360.org/dsg.aspx?Data_Set_Group_Id=233

3 International Diabetes Federation, 'Global Burden: Projections 2010 and 2030', www.diabetesatlas.org

4 See http://www.diabetes.org.uk/Professionals/Publications-reports-and-resources/Reports-statistics-and-case-studies/Reports/Diabetes-prevalence-2010/

5 See http://www.diabetes.org.uk/Documents/Reports/Diabetes_in_the_UK_2010.pdf

6 F. B. Hu et al., 'Diet, lifestyle, and the risk of type-2 diabetes mellitus in women', *New England Journal of Medicine*, 2001 Sep; 345:790–7

Part One

1 S. E. Nissen and K. Wolski, 'Effect of rosiglitazone on the risk of myocardial infarction and death from cardiovascular causes', *New England Journal of Medicine*, 2007 Jun; 356(24):2457–71

2 European Medicines Agency, 'European Medicines Agency recommends suspension of Avandia, Avandamet and Avaglim', press release, 23 Sep 2010

3 *Medical News Today*, 'Part of ACCORD study halted due to safety concerns, Canada', press release, 11 Feb 2008

4 DiabetesInControl.com, 'Insulin users have 50% higher cancer risk: Causes unclear', press release, 2 Sep 2010

5 S. L. Bowker, et al., 'Increased cancer-related mortality for patients with type-2 diabetes who use sulfonylureas or insulin', *Diabetes Care*, 2006 Feb:29(2); 254–8

6. D. Micic, et al., 'Metformin: Its emerging role in oncology', *Hormones*, 2011; 10(1):5–15.

7 G. Reaven, 'Role of insulin resistance in human disease', *Diabetes*, 1988; 37:1595–1607

8 E. Bonora, et al., 'Prevalence of insulin resistance in metabolic disorders: The Bruneck Study', *Diabetes*, 1998 Oct; 47(10):1643–9

9 A. Esteghamati, et al., 'Optimal threshold of homeostasis model assessment for insulin resistance in an Iranian population: The implication of metabolic syndrome to detect insulin resistance', *Diabetes Research and Clinical Practice*, 2009 Jun; 84(3):279–87; see also A. Esteghamati, et al.,'Optimal cut-off of homeostasis model assessment of insulin resistance (HOMA-IR) for the diagnosis of metabolic syndrome: Third national surveillance of risk factors of non-communicable diseases in Iran (SuRFNCD-2007)', *Nutrition and Metabolism*, 2010 Apr 7; 7:26; see also I. Madeira, et al., 'Cut-off point for Homeostatic Model Assessment for Insulin Resistance (HOMA-IR) index established from Receiver Operating Characteristic (ROC) curve in the detection of metabolic syndrome in overweight pre-pubertal children', *Arq Bras Endocrinol Metabol*, 2008 Dec; 52(9):1466–73; see also Z. Radikova, et al., 'Insulin sensitivity indices: A proposal of cut-off points for simple identification of insulin-resistant subjects', *Experimental and Clinical Endocrinology & Diabetes*, 2006 May; 114(5):249–56; see also B. Kuwana, et al., 'Reference value and cut-off value for diagnosis of insulin resistance in type-2 diabetes mellitus', *Rinsho Byori*, 2002 Apr; 50(4):398–403; see also J. Ascaso, et al., 'Insulin resistance quantification by fasting insulin plasma values and HOMA index in a non-diabetic population', *Medicina Clínica (Barc)*, 2001 Nov 3; 117(14):530–3

10 E. Selvin, et al., 'Glycated hemoglobin, diabetes, and cardiovascular risk in nondiabetic adults', *New England Journal of Medicine*, 2010 Mar 4; 362(9):800–11

11 D. Edelman, et al., 'Utility of hemoglobin A1c in predicting diabetes risk', *Journal of General Internal Medicine*, 2004; 19:1175–80

12 C. L. Rohlfing, et al., 'Use of GHb (HbA1c) in Screening for Undiagnosed Diabetes in the U.S. Population', *Diabetes Care*, 2000; 23:187–91

13 N. Sarwar, et al., 'Markers of dysglycaemia and risk of coronary heart disease in people without diabetes: Reykjavik prospective study and systematic review', *Public Library of Science Med*, 2010 May 25; 7(5):e1000278

14 R. M. Krauss, 'Carbohydrates raise LDL: Atherogenic lipoprotein phenotype and diet-gene interactions', *Journal of Nutrition*, 2001 Feb; 131(2):340S–3S

15 E. S. Ford, et al., 'Hypertriglyceridemia and its pharmacologic treatment among US adults', *Archives of Internal Medicine*, 2009; 169(6):572–8

16 E. J. Parks, et al., 'Dietary sugars stimulate fatty acid synthesis in adults', *Journal of Nutrition*, 2008 Jun; 138(6):1039–46

17 Dr. W. C. Willett, Symposium on Cancer Prevention, Annual meeting of the American Association for the Advancement of Science, March 2008

18 J. Ahn, et al., 'Adiposity, adult weight change, and postmenopausal breast cancer risk', *Archives of Internal Medicine*, 2007 Oct; 167(19):2091–102

19 M. J. Gunter, et al., 'Insulin, Insulin-Like Growth Factor-I, and Risk of Breast Cancer in Postmenopausal Women', *Journal of the National Cancer Institute*, 2009 Jan; 101(1):48–60

20 M. Pollak, et al., 'Insulin analogues and cancer risk: Cause for concern or cause celebre?', *International Journal of Clinical Practice*, 2010; 64:628–36

21 A. Tavani, et al., 'Consumption of sweet foods and breast cancer risk in Italy', *Annals of Oncology*, 2006 Feb; 17(2):341–5; and C. A. Krone and J. T. Ely, 'Controlling hyperglycemia as an adjunct to cancer therapy', *Integrative Cancer Therapies*, 2005 Mar; 4(1):25–31; and S. C. Larsson, et al., 'Glycemic load, glycemic index and breast cancer risk in a prospective cohort of Swedish women', *International Journal of Cancer*, 2009 July 1; 125(1):153–7; and W. Wen, et al., 'Dietary carbohydrates, fiber, and breast cancer risk in Chinese women', *American Journal of Clinical Nutrition*, 2009 Jan; 89(1):283–9; and S. Sieri, et al., 'Dietary glycemic index, glycemic load, and the risk of breast cancer in an Italian prospective cohort study', *American Journal of Clinical Nutrition*, 2007 Oct; 86(4):1160–6; and M. Lajous, et al., 'Carbohydrate intake, glycemic index, glycemic load, and risk of postmenopausal breast cancer in a prospective study of French women', *American Journal of Clinical Nutrition*, 2008 May; 87(5):1384–91; and S. E. McCann, et al., 'Dietary patterns related to glycemic index and load and risk of premenopausal and postmenopausal breast cancer in the Western New York Exposure and Breast Cancer Study', *American Journal of Clinical Nutrition*, 2007 Aug; 86(2):465–71 170.

22 M. L. Slattery, et al., 'Dietary sugar and colon cancer', *Cancer Epidemiology, Biomarkers and Prevention*, 1997 Sep; 6(9):677–85

23 S. A. Silvera, et al., 'Glycaemic index, glycaemic load and ovarian cancer risk: A prospective cohort study', *Public Health Nutrition*, 2007 Oct; 10(10):1076–81

24 S. A. Silvera, et al., 'Glycaemic index, glycaemic load and risk of endometrial cancer: A prospective cohort study', *Public Health Nutrition*, 2005 Oct; 8(7):912–19; and S. C. Larsson, et al., 'Carbohydrate intake, glycemic index and glycemic load in relation to risk of endometrial cancer: A prospective study of Swedish women', *International Journal of Cancer*, 2007 Mar; 120(5):1103–7

25 A. Tavani, et al., 'Consumption of sweet foods and breast cancer risk in Italy', *Annals of Oncology*, 2005 Oct; 17(2):341–5

26 M. Vanhala, et al., 'Depressive symptoms predispose females to metabolic syndrome: A 7-year follow-up study', *Acta Psychiatrica Scandinavica*, 2009 Feb; 119:137–42

27 L. Pulkki-Råback, et al., 'Depressive Symptoms and the Metabolic Syndrome in Childhood and Adulthood: A Prospective Cohort Study', *Health Psychology*, 2009 Jan; 28(1):108–16

28 A. Pan, et al., 'Bidirectional association between depression and type-2 diabetes mellitus in women', *Archives of Internal Medicine*, 2010; 170[21]:1884–91

29 A. Pan, et al., 'Insulin resistance and depressive symptoms in middle-aged and elderly Chinese: Findings from the Nutrition and Health of Aging Population in China Study', *Journal of Affective Disorders*, 2008 July; 109(1):75–82

30 R. S. McIntyre, et al., 'Should depressive syndromes be reclassified as "metabolic syndrome type II"?', *Annals of Clinical Psychiatry*, 2007 Oct–Dec; 19(4):257–64

31 H. Viinamäki, et al., 'Association of depressive symptoms and metabolic syndrome in men', *Acta Psychiatrica Scandinavica*, 2009 July; 120(1):23–9

32 L. Richardson, et al., 'Longitudinal effects of depression on glycemic control in veterans with type-2 diabetes', *General Hospital Psychiatry*, 2008 Nov; 30(6):509–14

33 R. S. McIntyre, et al. 'Should depressive syndromes be reclassified as "metabolic syndrome type II"?', *Annals of Clinical Psychiatry*, 2007 Oct–Dec; 19(4):257–64

34 T. Matsuzaki, et al., 'Insulin resistance is associated with the pathology of Alzheimer disease: The Hisayama study', *Neurology*, 2010 Aug; 75(9):764–70

35 K. Yaffe, 'The metabolic syndrome and development of cognitive impairment among older women', *Archives of Neurology*, 2009 Mar; 66(3):324–8

36 A. M. Kanaya, 'Total and Regional Adiposity and Cognitive Change in Older Adults: The Health, Aging, and Body Composition study', *Archives of Neurology*, 2009 March; 66(3):329–35

37 A. Kareinen, et al., 'Cardiovascular Risk Factors Associated With Insulin Resistance Cluster in Families With Early-Onset Coronary Heart Disease', *Arteriosclerosis Thrombosis and Vascular Biology*, 2001; 21:1346–52; see also K. Yaffe, et al., 'The Metabolic Syndrome and Development of Cognitive Impairment Among Older Women', *Archives of Neurology*, 2009; 66(3):324–8; see also S. Craft, 'The Role of Metabolic Disorders in Alzheimer Disease and Vascular Dementia: Two Roads Converged', *Archives of Neurology*, 2009; 66(3):300–5

38 I. Kyrou and C. Tsigos, 'Chronic stress, visceral obesity and gonadal dysfunction', *Hormones*, 2008; 7(4):287–93

39 J. Vrbíková, et al., 'Metabolic syndrome in adolescents with polycystic ovary syndrome', *Gynecological Endocrinology*, 2010 Sep [Epub ahead of print]

40 S. Kayaniyil, et al., 'Association of 25(OH)D and PTH with metabolic syndrome and its traditional and nontraditional components', *Journal of Clinical Endocrinology and Metabolism*, 2010 Oct 27 [Epub ahead of print]

41 A. H. Colagar, et al., 'Zinc levels in seminal plasma are associated with sperm quality in fertile and infertile men', *Nutrition Research*, 2009 Feb; 29(2):82–8; and M. Akmal, et al., 'Improvement in human semen quality after oral supplementation of vitamin C', *Journal of Medicinal Food*, 2006 Sep; 9(3):440–2; and A. Khosrowbeygia and N. Zarghami, http://www.plefa.com/article/S0952-3278%2807%2900103-2/abstract - aff2, 'Fatty acid composition of human spermatozoa and seminal plasma levels of oxidative stress biomarkers in subfertile males', *Prostaglandins, Leukotrienes and Essential Fatty Acids*, 2007 Aug; 77(2):117–21

42 S. Hexeberg and F. Lindberg, 'Insulin using woman with type-2 diabetes and weight problems', *Medisin Og Vitenskap Noe å lære av Tidsskr Nor Legeforen*, 2008; 128:443–5

43 G. Li, et al., 'The long-term effect of lifestyle interventions to prevent diabetes in the China Da Qing Diabetes Prevention Study: a 20-year follow-up study', *Lancet*, 2008 May; 371(9626):1783–9

44 D. R. Jacobs, et al., 'Association of 1-y changes in diet pattern with cardiovascular disease risk factors and adipokines: results from the 1-y randomized Oslo Diet and Exercise Study', *American Journal of Clinical Nutrition*, 2009 Feb; 89:509–17

45 K. J. Copell, et al., 'Nutritional intervention in patients with type-2 diabetes who are hyperglycaemic despite optimised drug treatment: Lifestyle Over and Above Drugs in Diabetes (LOADD) study: Randomised controlled trial', *British Medical Journal*, 2010 July; 341:c3337 (ISSN: 1468–5833)

46 J. Lindström, et al., 'The Finnish Diabetes Prevention Study (DPS): Lifestyle intervention and 3-year results on diet and physical activity', *Diabetes Care*, 2003; 26(12):3230–6

47 W. C. Knowler, 'Reduction in the incidence of type-2 diabetes with lifestyle intervention or metformin', *New England Journal of Medicine*, 2002 Feb 7; 346(6):393–403

48 T. Wu, et al., 'Associations of serum C-reactive protein with fasting insulin, glucose and glycosylated haemoglobin', *American Journal of Epidemiology*, 2002; 155:65–71

49 W. C. Knowler, et al., 'Diabetes in the Pima Indians: Incidence, risk factors and pathogenesis', *Diabetes and Metabolism Review*, 1990; 6:1–27

50 Dr Charles Clarke and Maureen Clarke, *Diabetes Revolution*, Vermilion, 2008

51 K. L. Mehers and K. M. Gillespie, 'The genetic basis for type-1 diabetes', *British Medical Bulletin*, 2008 Nov; 88(1):115–29

52 S. Eyre, 'Overlapping genetic susceptibility variants between three autoimmune disorders: Rheumatoid arthritis, type-1 diabetes and coeliac disease', *Arthritis Research and Therapy*, 2010 Sep 20; 12(5):R175 [Epub ahead of print]

53 C. C. Patterson, 'Incidence trends for childhood type-1 diabetes in Europe during 1989–2003 and predicted new cases 2005–20', *Lancet*, 2009 Jun; 373(9680):2027–33

54 F. W. Scott, et al., 'Milk and type-1 diabetes: Examining the evidence and broadening the focus', *Diabetes Care*, 1996; 19:379–83

55 E. Savilahti and K. M. Saarinen, 'Early infant feeding and type-1 diabetes', *European Journal of Nutrition*, 2009 Mar; 48(4):243–9

56 P. S. Clyne and A. Kulczycki, 'Human breast milk contains bovine IgG: Relationship to infant colic?', *Pediatrics*, 1991; 87:439–44

57 M. Nilsson, et al., 'Glycemia and insulinemia in healthy subjects after lactose equivalent meals of milk and other food proteins: The role of plasma amino acids and incretins', *American Journal of Clinical Nutrition*, 2004 Nov; 80(5):1246

58 M. Maglio, et al, 'The great majority of children with type-1 diabetes produce and deposit anti-tissue transglutaminase antibodies in the small intestine', *Diabetes*, 2009 Jul; 58(7):1578–84

59 D. Hansen, 'Clinical benefit of a gluten-free diet in type-1 diabetic children with screening-detected celiac disease: A population-based screening study with 2 years' follow-up', *Diabetes Care*, 2006 Nov; 29(11):2452–6

60 A. Grigorian, et al., 'Control of T Cell-mediated Autoimmunity by Metabolite Flux to N-Glycan Biosynthesis', *Journal of Biological Chemistry*, 2007 May; 282:20027–35

61 E. Hyppönen, et al., 'Intake of vitamin D and risk of type-1 diabetes: A birth-cohort study', *Lancet*, 2001 Nov; 358(9292):1500–3

62 S. J. Richardson, et al., 'The prevalence of enteroviral capsid protein vp1 immunostaining in pancreatic islets in human type-1 diabetes', *Diabetologia*, 2009 Jun; 52(6):1143–51

63 G. Dahlquist, 'Can we slow the rising incidence of childhood-onset autoimmune diabetes? The overload hypothesis', *Diabetologia*, 2006 Jan; 49(1):20–4

64 Editorial, 'Type-2 diabetes: Time to change our approach', *Lancet*, 2010 Jun; 375(9733):2193

65 M. Monami, et al., 'Metformin and cancer occurrence in insulin-treated type-2 diabetic patients', *Diabetes Care*, 2010 Oct [Epub ahead of print]; see also M. S. McFarland and R. Cripps, 'Diabetes Mellitus and Increased Risk of Cancer: Focus on Metformin and the Insulin Analogs', *Pharmacotherapy*, 2010; 30(11):1159–78

66 D. Buvat, 'Letter: Use of metformin is cause of vitamin B_{12} deficiency', *American Family Physician*, 2004 Jun; 69(2):264

67 J. Vidal-Alaball, 'Reduced serum vitamin B-12 in patients taking metformin', *British Medical Journal*, 2010 May; 40:c2198

68 A. D. Smith, et al., 'Homocysteine-lowering by B vitamins slows the rate of accelerated brain atrophy in mild cognitive impairment: A randomized controlled trial', *Public Library of Science One*, Published online ahead of print, doi: 10.1371/journal.pone.0012244

69 S. E. Nissen and K. Wolski, 'Effect of rosiglitazone on the risk of myocardial infarction and death from cardiovascular causes', *New England Journal of Medicine*, 2007 Jun; 356(24):2457–71

70 J. Burne, 'Should you still be taking Avandia? As the diabetes drug is linked to worrying side effects, some experts say there's a safer alternative', *Daily Mail*, July 26, 2010

71 P. D. Home, et al., 'Rosiglitazone evaluated for cardiovascular outcomes in oral agent combination therapy for type-2 diabetes (RECORD): A multicentre, randomised, open-label trial', *Lancet*, 2009 Jun 20; 373(9681):2125–35

72 Dr T. Marciniak, Food and Drug Administration, article in *New York Times* by G. Harris, 'Caustic government report deals blow to diabetes drug', July 9, 2010

73 D. DeNoon, 'Avandia Bares Changing FDA', *WebMD*, July 13, 2010. Accessed: http://blogs.webmd.com/breaking-news/2010/07/avandia-bares-changing-fda.html

74 S. E. Nissen and K. Wolski, 'Rosiglitazone revisited: an updated meta-analysis of risk for myocardial infarction and cardiovascular mortality', *Archives of Internal Medicine*, 2010 July; 170(14):1191–201

75 Article: 'European Medicines Agency recommends suspension of Avandia, Avandamet and Avaglim', European Medicines Agency, 23 September 2010

76 B. M. Psaty and C. D. Furberg, 'Rosiglitazone and cardiovascular risk', *New England Journal of Medicine*, 2007 Jun; 356(24):2522–4

77 N. Busso, et al., 'Circulating CD26 is negatively associated with inflammation in human and experimental arthritis', *American Journal of Pathology*, 2005; 166:433–42; C. McGuinness and U. V. Wesley, 'Dipeptidyl peptidase IV (DPPIV), a candidate tumor suppressor gene in melanomas is silenced by promoter methylation', *Frontiers in Bioscience*, 2008 Jan 1; 13:2435–43; M. R. Goldstein, 'DPP-4 inhibitors and cancer', *Annals of Internal Medicine*, 2007 Sep; Y. X. Sun, et al., 'CD26/dipeptidyl peptidase IV regulates prostate cancer metastasis by degrading SDF-1/CXCL12', *Clinical and Experimental Metastasis*, 2008; 25(7):765–76; U. V. Wesley, et al., 'Role for dipeptidyl peptidase IV in tumor suppression of human non small cell lung carcinoma cells', *Inernational Journal of Cancer*, 2004 May 10; 109(6):855–66

78 S. Bolen, et al., 'Systematic review: Comparative effectiveness and safety of oral medications for type-2 diabetes mellitus', *Annals of Internal Medicine*, 2007 Sep; 147(6):386–99

79 F. Ismail-Beigi, et al., 'Effect of intensive treatment of hyperglycaemia on microvascular outcomes in type-2 diabetes: An analysis of the ACCORD randomized trial', *Lancet*, 2010 Aug; 376(9739):419–30

80 S. Stiles, 'Standard CV risk factors don't explain the doubling of vascular disease risk in diabetics', Heart.org, June 20, 2010. Accessed: http://www.theheart.org/article/1092043.do

81 DiabetesInControl.com, 'Insulin users have 50% higher cancer risk; causes unclear', Press Release, 2 September 2010. Accessed: http://www.diabetesincontrol.com/articles/diabetes-news/9766-insulin-users-have-50-higher-cancer-risk-causes-unclear

82 S. L. Bowker, et al., 'Glucose-lowering agents and cancer mortality rates in type-2 diabetes: assessing effects of time-varying exposure', *Diabetologia*, 2010 Aug; 53(8):1631–7

83 T. Orchard, et al, 'The effect of metformin and intensive lifestyle intervention on the metabolic syndrome: the Diabetes Prevention Program randomized trial', *Annals of Internal Medicine*, 2005; 142(8):611–19

84 J. Wylie-Rosett, et al., 'Lifestyle intervention to prevent diabetes: Intensive AND cost effective', *Current Opinion Lipidology*, 2006; 17(1):37–44

85 W. C. Knowler, et al., 'Reduction in the incidence of type-2 diabetes with lifestyle intervention or metformin', *New England Journal of Medicine*, 2002; 246:393–403

86 P. Wursch and F. X. Pi-Sunyer, 'The role of viscous soluble fiber in the metabolic control of diabetes: A review with special emphasis on cereals rich in beta-glucan', *Diabetes Care*, 1997; 20(11):1774–80; L. Tappy, et al., 'Effects of breakfast cereals containing various amounts of beta-glucan fibers on plasma glucose and insulin responses in NIDDM subjects', *Diabetes Care*, 1996 Aug; 19(8):831–4

87 E. Balk, et al., 'Effect of chromium supplementation on glucose metabolism and lipids: A systematic review of randomized controlled trials', *Diabetes Care*, 2007; 30(9): e103

88 D. M. Zulman, et al., 'Patient-provider concordance in the prioritization of health conditions among hypertensive diabetes patients', *Journal of General Internal Medicine*, 2010 May; 25(5):408–14

Part Two

1 I. Sluijs, et al., 'Carbohydrate quantity and quality and risk of type-2 diabetes in the European Prospective Investigation into Cancer and Nutrition-Netherlands (EPIC-NL) study', *American Journal of Clinical Nutrition*, 2010 Oct; 92(4):905–11

2 K. Esposito, et al., 'Dietary glycemic index and glycemic load are associated with metabolic control in type-2 diabetes: The CAPRI experience', *Metabolic Syndrome and Related Disorders*, 2010 Jun; 8(3):255–61

3 C. K. Roberts and S. Liu, 'Effects of glycemic load on metabolic health and type-2 diabetes mellitus', *Journal of Diabetes Science and Technology*, 2009 Jul; 3(4):697–704

4 D. Thomas and E. J. Elliott, 'Low glycemic index, or low glycemic load, diets for diabetes mellitus', *Cochrane Database Systematic Review*, 2009 Jan; (1):CD006296

5 M. A. Martínez-González, et al., 'Adherence to Mediterranean diet and risk of developing diabetes: Prospective cohort study', *British Medical Journal*, 2008 May; 336:1348

6 A. Elhayani, et al., 'A low carbohydrate Mediterranean diet improves cardiovascular risk factors and diabetes control among overweight patients with type-2 diabetes mellitus: A one-year prospective randomised intervention study', Conference report, IDOF 2010, Athens

7 Y. Granfeldt, et al., 'On the importance of processing conditions, product thickness and egg addition for the glycemic and hormonal responses to pasta: A comparison of bread made with "pasta ingredients"', *European Journal of Clinical Nutrition*, 1991; 45:489–99

8 J. S. Lim, et al., 'The role of fructose in the pathogenesis of NAFLD and the metabolic syndrome', *Nature Reviews: Gastroenterology and Hepatology*, 2010 May; 7(5):251–64

9 M. K. Hellerstein, et al., 'Regulation of hepatic de novo lipogenesis in humans', *Nutrition*, 1996 Jul; 16:523–57

10 E. J. Parks, et al., 'Dietary sugars stimulate fatty acid synthesis in adults', *Journal of Nutrition*, 2008 Jun; 38(6):1039–46

11 P. Mitrou, et al., 'Vinegar decreases postprandial hyperglycemia in patients with type-1 diabetes', *Diabetes Care*, 2010 Feb; 33(2):e27

12 S. Liatis, et al., 'Vinegar reduces postprandial hyperglycaemia in patients with type II diabetes when added to a high, but not to a low, glycemic index meal', *European Journal of Clinical Nutrition*, 2010 Jul; 64(7):727–32

13 J. Uribarri, et al., 'Advanced glycation end products in foods and a practical guide to their reduction in the diet', *Journal of the American Dietetic Association*, 2010 Jun; 110(6):911–16. e12.

14 D. Jenkins, et al., 'Glycemic index of foods: A physiological basis for carbohydrate exchange', *American Journal of Clinical Nutrition*, 1980; 34:362–6

15 T. Solomon, et al., 'Exercise and diet enhance fat oxidation and reduce insulin resistance in older obese adults', *Journal of Applied Physiology*, 2008; 104(5):1313–19

16 A. Shapiro, et al., 'Fructose induced leptin resistance exacerbates weight gain in response to subsequent high-fat feeding', *AJP- Regulatory, Integrative and Comparative*, 2008 Nov; 295(5):R1370–R1375

17 J. L. Ivy, 'Role of exercise training in the prevention and treatment of insulin resistance and non-insulin-dependent diabetes mellitus', *Sports Medicine*, 1997 Nov; 24(5):321–36

18 P. Salmon, 'Effects of physical exercise on anxiety, depression, and sensitivity to stress: A unifying theory', *Clinical Psychology Review*, 2001 Feb; 21(1):33–61

19 S. Thornley, et al., 'The Obesity Epidemic: Is glycemic index the key to unlocking a hidden addiction?', *Medical Hypotheses*, 2008 Nov; 71(5):709–14

20 B. Spring, et al., 'Abuse potential of carbohydrates for overweight carbohydrate cravers', *Psychopharmacology*, 2008; 197:637–47

21 A. Geliebter, 'Night-eating syndrome in obesity', *Nutrition*, 2001 Jun; 17(6):483–4.

22 M. S. Bray and M. E. Young, 'Circadian rhythms in the development of obesity: Potential role for the circadian clock within the adipocyte', *Obesity Review*, 2007 Mar; 8(2):169–81; S. Taheri, et al., 'Short sleep duration is associated with reduced leptin, elevated ghrelin, and increased body mass index', *PLoS Medicine*, 2004 Dec; 1(3):e62

23 Article: 'Beta glucan Key to Cardiovascular Health Benefits', *Medscape Medical News*, 2000 May

24 Y. T. Ko and Y. L. Lin, '1,3-beta-glucan quantification by a fluorescence microassay and analysis of its distribution in foods', *Journal of Agricultural and Food Chemistry*, 2004 Jun 2; 52(11):3313–18. See www.ncbi.nlm.nih.gov/pubmed/15161189

25 M. Ulmius, et al., 'The influence of dietary fibre source and gender on the postprandial glucose and lipid response in healthy subjects', *European Journal of Nutrition*, 2009 Oct; 48(7):395–402

26 P. Kallio, et al., 'Dietary carbohydrate modification induces alterations in gene expression in abdominal subcutaneous adipose tissue in persons with the metabolic syndrome: the FUNGENUT Study', *American Journal of Clinical Nutrition*, 2007 May; 85(5):1417–27; see also M. Lankinen, et al., 'Dietary carbohydrate modification alters serum metabolic profiles in individuals with the metabolic syndrome', *Nutrition, Metabolism and Cardiovascular Disease*, 2010 May; 20(4):249–57

27 Article: 'Beta glucan key to cardiovascular health benefits', *Medscape Medical News*, 2000 May; article no. 411884

28 V. Vuksan, et al., 'Supplementation of conventional therapy with the novel grain salba (Salvia hispanica L.) improves major and emerging cardiovascular risk factors in type-2 diabetes: Results of a randomized controlled trial', *Diabetes Care*, 2007; 30:2804–10

29 Y. Ma, et al., 'Effects of walnut consumption on endothelial function in type-2 diabetes: A randomized, controlled, crossover trial', *Diabetes Care*, 2010 Feb; 33(2):227–32

30 T. Xia and Q. Wang, 'Hypoglycemic role of Cucurbita ficifolia (Cucurbitaceae) fruit extract in streptozotocin-induced diabetic rats', *Journal of the Science of Food and Agriculture*, 2007; 87:1753–7

31 A. J. Stull, et al., 'Bioactives in blueberries improve insulin sensitivity in obese, insulin-resistant men and women', *Journal of Nutrition*, 2010 Aug; 140 (10):1764–8

32 A. Khan, et al., 'Cinnamon improves glucose and lipids of people with type-2 diabetes', *Diabetes Care*, 2003; 26(12):3215–18

33 H. G. Preuss, et al., 'Whole cinnamon and aqueous extracts ameliorate sucrose-induced blood pressure elevations in spontaneously hypertensive rats', *Journal of the American College of Nutrition*, 2006 Apr; 25(2):144–50

34 E. J. Verspohl, et al., 'Antidiabetic effect of cinnamoncassia and cinnamomum zeylanicum in vivo and in vitro', *Phytotherapy Research*, 2005; 19(3):203–6

35 S. H. Kim, et al., 'Anti-diabetic effect of cinnamon extract on blood glucose in db/db mice', *Journal of Ethnopharmacology*, 2006; 104(1–2):119–23

36 T. N. Ziegenfuss, et al., 'Effects of a Water-Soluble Cinnamon Extract on Body Composition and Features of the Metabolic Syndrome in Pre-Diabetic Men and Women', *Journal of the International Society of Sports Nutrition*, 2006; 3(2):45–53

37 A.-M. Roussel, et al., 'Antioxidant effects of a cinnamon extract in people with impaired fasting glucose that are overweight or obese', *Journal of the American College of Nutrition*, 2009; 28:16–21

38 Z. T. Bloomgarden, et al., 'Lower baseline glycemia reduces apparent oral agent glucose-lowering efficacy: A meta-regression analysis', *Diabetes Care*, 2006; 29:2137–9

39 S. Chearskul, et al., 'Glycemic and lipid responses to glucomannan in Thais with type-2 diabetes mellitus', *Journal of the Medical Association of Thailand*, 2007 Oct; 90(10):2150–7

40 M. Yoshida, et al., 'Effect of plant sterols and glucomannan on lipids in individuals with and without type II diabetes', *European Journal of Clinical Nutrition*, 2006 Apr; 60(4):529–37; see also H. L. Chen, et al., 'Konjac supplement alleviated hypercholesterolemia and hyperglycemia in type-2 diabetic subjects: A randomized double-blind trial', *Journal of the American College of Nutrition*, 2003 Feb; 22(1):36–42.

41 V. Vuksan, et al., 'Beneficial effects of viscous dietary fiber from Konjac-mannan in subjects with the insulin resistance syndrome: Results of a controlled metabolic trial', *Diabetes Care*, 2000 Jan; 23(1):9–14; see also V. Vuksan, et al., 'Konjac-mannan (glucomannan) improves glycemia and other associated risk factors for coronary heart disease in type-2 diabetes: A randomized controlled metabolic trial', *Diabetes Care*, 1999 Jun; 22(6):913–19

42 A. Mito, data held in ION library, source unknown

43 D. Walsh, 'Effect of glucomannan on obese patients', *International Journal of Obesity*, 1984; 8:289–93

44 P. Holford, 'The Effects of Glucomannan on Weight Loss', ION (1983)

45 J. Keithley and B. Swanson, 'Glucomannan and obesity: A critical review', *Alternative Therapies in Health and Medicine*, 2005 Nov–Dec; 11(6):30–4

46 M. Lyon and R. Reichert, 'The effect of a novel viscous polysaccharide along with lifestyle changes on short-term weight loss and associated risk factor of overweight and obese adults', *Alternative Medicine Review*, 2010; 115(1):68–75

47 J. Brand-Miller, et al., 'Effects of PGX, a novel functional fibre, on acute and delayed postprandial glycaemia', *European Journal of Clinical Nutrition*, 2010 Oct, advance online publication

48 A. L. Jenkins, et al., 'Reduction of postprandial glycemia by the novel viscous polysaccharide PGX, in a dose-dependent manner, independent of food form', *Journal of the American College of Nutrition*, 2010 Oct; 29(2):92–8

49 A. L. Jenkins, et al., 'Effect of adding the novel fiber, PGX®, to commonly consumed foods on glycemic response, glycemic index and GRIP: a simple and effective strategy for reducing post prandial blood glucose levels: A randomized, controlled trial', *Nutrition Journal*, 2010; 9:58

50 V. Vuksan, 'Viscosity of fiber preloads affects food intake in adolescents', *Nutrition, Metabolism and Cardiovascular Diseases*, 2009 Sep; 19(7):498–503

51 G. J. Grover, 'Effects of the soluble fiber complex PolyGlycopleX® on insulin and glucose homeostasis and body weight in zucker diabetic rats' (unpublished)

52 T. L. Halton, et al., 'Low-carbohydrate-diet score and risk of type-2 diabetes in women', *American Journal of Clinical Nutrition*, 2008 Feb; 87(2):339–46

53 P. W. Siri-Tarino, et al., 'Meta-analysis of prospective cohort studies evaluating the association of saturated fat with cardiovascular disease', *American Journal of Clinical Nutrition*, 2010 Mar; 91(3):535–46

54 I. Shai, et al., 'Weight loss with a low-carbohydrate, Mediterranean, or low-fat diet', *New England Journal of Medicine*, 2008 Jul; 359(3):229–41

55 S. A. LaHaye, et al., 'Comparison between a low glycemic load diet and a Canada Food Guide diet in cardiac rehabilitation patients in Ontario', *Canadian Journal of Cardiology*, 2005; 21(6):489–94

56 I. Shai, et al., 'Weight loss with a low-carbohydrate, Mediterranean, or low-fat diet', *New England Journal of Medicine*, 2008 Jul; 359(3):229–41

57 M. Moyer, 'Carbs against cardio: more evidence that refined carbohydrates, not fats, threaten the heart', *Scientific American*, April 27, 2010

58 For a full discussion of the links between diabetes, metabolic syndrome, testosterone and the andropause read Dr Malcolm Carruthers, *Androgen Deficiency in the Adult Male: Causes, Diagnosis and Treatment*, Taylor and Francis, 2004

59 L. A. Baur, et al., 'The fatty acid composition of skeletal muscle membrane phospholipid: Its relationship with the type of feeding and plasma glucose levels in young children', *Metabolism*, 1998; 47:106–12

60 S. O. E. Ebbesson, et al., 'Omega-3 fatty acids improve glucose tolerance and components of the metabolic syndrome in Alaskan Eskimos: The Alaska–Siberia Project', *International Journal of Circumpolar Health*, 2005 Sep; 64(4):396–408

61 K. Esposito, et al., 'Effect of a Mediterranean-style diet on endothelial dysfunction and markers of vascular inflammation in the metabolic syndrome a randomized trial', *Journal of the American Medical Association*, 2004, Sep; 292:1440–6; V. R. Sreeraman, 'Secret behind fish oils' effect on diabetes unlocked', *Diet and Nutrition News*, Sep 4, 2010

62 G. Riccardi, et al., 'Dietary fat, insulin sensitivity and the metabolic syndrome', *Clinical Nutrition*, 2004 Aug; 23(4):447–56; B. Vessby, et al., 'Substituting dietary saturated for monounsaturated fat impairs insulin sensitivity in healthy men and women: The KANWU study', *Diabetologia*, 2001; 44:312–19

63 B. B. Duncan, et al., 'Adiponectin and the development of type-2 diabetes', *Diabetes*, 2004; 53(9):2473–8

64 L. M. Browning, et al., 'The impact of long chain n-3 polyunsaturated fatty acid supplementation on inflammation, insulin sensitivity and CVD risk in a group of overweight women with an inflammatory phenotype', *Diabetes, Obesity and Metabolism*, 2007; 9:70–80

65 A. Bener, et al., 'High prevalence of vitamin D deficiency in type-1 diabetes mellitus and healthy children', *Acta Diabetologia*, 2008 Oct 10 [Epub ahead of print]; E. Hyppönen, et al., 'Intake of vitamin D and risk of type-1 diabetes: A birth-cohort study', *Lancet*, 2001, Nov; 358(9292):1500–3

66 A. G. Pittas, et al., 'The role of vitamin d and calcium in type-2 diabetes: A systematic review and meta-analysis', *Journal of Clinical Endocrinology and Metabolism*, 2007; 92(6):2017–20

67 A.-M. Borissova, et al., 'The effect of vitamin D_3 on insulin secretion and peripheral insulin sensitivity in type-2 diabetic patients', *International Journal of Clinical Practice*, 2003; 57(4):258–61

68 J. R. Greenfield, et al., 'Oral glutamine increases circulating glucagon-like peptide 1, glucagon and insulin concentrations on lean, obese and type-2 diabetic subjects', *American Journal of Clinical Nutrition*, 2009; 89:106–13

69 A.-H. Harding, et al., 'Plasma Vitamin C Level, Fruit and Vegetable Consumption, and the Risk of New-Onset Type-2 Diabetes Mellitus. The European Prospective Investigation of Cancer–Norfolk Prospective Study', *Archives of Internal Medicine*, 2008; 168(14):1493–9

70 M. Afkhami-Ardekani and A. Shojaoddiny-Ardekani, 'Effect of vitamin C on blood glucose, serum lipids and serum insulin in type-2 diabetes patients', *Indian Journal of Medical Research*, 2007 Nov; 126(5):471–4

71 P. Carter, et al., 'Fruit and vegetable intake and incidence of type-2 diabetes mellitus: Systematic review and meta-analysis', *British Medical Journal*, 2010 Aug; 341:c4229

72 J. S. Vinson, et al., 'In vitro and in vivo reduction of erythrocyte sorbitol by ascorbic acid', *Diabetes*, 1989 Aug; 38(8):1036–41

73 J. G. Regensteiner, et al., 'Oral L-arginine and vitamins E and C improve endothelial function in women with type-2 diabetes', *Vascular Medicine*, 2003; 8(3):169–75

74 P. Gaede, et al., 'Double-blind, randomised study of the effect of combined treatment with vitamin C and E on albuminuria in type-2 diabetic patients', *Diabetes Medicine*, 2001 Sep; 18(9):756–60

75 P. Gaede, et al., 'Multifactorial intervention and cardiovascular disease in patients with type-2 diabetes', *New England Journal of Medicine*, 2003 Jan; 348(5):383–93

76 J. M. Hodgson, et al., 'Coenzyme Q10 improves blood pressure and glycemic control: A controlled trial in subjects with type-2 diabetes', *European Journal of Clinical Nutrition*, 2002 Nov; 56(11):1137–42

77 S. J. Hamilton, et al., 'Coenzyme Q10 improves endothelial dysfunction in statin-treated type-2 diabetic patients', *Diabetes Care*, 2009 May; 32(5):810–12

78 U. Singh and I. Jialal, 'Alpha-lipoic acid supplementation and diabetes', *Nutrition Reviews*, 2008 Nov; 66(11):646–57; L. Packer, et al., 'Lipoic acid as a biological antioxidant', *Free Radical Biology and Medicine*, 1995 Aug; 19:227–50

79 P. Kamenova, 'Improvement of insulin sensitivity in patients with type-2 diabetes mellitus after oral administration of alpha-lipoic acid', *Hormones* (Athens), 2006 Oct–Dec; 5(4):251–8

80 G. S. Mijnhout, et al., 'Alpha lipoic acid: A new treatment for neuropathic pain in patients with diabetes?', *Netherlands Journal of Medicine*, 2010 Apr; 68(4):158–62

81 B. B. Heinisch, et al., 'Alpha-lipoic acid improves vascular endothelial function in patients with type-2 diabetes: A placebo-controlled randomized trial', *European Journal of Clinical Investigation*, 2010 Feb; 40(2):148–54

82 D. Ziegler, et al., 'Treatment of symptomatic diabetic peripheral neuropathy with the anti-oxidant alpha-lipoic acid: A 3-week multicentre randomized controlled trial (ALADIN Study)', *Diabetologia*, 1995 Dec; 38(12):1425–33; M. Reljanovic, et al., 'Treatment of diabetic polyneuropathy with the antioxidant thioctic acid (alpha-lipoic acid): A two year multicenter randomized double-blind placebo-controlled trial (ALADIN II). Alpha Lipoic Acid in Diabetic Neuropathy', *Free Radical Research*, 1999 Sep; 31(3):171–9; D. Ziegler, et al., 'Treatment of symptomatic diabetic polyneuropathy with the antioxidant alpha-lipoic acid: A 7-month multicenter randomized controlled trial (ALADIN III Study). ALADIN III Study Group. Alpha-Lipoic Acid in Diabetic Neuropathy', *Diabetes Care*, 1999 Aug; 22(8):1296–301; D. Ziegler, et al., 'Effects of treatment with the antioxidant alpha-lipoic acid on cardiac autonomic neuropathy in NIDDM patients: A 4-month randomized controlled multicenter trial (DEKAN Study). Deutsche Kardiale Autonome Neuropathies', *Diabetes Care*, 1997 Mar; 20(3):369–73; A. S. Ametov, et al., 'The sensory symptoms of diabetic polyneuropathy are improved with alpha-lipoic acid: The SYDNEY trial', *Diabetes Care*, 2003 Mar; 26(3):770–6

83 R. V. Sekhar, et al., 'Glutathione synthesis is diminished in patients with uncontrolled diabetes and restored by dietary supplementation with cysteine and glycine', *Diabetes Care*, 2010 Oct 7 [Epub ahead of print]

84 J. A. Baur, et al., 'Resveratrol improves health and survival of mice on a high-calorie diet', *Nature*, 2006 Nov; 444:337–42; see also P. Brasnyo, et al., 'Resveratrol improves insulin sensitivity in type-2 diabetic patients', *British Journal of Nutrition*, 2011 March 9; 1–7; and a pilot study presented at the American Diabetes Associations annual scientific meeting, http://www.diabetes.org by J. Crandall

85 Mario Barbagallo, et al., 'Role of magnesium in insulin action, diabetes and cardio-metabolic syndrome X', *Molecular Aspects of Medicine*, 2003 Feb; 24(1–3):39–52; see also S. O. Emdin, et al., 'Role of zinc in insulin bisynthesis', *Diabetologia*, 2008; 19(3):174–82

86 Q. Sun, et al., 'Prospective study of zinc intake and risk of type-2 diabetes in women', *Diabetes Care*, 2009 Apr; 32(4):629–34

87 J. Ma, et al., 'Associations of serum and dietary magnesium with cardiovascular disease, hypertension, diabetes, insulin, and carotid arterial wall thickness in the ARIC study', *Journal of Clinical Epidemiology*, 1995; 48:927–40

88 B. N. Hopping, et al., 'Dietary fiber, magnesium, and glycemic load alter risk of type-2 diabetes in a multiethnic cohort in Hawaii', *Journal of Nutrition*, 2010 Jan; 140(1):68–74

89 M. Rodríguez-Morán and F. Guerrero-Romero, 'Oral magnesium supplementation improves insulin sensitivity and metabolic control in type-2 diabetic subjects', *Diabetes Care*, 2003 Apr; 26(4):1147–52

90 M. Velussi, et al., 'Long-term (12 months) treatment with an anti-oxidant drug (silymarin) is effective on hyperinsulinemia, exogenous insulin need and malondialdehyde levels in cirrhotic diabetic patients', *Journal of Hepatology*, 1997; 26:871–9; H. F. Huseini, et al., 'The efficacy of Silybum marianum (L.) Gaertn. (silymarin) in the treatment of type II diabetes: A randomized, double blind, placebo-controlled, clinical trial', *Phytotherapy Research*, 2006; 20:1036–9; S. A.-R. Hussain, et al., 'Silymarin as an adjunct to glibenclamide therapy improves long-term and postprandial glycemic control and body mass index in type-2 diabetes', *Journal of Medicinal Food*, 2007; 10:543–7

91 E. R. B. Shangmugasundaram, et al., 'Use of gymnema sylvestre leaf extract in the control of blood glucose in insulin-dependent diabetes mellitus', *Journal of Ethnopharmacology*, 1990; 30:281–94; K. Baskaran, et al., 'Antidiabetic effect of a leaf extract from Gymnema sylvestre in non-insulin-dependent diabetes mellitus patients', *Journal of Ethnopharmacology*, 1990; 30:295–306

92 A. A. House, et al., 'Effect of B-vitamin therapy on progression of diabetic nephropathy: A randomized controlled trial', *Journal of the American Medical Association*, 2010; 303(16):1603–9

93 S. M. Grundy, et al., 'Efficacy, safety, and tolerability of once-daily niacin for the treatment of dyslipidcmia associatcd with typc-2 diabetes: Results of the assessment of diabetes control and evaluation of the efficacy of niaspan trial', *Archives of Internal Medicine*, 2002 Jul; 162(14):1568–76

94 E. Balk, et al, 'Effect of chromium supplementation on glucose metabolism and lipids: A systematic review of randomized controlled trials', *Diabetes Care*, 2007; 30(8):2154–63

95 R. A. Anderson, et al., 'Elevated intakes of supplemental chromium improve glucose and insulin variables in individuals with type-2 diabetes', *Diabetes*, 1997; 46:1786–91

96 N. Cheng, et al., 'Follow-up survey of people in China with type-2 diabetes mellitus consuming supplemental chromium', *Journal of Trace Elements in Experimental Medicine*, 1999 May; 12:55–60

97 H. Rabinovitz, et al., 'Effect of chromium supplementation on blood glucose and lipid levels in type-2 diabetes mellitus elderly patients', *International Journal for Vitamin and Nutrition Research*, 2004 May; 74:178–82

98 S. Anton, et al., 'Effects of chromium picolinate on food intake and satiety', *Diabetes Technology and Therapeutics*, 2008 Oct; 10(5):405–12

99 Food Standards Agency, 'Agency revises chromium picolinate advice', 13 December 2004, http://www.food.gov.uk/news/newsarchive/2004/dec/chromiumupdate

100 S. Anton, et al., 'Effects of chromium picolinate on food intake and satiety', *Diabetes Technology and Therapeutics*, 2008 Oct; 10(5):405–12

101 A. Ravina, et al., 'Clinical use of the trace element chromium (III) in the treatment of diabetes mellitus', *Journal of Trace Elements in Experimental Medicine* 1995; 8:183–190; also see R. A. Anderson, et al., 'Elevated intakes of supplemental chromium improve glucose and insulin variables in individuals with type-2 diabetes', *Diabetes*, 1997; 46:1786–91

102 P. Holford, et al., 'The effects of a low glycemic load diet on weight loss and key health risk indicators', *Journal of Orthomolecular Medicine*, 2006; 21(2):71–8

103 M. S. Westerterp-Plantenga and E. M. Kovacs, 'The effect of hydroxycitrate on energy intake and satiety in overweight humans', *International Journal of Obesity Related Metabolic Disorders*, 2002; 26(6):870–2

104 H. Preuss, et al., 'An overview of the safety and efficacy of a novel, natural hydroxycitric acid extract (HCA-SX) for weight management', *Journal of Medicine*, 2004; 35(1–6):33–48

105 C. Cangiano, et al., 'Eating behavior and adherence to dietary prescriptions in obese adult subjects treated with 5-hydroxytryptophan', *American Journal of Clinical Nutrition*, 1992; 56(5):863–7

106 C. Cangiano, et al., 'Effects of oral 5-hydroxy-tryptophan on energy intake and macronutrient selection in non-insulin dependent diabetic patients', *International Journal of Obesity Related Metabolic Disorders*, 1998; 22(7):648–54

107 E. J. Hendricks, et al., 'How physician obesity specialists use drugs to treat obesity', *Obesity*, 2009 Sep; 17(9):1730–5

108 J. R. Palmer, et al., 'Sugar-sweetened beverages and incidence of type-2 diabetes mellitus in African American women', *Archives of Internal Medicine*, 2008; 168(14):1487–92

109 W. Nseir, et al., 'Soft drinks consumption and nonalcoholic fatty liver disease', *World Journal of Gastroenterology*, 2010 Jun; 16(21):2579–88

110 H. K. Choi and G. Curhan, 'Soft drinks, fructose consumption, and the risk of gout in men: Prospective cohort study', *British Medical Journal*, 2008 Feb 9; 336(7639):309–12

111 A. R. Gaby, 'Adverse effects of dietary fructose', *Alternative Medicine Review*, 2005 Dec; 10(4):294–306

112 H. Vlassara, et al., 'Inflammatory mediators are induced by dietary glycotoxins, a major risk factor for diabetic angiopathy', *Proceedings of the National Academy of Science USA*, 2002 Nov; 99(24):15596–601

113 A. Ferland, et al., 'Is aspartame really safer in reducing the risk of hypoglycemia during exercise in patients with type-2 diabetes?', *Diabetes Care*, 2007 Jul; 30(7):e59

114 R. Huxley, et al., 'Coffee, decaffeinated coffee, and tea consumption in relation to incident type-2 diabetes mellitus: A systematic review with meta-analysis', *Archives of Internal Medicine*, 2009 Dec 14; 169(22):2053–63

115 T. Wu, et al., 'Caffeinated coffee, decaffeinated coffee, and caffeine in relation to plasma C-peptide levels, a marker of insulin secretion, in U.S. women', *Diabetes Care*, 2005 Jun; 28(6):1390–6; R. C. Loopstra-Masters, et al., 'Associations between the intake of caffeinated and decaffeinated coffee and measures of insulin sensitivity and beta cell function', *Diabetologia*, 2010 Nov [Epub ahead of print]

116 J. A. Greenberg, et al., 'Coffee, diabetes, and weight control', *American Journal of Clinical Nutrition*, 2006 Oct; 84(4):682–93

117 L. Moisey, et al., 'Caffeinated coffee consumption impairs blood glucose homeostasisin response to high and low glycemic index meals in healthy men', *Journal of Clinical Nutrition*, 2008; 87:1254–61

118 J. A. Greenberg, et al., 'Coffee, diabetes, and weight control', *American Journal of Clinical Nutrition*, 2006 Oct; 84(4):682–93; see also J. Geleijnse, 'Habitual coffee consumption and blood pressure: An epidemiological perspective', *Vascular Health Risk Management*, 2008 Oct; 4(5):963–70

119 M. J. Grubben, et al., 'Unfiltered coffee increases plasma homocysteine concentrations in healthy volunteers: A randomized trial', *American Journal of Clinical Nutrition*, 2000 Feb; 71(2):480–4; see also P. Verhoef, et al., 'Contribution of caffeine to the homocysteine-raising effect of coffee: A randomized controlled trial in humans', *American Journal of Clinical Nutrition*, 2002 Dec; 76(6):1244–8

120 P. Holford, et al., 100% Health Survey, published by Holford and Associates, 2010

121 A. Peters, 'The selfish brain: Competition for energy resources', *American Journal of Human Biology*, 2010 Nov [Epub ahead of print]

122 K. D. Laugero, et al., 'Relationship between perceived stress and dietary and activity patterns in older adults participating in the Boston Puerto Rican Health Study', *Appetite*, 2010 Nov 8 [Epub ahead of print]

123 B. McEwen and R. Sapolsky, 'Patient information page from The Hormone Foundation Stress and Your Health', *Journal of Clinical Endocrinology and Metabolism*, 91(2):735

124 P. Holford, et al., 'The effects of a low glycemic load diet on weight loss and key health risk indicators', *Journal of Orthomolecular Medicine*, 2006; 21(2):71–8

125 R. McCraty, et al., 'The coherent heart heart–brain interactions, psychophysiological coherence, and the emergence of system-wide order', *Integral Review*, 2009 Dec; 5(2):11–15

126 R. McCraty and D. Childre, 'Coherence: Bridging personal, social, and global health', *Alternative Therapies in Health and Medicine*, 2010; 16(4):10–24

127 R. McCraty, et al., 'The impact of a new emotional self-management program on stress, emotions, heart rate variability, DHEA and cortisol', *Integrative Physiological and Behavioural Science*, 1988 Apr–Jun; 33:151–70

128 R. McCraty and D. Tomasino, 'Emotional stress, positive emotions and psychophysiological coherence', in *Stress in Health and Disease* (2006), Wiley, pp. 342–65

129 R. McCraty, M. Atkinson and L. Lipensthal, *Emotional Self-Regulation Program Enhances Psychological Health and Quality of Life in Patients With Diabetes*, Boulder Creek, CA: HeartMath Research Center, Institute of HeartMath, Publication no. 00–006 (2000)

130 K. Katsumata, et al., 'High incidence of sleep apnea syndrome in a male diabetic population', *Diabetes Research and Clinical Practice*, 1991; 13:45–51

131 A. Pandey, et al., 'Sleep apnea and diabetes: Insights into the emerging epidemic', *Current Diabetes Reports*, 2010 Nov 11 [Epub ahead of print]; see also S. Fendri, et al., 'Nocturnal hyperglycaemia in type-2 diabetes with sleep apnoea syndrome', *Diabetes Research in Clinical Practice*, 2010 Oct 21 [Epub ahead of print]

132 G. Mugnai, 'Pathophysiological links between obstructive sleep apnea syndrome and metabolic syndrome', *Giornale Italiano di Cardiologia*, 2010 Jun; 11(6):453–9

133 N. J. Pearson, et al., 'Insomnia, trouble sleeping, and complementary and alternative medicine: Analysis of the 2002 National Health Interview Survey Data', *Archives of Internal Medicine*, 2006 Sep; 166:1775–82

134 'Common ones include "daytime sedation, motor incoordination, cognitive impairments (anterograde amnesia), and related concerns about increases in the risk of motor vehicle accidents and injuries from falls', M. J. Sateia and P. D. Nowell, 'Insomnia', *Lancet*, 2004 Nov; 364 (9449):1959–73

135 Editorial, 'Treating insomnia: Use of drugs is rising despite evidence of harm and little meaningful benefit', *British Medical Journal*, 2004 Nov; 329:1198–9

136 S. Saul, 'Sleep drugs found only mildly effective but wildly popular', *New York Times*, 23 October 2007

137 P. Lemoine, et al., 'Prolonged release melatonin improves sleep quality and morning alertness in insomnia patients aged 55 years and older and has no withdrawal effects', *Journal of Sleep Research*, 2007 Dec; 16(4):372–80

138 A. Prentice and S. Jebb, 'Obesity in Britain: Gluttony or sloth?', *British Medical Journal*, 1995; 311:437–9

139 W. McArdle, chapter in J. Bland's *Medical Aspects of Clinical Nutrition*, Keats Publishing (1983)

140 S. P. Helmrich, et al., 'Physical activity and reduced occurrence of non-insulin-dependent diabetes mellitus', *New England Journal of Medicine*, 1991 Jul; 325:147–52

141 D. Broughton, et al., 'Review: Deterioration of glucose tolerance with age: The role of insulin resistance', *Age and Ageing*, 1991; 20:221–5

142 J. E. Manson, et al., 'Physical activity and incidence of non-insulin-dependent diabetes mellitus in women', *Lancet*, 1991; 338(8770):774–8

143 C. Hollenbeck, et al., 'Effect of habitual exercise on regulation of insulin stimulated glucose disposal in older males', *Journal of the American Geriatric Society*, 1986; 33:273–7

144 P. Ebelin, et al., 'Mechanism of enhanced insulin sensitivity in athletes', *American Society for Clinical Investigations*, 1993; 92:1623–31

145 S. Balducci, et al., 'Effect of an intensive exercise intervention strategy on modifiable cardiovascular risk factors in subjects with type-2 diabetes mellitus: A randomized controlled trial: The Italian Diabetes and Exercise Study (IDES)', *Archives of Internal Medicine*, 2010 Nov; 170(20):1794–803

146 C. J. Kim, et al., 'Effects of a Cardiovascular Risk Reduction Intervention With Psychobehavioral Strategies for Korean Adults With Type-2 Diabetes and Metabolic Syndrome', *Journal of Cardiovascular Nursing*, 2010 Nov [Epub ahead of print]

147 T. P. Solomon, et al., 'A low-glycemic index diet combined with exercise reduces insulin resistance, postprandial hyperinsulinemia, and glucose dependent insulinotropic polypeptide responses in obese prediabetic humans', *American Journal of Clinical Nutrition*, 2010 Oct [Epub ahead of print]

148 R. Sigal and G. Kenny, 'Combined aerobic and resistance exercise for patients with type-2 diabetes T', *Journal of the American Medical Association*, 2010; 304[20]:2298–9

149 R. Alleyne, science correspondent, 'Doctors pinpoint genes connected to type-2 diabetes', *Daily Telegraph*, June 28, 2010

150 J. B. Johnson, et al., 'Alternate day calorie restriction improves clinical findings and reduces markers of oxidative stress and inflammation in overweight adults with moderate asthma', *Free Radical Biology and Medicine*, 2007 Mar; 42(5)1:665–74

151 J. B. Johnson, *The Alternate Day Diet*, Putnam Adult (2008)

152 K. A.Varady, et al., 'Improvements in body fat distribution and circulating adiponectin by alternate-day fasting versus calorie restriction', *Journal of Nutrition and Biochemistry*, 2010 Mar; 21(3):188–95

153 D. Kim, et al., 'SIRT1 deacetylase protects against neurodegeneration in models for Alzheimer's disease and amyotrophic lateral sclerosis' *EMBO Journal*, 2007 Jun; 26:3169–79; see also R. R. Alcendor, et al., 'Sirt1 regulates aging and resistance to oxidative stress in the heart', *Circulation Research*, 2007; 100:152; see also S. Imaiand and W. Kiess, 'Therapeutic potential of SIRT1 and NAMPT-mediated NAD biosynthesis in type-2 diabetes', *Front Biosci*, 2009 Jan; 14:2983–95

154 Y. H. Yu, 'The function of porcine PPARγ and dietary fish oil effect on the expression of lipid and glucose metabolism related genes', *Journal of Nutritional Biochemistry*, 2010 Oct [Epub ahead of print]

155 Y. Oh da Y and S. Talukdar, 'GPR120 is an omega-3 fatty acid receptor mediating potent anti-inflammatory and insulin-sensitizing effects', *Cell*, 2010 Sep 3; 142(5):687–98

156 M. C. Zilikens and J. B. van Meurs, 'SIRT1 genetic variation and mortality in type 2 diabetes: interaction with smoking and dietary niacin', *Free Radical Biology and Medicine*, 2010 Mar 15; 46(6):836–41

157 K. A. Varady, et al., 'Acute effects of weight lifting on plasma adiponectin in trained versus untrained individuals', *Federation of American Societies for Experimental Biology Journal*, 2009 Apr; Meeting Abstract Supplement LB451

158 S. F. Ng, et al., 'Chronic high-fat diet in fathers programs beta-cell dysfunction in female rat offspring', *Nature*, 2010 Oct; 467(7318):963–6

Part Three

1 J. Warren, et al., 'Low glycemic index breakfasts and reduced food intake in preadolescent children', *Pediatrics*, 2003; 112(5):414

2 D. Ludwig, 'Dietary glycemic index and regulation of body weight', *Lipids*, 2003; 38(2):117–21

3 K. Heaton, et al., 'Particle size of wheat, maize and oat test meals: Effects on plasma glucose and insulin responses and on the rate of starch digestion in vitro', *American Journal of Clinical Nutrition*, 1988; 47:675–82

4 E. Cheraskin, 'The Breakfast/Lunch/Dinner Ritual', *Journal of Orthomolecular Medicine*, 1993; 8(1):6–10

5 J. T. Braaten, et al., 'High beta-glucan oat bran and oat gum reduce postprandial blood glucose and insulin in subjects with and without type 2 diabetes', *Diabetic Medicine*, 1994; 11(3):312–18

6 J. Uribarri, et al., 'Advanced glycation end products in foods and a practical guide to their reduction in the diet', *Journal of the American Dietetic Association*, 2010 Jun; 110(6):911–16. e12

7 M. S. Bray and M. E. Young, 'Circadian rhythms in the development of obesity: Potential role for the circadian clock within the adipocyte', *Obesity Reviews*, 2007 Mar; 8(2):169–81; S. Taheri, et al., 'Short sleep duration is associated with reduced leptin, elevated ghrelin, and increased body mass index', *PLoS Medicine*, 2004 Dec; 1(3):e62

8 R. J. Sigal, et al., 'Physical Activity/Exercise and Type 2 Diabetes', *Diabetes Care*, 2004 Oct; 27(10):2518–39

Recommended Reading

PART 1
Patrick Holford, *The Low-GL Diet Bible*, Piatkus (2009)
Dr Charles Clarke and Maureen Clark, *The Diabetes Revolution*, Vermilion (2008)
Dr Neal Barnard, *The Reverse Diabetes Diet*, Rodale (2007)
Antony Haynes, *The Insulin Factor*, Thorsons (2004)
Dr Alan Rubin and Dr Sarah Jarvis, *Diabetes for Dummies*, John Wiley & Sons (2007)

PART 2
Professor Lustig, *Sugar, the Bitter Truth*, YouTube seminar: www.you tube.com/watch?v=dBnniua6-oM
Patrick Holford and Fiona McDonald Joyce, *The Holford 9-Day Liver Detox*, Piatkus (2007)
Dr Malcolm Carruthers, *The Testosterone Revolution*, Thorsons (2005)
Phil Campbell, *Ready Set Go!*, Pristine Publishers (2002)

PART 4
Patrick Holford and Fiona McDonald Joyce, *Food GLorious Food*, Piatkus (2008)
Patrick Holford and Fiona McDonald Joyce, *The Low-GL Diet Cookbook*, Piatkus (2010)

Resources

The Institute for Optimum Nutrition (ION) offers a three-year foundation degree course in nutritional therapy. Visit www.ion.ac.uk, address: Avalon House, 72 Lower Mortlake Road, Richmond TW9 2JY, UK, tel.: +44 (0)208 614 7800.

Nutritional therapy and consultations To find a nutritional therapist near you whom I recommend, visit www.patrickholford.com. This service gives details on who to see in the UK as well as internationally. If there is no one available nearby, you can always take an on-line assessment – see below.

On-line 100% Health Programme Are you 100 per cent healthy? Find out with our FREE health check and comprehensive 100% Health Programme giving you a personalised action plan, including diet and supplements. Visit www.patrickholford.com.

The Centre For Men's Health Dr Malcolm Carruthers' clinic provides testosterone treatment for a variety of male sexual-health concerns and offers a prostate health programme. Visit www.centre formenshealth.co.uk/. Address: 20 Harley Street, London W1G 9PH, tel.: +44 (0)207 636 8283.

The HeartMath stress-relieving **EM-Wave Monitor** is available from the HeartMath website. For more information visit www.heartmath store.com. In the UK you can attend workshops called 'Transforming Stress into Resilience', see www.patrickholford.com/heartmath for more details on these products and workshops.

The National Institute of Medical Herbalists (www.nimh.org.uk/index.html) can be contacted for advice on sleep-inducing herbs.

Resistance-training exercises Visit www.holforddiet.com for information on fatburning exercises (see the right-hand side of the home page) that can be easily included in your exercise plan.

Also, to see the video of Dr Joseph Mercola's Peak 8 system visit http://fitness.mercola.com/sites/fitness/archive/2010/11/13/phil-campbell-on-peak-8-exercises.aspx or find out more at his website www.readysteadygofitness.com.

Sleep CDs Dr John Levine's CDs, *Silence of Peace* and *Orange Grove Siesta* are available from www.patrickholford.com/CD.

Zest4Life is a health and nutrition club, based on low-GL principles, that provides advice, coaching and support for losing weight and gaining health through a series of weekly meetings. For more information, visit www.zest4life.eu.

Laboratory tests

Food Allergy (IgG ELISA), Homocysteine, GLCheck (measures your level of glycosylated haemoglobin, also called HbA1C) and LiverCheck tests are available through YorkTest Laboratories, using a home test kit where you can take your own pin-prick blood sample and return it to the lab for analysis. Visit www.yorktest.com, or call freephone (UK) 0800 074 6185. These test kits are also available from www.totallynourish.com or call freephone (UK) 0800 085 7749.

In Canada, CanLabs Inc. is the exclusive provider of the YorkTest FoodScan food intolerance test. The simple finger-prick blood collection method allows you to conduct a test without a prescription. For more information visit www.canlabs.ca or call toll-free on 1 855 854 8644.

BioCard Celiac Test A home test kit that provides results in less than 10 minutes. Available through Totally Nourish (www.totallynourish.com) or call freephone (UK) 0800 085 7749.

Other Tests You may also want to measure your **C-reactive protein (CRP)** or **Vitamin B$_{12}$ levels**. Speak to your nutritional therapist, healthcare professional or doctor who can arrange for these tests to be carried out.

Health products

Cherry Active is sold in a highly concentrated juice format. Mix a 30ml (2 tbsp) serving with 250ml (9fl oz) water to make a deliciously healthy, low-GL cherry juice. Each 946ml bottle contains the juice from over 3,000 cherries – that's half a tree's worth – and contains a month's supply. Cherry Active is also available as a dried cherry snack and in capsules. For more information and to order, visit www.totally nourish.com or call freephone (UK) 0800 085 7749.

Chia Seeds, the highest vegetarian source of omega-3, are available from Totally Nourish, www.totallynourish.com. If you'd like to find out more, here are two useful websites – www.eatchia.com and www.drcoateschia.com.

Essential Balance and **Udo's Choice** are two good seed oil blends that are available in health-food stores.

Get Up & Go, my low-GL breakfast shake powder, is made by BioCare and is available in most health-food stores or by mail order from www.totallynourish.com, or call freephone (UK) 0800 085 7749.

Glucomannan and **Konjac Fibre** are available in health-food stores and from www.totallynourish.com or call freephone (UK) 0800 085 7749. **PGX** is available on-line from the US.

Sugar alternative – XyloBrit (xylitol) is a low-GL natural sugar alternative – available in health-food stores and from www.totally nourish.com or call freephone (UK) 0800 085 7749.

Supplements

Finding your own perfect supplement programme can be confusing, but my website, www.patrickholford.com, offers useful guidance. See the section on 'supplements'.

The backbone of a good supplement programme is:

- An 'optimum nutrition' high-strength multivitamin–mineral
- An essential-fat supplement containing omega-3 and omega-6 oils
- Extra vitamin C, plus other immune-boosting nutrients

In this section are examples of supplements that provide the herbs and nutrients at the levels discussed in this book. The addresses of the companies whose products I've referred to are given at the end.

Multivitamin and mineral supplements

Supplementing the right multivitamin is the most important supplement decision you make. Most multis are based on RDA levels of nutrients, which are not the same as optimum nutrition levels. A good multivitamin based on optimum nutrition levels is BioCare's Advanced Optimum Nutrition Formula. Another is Solgar's Formula VM2000. Both of these recommend taking two tablets a day. Advanced Optimum Nutrition Formula has higher mineral levels, especially for calcium and magnesium. If you are taking metformin, remember to ensure that your multi contains at least 20mg of B_6, 10mcg of B_{12} and 200mcg of folic acid. Ideally, take a multivitamin–mineral with at least an extra 1g of vitamin C.

Essential fats and fish oil supplements

The most important omega-3 fats are EPA, DPA and DHA, found both in oily fish and in cod liver oil. The most important omega-6 fat is GLA, the richest source being borage (also known as starflower) oil. In all, you are looking for at least 600mg of combined EPA, DPA and DHA a day.

Try BioCare's Essential Omegas, which provides a highly concentrated mix of EPA, DHA, DPA and GLA. They also produce Mega-EPA, a high-potency omega-3 fish oil supplement. Seven Seas produce Extra High Strength Cod Liver Oil.

Vitamin C

You want to supplement 2g of vitamin C a day. You can take a single supplement or look for one which contains synergistic antioxidant nutrients such as zinc, black elderberry extracts and anthocyanidins. Complexes of vitamin C with bioflavonoids are available from both BioCare and Solgar.

Antioxidant complex

A good all-round antioxidant complex should provide glutathione or N-acetyl cysteine (NAC), alpha lipoic acid, vitamin E, vitamin C (not so essential since in the basics), CoQ_{10}, resveratrol, anthocyanidins of berry extracts, zinc, selenium, carotenoids and vitamin A. Two products that fulfil these criteria are BioCare's AGE Antioxidant and Solgar's Advanced Antioxidant Nutrients.

Sugar balance and weight maintenance

Look for a product that contains 200mcg of chromium, either as chromium polynicotinate or chromium picolinate, ideally with a cinnamon high in MCHP (Cinnulin PF® is the name of a concentrated extract of cinnamon that is especially high in MCHP). Try BioCare's Cinnachrome which combines chromium, cinnamon extract and niacin. Chromium may also be supplied with either *Garcinia cambogia* (high in HCA) or 5-HTP which are primarily included to help weight. GL Support by BioCare combines these with B vitamins.

Liver support

BioCare's Milk Thistle provides 250mg of 80 per cent silymarin per dose. You want to supplement 600mg a day.

9 Day Detox Pack by mail order from Totally Nourish (www.totallynourish.com).

Optional extras

Other supplements that you might want to try include alpha lipoic acid, CoQ_{10}, *Gymnema sylvestre*, homocysteine-lowering B vitamins (containing at least B_{12} 500mcg, folic acid 500mcg and B_6 20mg), 5-HTP, glutamine powder and high dose niacin. These are available from the companies listed below.

Supplement suppliers

The following companies produce good-quality supplements that are widely available in the UK.

BioCare offers an extensive range of nutritional and herbal supplements, including daily 'packs', which are good for travelling or when you are away from home. Their products are stocked by most good health-food shops. Visit www.biocare.co.uk, tel.: +44 (0)121 433 3727. They are also available by mail order from Totally Nourish (www.totallynourish.com) – see below.

Totally Nourish is an 'e'-health shop that stocks many high-quality health products, including home test kits and supplements. Visit www. totallynourish.com, call freephone (UK) 0800 085 7749.

Solgar Available in most independent health-food stores or visit www. solgar-vitamins.co.uk, tel.: +44 (0) 1442 890355.

And in other regions

South Africa

The original Patrick Holford vitamin and supplement brand from the UK is now available in South Africa through leading health-food stores, Dis-Chem and Clicks retail pharmacies. They are also available on-line direct from www.holforddirect.co.za or phone 011 2654 554 and are delivered by post or by courier direct to your door.

Australia

Solgar supplements are available in Australia. Visit www.solgar. com.au, tel.: 1800 029 871 (free call) for your nearest supplier. Another good brand is **Blackmores**.

New Zealand

BioCare products (see above) are available in New Zealand through Pacific Health, PO Box 56248, Dominion Road, Auckland 1446. Visit www.pachealth.co.nz, tel.: 0064 9815 0707.

Singapore

BioCare (see above) and **Solgar** products are available in Singapore through Essential Living. Visit www.essliv.com, tel.: 6276 1380.

UAE

BioCare supplements (see above) are available in Dubai and the UAE from Organic Foods & Café, PO Box 117629, Dubai, United Arab Emirates; tel.: +971 44340577.

Index

(page numbers in italics indicate graphs and tables)

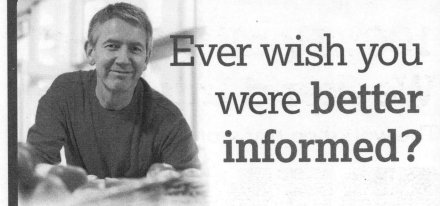

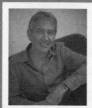

Say NO to Diabetes
The Fast Track Back to Health Programme

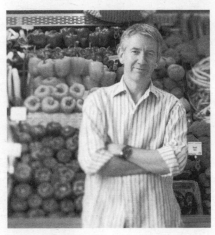

Patrick Holford invites you to follow the zest4life programme to achieve the same results achieved by those on our trial*. Take control of your health, and learn how to stay well through simple dietary and lifestyle changes. Now you can get the expert support you need with zest4life.

Are you unsure how you can achieve optimum health and avoid getting ill?

Do you find it difficult to lose weight or improve your diet and lifestyle on your own?

zest4life group (or private) sessions are led by health and nutrition experts.

They provide a fun, educational & stimulating environment where you can achieve life changing results.

Let us show you how to take responsibility for your health, lose weight intelligently and say **NO** to Diabetes.

In addition to collectively losing 21 stone with a low GL diet and exercise, the blood test results for the trial group of 21 participants showed that their risk factors for diabetes/ heart disease had substantially reduced. For some this will mean that medication will not be required and for others it has meant that they can begin to reduce the level of medication, under close GP supervision. As well as reduced blood pressure, cholesterol and blood sugar levels, participants rated themselves as having much more energy, reduced cravings, better sleep and more stable moods.

Visit our website to find out more about joining a zest4life programme:
www.zest4life.com

Patrick **Holford's**
zest4life
nutrition & weightloss